Symptoms After 40

Symptoms After 40

KENNETH ANDERSON

A Stonesong Press Book

ARBOR HOUSE   NEW YORK

Manufactured in the United States of America

10 9 8 7 6 5 4 3 2 1

Library of Congress Cataloging in Publication Data

Anderson, Kenneth, 1921–
Symptoms after 40.

"A Stonesong Press book."
1. Symptomatology—Dictionaries.   2. Middle age—
Health and hygiene—Dictionaries.   I. Title.   II. Title:
Symptoms after forty.   [DNLM: 1. Geriatrics—
encyclopedias—popular works.   WT 13 A547s]
RC69.A53   1987   616.07′2   86–32242
ISBN 0–87795–879–3

FOREWORD

As people age, their bodies change, but all too often people confuse changes caused by the "normal" aging process with signs of illness—and vice versa. Whether they consult a doctor with their problems or wait for the symptoms to disappear, their failure to distinguish between what is normal and what isn't often results in adults being treated unnecessarily for conditions that need no attention or in their not being treated at all for conditions that require prompt attention. Furthermore, even after a problem has been evaluated and treated by a physician, many people remain confused about how they were treated and exactly for what.

Symptoms After 40 will fill these gaps. In addition, it will encourage each of us to take responsibility for our own and our family's well-being and health care. A lifetime of optimal health and functioning begins at home. Only then can we help our physicians work most effectively with us to ensure ourselves of the best possible prognoses and health care.

Although this book is designed to be most useful to the millions of Americans who are over forty, it is important to note that many of the symptoms, signs, conditions, and procedures covered in this book can and do occur at other ages. In fact, we all age in two ways: chronologically, based on the date on our birth certificates; and physiologically, based on the ways in which our bodies function. These two ages do not necessarily coincide; all of us have known people in their forties and fifties who seem "old" to us and others in their seventies and eighties whose vitality and zest match those of people decades younger. Much of the information in these pages will be useful to you regardless of the date on which you were born.

Nevertheless, it is a fact that there are numerous changes in body structure and function that accompany the aging process. Ignorance of these changes can cause unwarranted worry; knowledge of them can enhance the likelihood of adapting to them in useful ways and, often, of preventing problems from developing in the first place. Whether for ourselves or on behalf of older members of our families, the better we recognize and understand the realities of growing older, both physically and mentally, the more satisfying our lives will be.

The entries in *Symptoms After 40* have been presented in a form designed for clarity of content and ease of use. They have been reviewed for scientific validity by a medical advisory board comprised of leading authorities, and they represent state-of-the-art medical information. Of course, no book should ever substitute for the advice and recommendations of a physician. But consulted often and used wisely, *Symptoms After 40* will prove a welcome and invaluable addition to your home library—and your good health.

Steven R. Gambert, M.D., F.A.C.P.
Professor of Medicine
Director, The Center for Aging and
Adult Development
New York Medical College

A

A A prefix derived from the Greek language, indicating *not, without,* or other negative meanings. It is commonly used, without a hyphen, in medical terms to suggest an absence of something, as in *arrhythmia,* meaning absence of (normal heart) rhythm, or *amenorrhea,* the absence of menstruation in women.

Abdominal dropsy See **Ascites.**

Abdominal hernia The protrusion of an internal structure, such as a loop of intestine (bowel) or a portion of the stomach, the liver, or the membrane lining the abdominal cavity, through a weak point or defect in the muscle layer of the abdominal wall. The hernia appears as an abnormal bulge under the skin of the abdomen. An abdominal hernia often occurs at the site of a surgical scar where tissues under the skin have not healed properly. The hernia may not be visible when the person is lying down on his or her back, or when the abdominal muscles are relaxed. But when the supine person raises the head, which usually requires a tightening of the abdominal muscles, the bulge can be seen under the scar.

An abdominal hernia also may appear along the center line (the *linea alba,* a Latin term for "white line,") of the abdomen that runs from the breastbone to the genital area. Muscle tissue on the left and right sides of the body is joined along this midline by white connective tissue, so the abdominal wall is weakened at this point. The bulge of a midline abdominal hernia may contain a fat deposit. The hernia may appear only in a standing position because it is usually reducible, that is, when

1

the person is supine the contents of the bulge fall back into the abdominal cavity.

A hernia that is not reducible may become trapped, or incarcerated, in the abdominal wall. This is called a *strangulated hernia* and is a life-threatening emergency because blood circulation to the incarcerated portion of the intestine is blocked. Immediate surgery is required to prevent the formation of potentially fatal gangrene. *See also* **Hernia.**

Abdominal pain   Any pain that is felt in the region between the bottom of the chest and the base of the pelvis. The abdomen contains a number of major organs, including the stomach, small and large intestines, kidneys, liver, spleen, pancreas, gallbladder, urinary bladder, the prostate gland (in the male), and the uterus, ovaries, and fallopian tubes (in the female). In addition, there are blood vessels, nerves, membranes, and other tissues. Any of these, or the abdominal wall itself, may be the source of pain. The cause may be inflammation, infection, obstruction, or other problems.

The pain also can be a **referred pain**, that is, one that originates in another part of the body than the site in which it is felt. An example is an injury to the spleen, which may be felt as a pain in the right shoulder. Nevertheless, in diagnosing the source of the problem, the doctor relies a great deal on the location of the pain and the resulting degree of tenderness. The pain also may move about, as in appendicitis, which may be felt in the area above the navel at the beginning of an attack and in the lower right side later in the attack.

The nature of a pain may change, depending on whether one is lying down, standing, or walking about. A pain in the upper abdomen, between the base of the breastbone and the navel, could be a sign of inflammation of the pancreas, a heart attack, an intestinal obstruction, a severe stomach irritation, or the start of appendicitis. A chronic dull pain or a sudden severe one in the same area could also be a sign of peptic ulcer. The pain of a pancreas inflammation may radiate from the upper abdomen to the lower back, and in some cases, by irritating a nerve, it might become a referred pain felt in the left shoulder. The pain of an inflamed pancreas often is relieved somewhat if the person assumes a sitting position and leans forward.

A gallbladder attack frequently is marked by a pain in the upper right side of the abdomen that radiates to the right shoulder. In addition, the upper right abdomen is constantly tender. Gallstones may block one of the bile ducts or perforate the wall of the gallbladder, also causing severe pain in the upper right abdomen. The pain comes in waves that may be so acute as to cause the person to double up.

Pleurisy, in which the pleural membrane that covers the lungs and diaphragm becomes inflamed, may cause pain in the upper abdomen with breathing, so the person with pleurisy often takes shallow breaths.

Pain caused by an obstruction in the intestine occurs in spasms as the intestine itself tries to overcome the problem with waves of muscle contractions. Generally, the obstruction can be located by the doctor with the help of certain signs, such as the intensity of the pain. For example, the pain is usually most severe if the obstruction is high in the small intestine and less severe if the obstruction is at the lower end of the digestive tract, in the colon.

Because vomiting usually accompanies the pain of an obstruction, the contents of the vomitus can provide clues as to the location of the obstruction. The presence of bile, for example, indicates that the problem is below the point where bile from the gallbladder enters the intestine. A frequent cause of an intestinal obstruction is an abdominal hernia that traps a loop of intestine in the abdominal wall.

Other causes of abdominal pain can be a sharp blow to the abdomen resulting in damage to the urinary bladder, liver, kidneys, or spleen.

Food poisoning, chemical poisoning, diabetic acidosis, sickle cell anemia, rupture or obstruction of a major artery, diverticulitis, or an ectopic (misplaced) pregnancy are among the many other possible causes of abdominal pain, also called "acute abdomen." *See also* **Abdominal hernia, Pelvic pain.**

Abiotrophy   A term used to describe the premature loss of vitality or the deterioration of cells or tissues as a result of a degenerative disease or a nutritional defect. The condition is often associated with a disorder of the body's immune system and may be marked by a failure of resistance or a loss of endurance. *See also* **Immune deficiency.**

Abscess   An accumulation of pus produced by a bacterial infection, usually within an area of inflamed tissue. Pus is a thick yellowish fluid comprised of cellular debris, bacteria, and white blood cells (leukocytes). The infection may be located at the site of the abscess or in another part of the body; the infectious material is often transported from one area to another by blood or lymph. An abscess may continue to expand due to the ongoing destruction of surrounding cells until the pus is drained and the infection controlled.

An abscess can develop in almost any part of the body, but it is most visible when in the skin or the tissues beneath the skin, where it produces symptoms of heat, swelling, and tenderness. The skin over the abscess is red, a sign of inflammation. An abscess deep within the body is characterized by pain, fever, and often fatigue and a loss of appetite. Although a small abscess will sometimes rupture, releasing the pus and draining spontaneously as the underlying infection heals without further treatment, it is usually advisable to have the abscess treated by a physician, who can drain it and administer an appropriate antibiotic.

Untreated, an abscess can rupture into adjoining tissues or organs, cause bleeding by eroding the walls of blood vessels, or interfere with the normal functioning of a vital organ system.

Acalculia A form of **aphasia** in which a person loses the ability to perform calculations or arithmetic, usually due to damage resulting from a stroke, a tumor, or an injury to the upper left side of the brain in right-handed adults. Although there are several different types of acalculia, all are related to a central nervous system dysfunction in the region of the brain that controls the use of language. Also called "number blindness."

Acanthosis nigricans An inflammatory skin disease characterized by the appearance of darkly pigmented pimplelike eruptions with a velvety surface. They tend to appear in the armpits, the groin, the lower abdomen, and the back. The eruptions are sometimes associated with cancers of internal organs, although the precise relationship is not clear.

Accommodation The process of adjusting or adapting. The term is commonly used to describe the adjustment of the lens of the eye to near or far vision. Visual accommodation involves the contraction or relaxation of the ciliary muscle inside the eyeball, and begins to diminish after the age of forty, as the ciliary muscle starts to atrophy. The closest distance at which one can see clearly begins to recede, and eyeglasses or contact lenses are needed to improve near vision. The condition is usually complicated by an accumulation of old fibers in the lens of the eye. The lens becomes harder and more compact, resulting in an increase in its refractive power.

The loss of near vision associated with normal aging is called **presbyopia**.

Acetylcholine A neurotransmitter chemical found in nerve endings in many parts of the body, which helps conduct nerve impulses across the gap (synapse) between nerve fibers. It is also released from the endings of nerve fibers in the autonomic nervous system, which controls the automatic functions of the body's organs. Acetylcholine is involved in such body functions as the rate of the heartbeat, the dilation of blood vessels, and activity of the digestive tract. The chemical is sometimes used as a drug, as in eye surgery when it is given to constrict the pupil. A deficiency of acetylcholine is associated with several disorders of the brain and nervous system, including Alzheimer's disease. *See also* **Alzheimer's disease.**

Acetylcholinesterase An enzyme present in brain tissues, red blood cells, and skeletal muscles, whose main function is to break down molecules of acetylcholine, a substance that aids in the transmission of nerve impulses. By controlling the amount of acetylcholine in the body, the enzyme prevents unnecessary nervous system activity, such as unwanted automatic muscle contractions. Some nerve poisons block the enzyme's action, producing symptoms of tremors, muscle twitching, and other kinds of inappropriate muscle contractions. *See* **Acetylcholine.**

Achalasia A failure of a ringlike group of sphincter muscle fibers to relax. The term is most commonly applied to a disorder of the digestive tract in which the muscles at the lower end of the esophagus fail to relax, interfering with the passage of swallowed food into the stomach. There is usually difficulty in swallowing and regurgitation of food. (Inhalation of regurgitated food can lead to pneumonia and lung abscesses.) The esophagus may become elongated, wide, and weak. There may be some chest pain, experienced as "heartburn." The condition can be aggravated by anxiety or emotional upsets.
   The exact cause of achalasia is unknown, but it is believed to involve a failure of nerve cells near the cardiac sphincter, the circular muscle that controls the emptying of the esophagus into the stomach. Because this muscle junction between the esophagus and the stomach is located near the heart, attacks are sometimes mistaken for a heart problem. Also called "cardiospasm."

Achard-Thiers syndrome A hormone disorder that may affect diabetic women after the menopause. It is caused by a malfunction of the adrenal gland, a source of androgen production in women, and results in the growth of body hair distributed in the pattern of male body hair. Other effects include atrophy of the breast and increased blood pressure. The condition is treated by bleaching, mechanical hair removal, and by hormone treatments or surgery to remove adrenal gland tissue.

Achlorhydria A lack of hydrochloric acid in the gastric juice of the stomach. The condition is associated with stomach cancer, pernicious anemia, and iron-deficiency anemia. The person with achlorhydria often has trouble digesting proteins and may associate the problem with eating meat or other high-protein foods. Because the enzymes in other

parts of the digestive system continue to function normally, digestion
of other foods may not be impaired. Achlorhydria is believed to be due
to atrophy of glands in the stomach that secrete hydrochloric acid.
There is a wide range in what is considered a "normal" degree of acidity
in the stomach, and laboratory tests are needed to determine if achlorhydria is the source of a person's digestive problems.

Acid-base balance   The balance between the acid and alkaline (base)
constituents in blood and other body fluids. It is generally measured
during analysis of a person's urine, which is ordinarily slightly acid.
Increasing acidity is usually a sign of a health disorder that has upset
the body's chemical equilibrium. Excess of acidity leads to an abnormal
condition called *acidosis,* while an excess of alkalinity results in a
disorder known as *alkalosis.* The urine of an adult may be slightly
more acidic or more alkaline depending upon, among other factors,
the kinds of foods eaten. Protein-rich foods, particularly meat, tend to
increase acidity, while milk and most fruits and vegetables have an
alkaline influence on the urine. The acid-base balance also may shift
during the day, becoming temporarily alkaline following a meal. *See
also* **Acidosis, Alkalosis.**

Acidosis   A serious, abnormal condition of an excessive level of acidic
chemical molecules in the body tissues. There are several different kinds
of acidosis and many causes. A common form is *diabetic acidosis* that
results from an accumulation of substances (ketones) formed in the
body because of its inability to metabolize carbohydrates effectively.
Because carbohydrates are not utilized properly, the body uses fatty
acids instead as a source of energy. The end products are ketones,
which are acids. The accumulation of ketones causes adverse effects,
including mental confusion, breathlessness, nausea, vomiting, dehydration, weight loss, and, if untreated, loss of consciousness and
death. A similar type of acidosis can be caused by starvation, certain
crash diets, or other situations in which an inadequate intake of protein and carbohydrates leads to rapid burning of fats in the body.
Among other causes of acidosis are kidney failure, use of certain
drugs, poisons such as wood alcohol, and conditions like diarrhea
that may result in an excessive loss of alkaline substances, thereby
tilting the acid-base balance toward the acid side.

Acid perfusion test   A test of the sensitivity of the esophagus to acids.
The test may be done when there is inflammation and regurgitation of
the stomach contents into the esophagus (reflux esophagitis). A mildly
acid solution and a neutral salt solution are dripped alternately into the

esophagus. The patient is not told which solution is being used, but the reaction is recorded. In a similar test, the patient is asked to swallow alternately samples of a barium solution, one sample of which has been made slightly acid. The swallowing is observed on a fluoroscope, an X-ray device that reveals spasms in the esophagus if the person is acid-sensitive. If the tests reproduce the symptoms of reflux esophagitis, this is interpreted as a sign that the person suffers from this condition. *See also* **Achalasia.**

Acid therapy   A technique for removing warts by applying drops of a mild acid, usually salicylic or lactic acid, or a dressing impregnated with acid.

Acousma   The sensation of "hearing" a sound in the absence of a stimulus. An acousma may be experienced as a buzzing, ringing, or roaring sound (tinnitus). It is sometimes regarded as an auditory hallucination, particularly when no organic cause can be found. *See also* **Tinnitus.**

Acoustic neuroma   A tumor that originates in the acoustic or auditory nerve and spreads into the surrounding cranial nerves and brain tissues. The initial symptoms are a loss of hearing and a "ringing" (tinnitus) in the ear. Because the sense of balance is also affected, the person may feel dizzy and unsteady on his feet. If untreated, the tumor affects the facial nerve and compresses the brain stem. The tumor is removed by surgery, the approach depending upon the precise location of the tumor and how much of the person's useful hearing has been destroyed. Also called "acoustic neurinoma."

Acoustic trauma   Hearing loss due to damage to the inner ear from exposure to intense noise levels. The condition may result from a sudden nearby loud noise, such as gunfire or blasting. The hearing loss may be temporary or permanent, depending upon individual factors. *See also* **Hearing loss.**

Acrocyanosis   A condition of spasms of the small blood vessels of the hands, resulting in a bluish (cyanotic) discoloration of the hands. The hands may also feel cold but sweaty. Sometimes the feet are affected in the same way. Acrocyanosis is often triggered by exposure to cold temperatures but also may be associated with emotional stress. The condition is painless and is not associated with any serious circulatory disorder. There is no specific treatment. *See also* **Raynaud's phenomenon.**

Acro-osteolysis A disorder characterized by the loss of bone tissue in the hands and fingers, accompanied by symptoms of **Raynaud's phenomenon,** in which exposure to cold temperatures causes spasms of the small arteries supplying blood to the fingers. It can be an occupational disease affecting those who work with polyvinyl chloride plastics. There is also a nonoccupational form of the disease. Unlike true **Raynaud's disease,** in which the person experiences feelings of numbness and skin color changes, from blanching through redness to a bluish (cyanotic) shade, the blood vessel spasms in acro-osteolysis are accompanied by rheumatoid pain.

The loss of bone tissue is usually detected by X-ray films. In the occupational form of the disease, calcium is redeposited in the finger bones after the workers are no longer exposed to PVC. However, calcium loss is permanent in the hereditary form of acro-osteolysis.

Acroparesthesia A feeling of numbness, prickling, or a similar sensation in the hands or feet, resulting from a compressed or damaged nerve. The medical term is derived from the Greek words *acro,* meaning "the end," *para,* meaning "near," and *esthesia,* for "feelings" or "sensations." Because different nerve branches can be involved, the sensation varies from person to person. Some individuals describe the sensation as one of "pins and needles." Others report a feeling of "insects crawling on the skin," or cold, warmth, pressure, or pain.

In most cases, the cause can be traced to a compressed or damaged nerve in the area of the body where the feeling is experienced. When acroparesthesia occurs in the hand, the problem usually involves one of three major nerve branches that extend from spinal cord connections in the neck or upper chest area to the hand. The median nerve branch, which passes under a tunnel of ligaments in the wrist, is the branch most commonly affected. This carpal tunnel contains tendons that move the fingers. It is small, with barely enough room for the ligaments, nerves, and other tissues that pass through it. Any stress, injury, or abnormal growth, such as a tumor, will result in a swelling of the tissues crowded within the tunnel and compression of the nerve.

More than a dozen different factors can contribute to the acroparesthesia that accompanies the condition, often called **carpal tunnel syndrome.** Acroparesthesia of the hand can also be caused by compression or injury to a second nerve branch in the arm, that of the ulnar nerve. The ulnar nerve passes through two tunnels, the cubital tunnel at the elbow and the ulnar tunnel in the wrist. Compression of the ulnar nerve can result from arthritis, from leaning on the elbows, or from work, such as carpentry, that requires repeated movement of the elbow. The third nerve branch in the arm, the radial nerve, is rarely a cause of acroparesthesia, though the condition can occur as a result of wearing a tight wristband while golfing or playing tennis.

Acroparesthesia of the legs and feet can be caused by simply crossing the legs, an act that may compress the peroneal nerve. Long periods of sleep or prolonged confinement in bed because of an illness or injury can have a similar nerve compression effect, though the sleeping or seated person may not notice the numbness in the legs until standing or walking is required. The legs also contain a counterpart to the carpal tunnel: the tarsal tunnel, through which a nerve passes with fibers to various areas of the foot. The nerve may be compressed by arthritis, a foot injury, or an accumulation of fluid in the legs. Treatment involves eliminating the cause of nerve compression, application of warmth, and massage. In cases that do not respond to simple measures, surgery may be required. *See also* **Burning feet syndrome, Causalgia, Honeymoon paralysis.**

ACTH An abbreviation for adrenocorticotropic hormone, a hormone secreted by the pituitary gland at the base of the brain. It stimulates production of hormones by the cortex or outer portion of the adrenal gland. *See also* **Adrenal gland.**

Actinic keratosis A skin lesion that often begins as a faint red patch and gradually evolves into a flat or slightly elevated grayish or brown scale. An actinic keratosis is associated with exposure to sunlight and tends to occur on a skin surface usually not covered by protective clothing, such as the neck, face, and hands, of people who work or play outdoors. Men are more likely to be affected than women, and farmers and sailors are among the most frequent victims. There also appears to be a hereditary factor, since those with blue eyes, light hair, and thin skin are more susceptible. Persons with actinic keratoses feel a stinging or burning sensation around the sores, or lesions.

Early treatment is recommended because actinic keratoses may progress to cancers if untreated. Treatment may involve freezing the lesions with liquid nitrogen or chemotherapy by application of ointments or lotions. The exact form of treatment depends upon the size and location of the keratosis, as well as cosmetic considerations when the lesion occurs on the face or neck. Because the risk of developing actinic keratoses increases as one grows older, the growth is sometimes called a **senile wart**. Any sudden growth in one of the lesions, either over a larger area or deeper into the skin layers, may be a sign that an actinic keratosis is developing into a **squamous cell carcinoma**.

Activities of daily living (ADL)   The normal daily functions of most people, such as getting out of bed at the start of a new day; dressing; preparing a meal; eating; taking a bath and using the toilet; performing other personal grooming tasks; using household furniture, appliances, utensils, and tools; and performing productive work of some kind.

Although such activities are taken for granted by most adults, many older people are eventually faced with a disability that requires the relearning of one or more activities of daily living in a different manner and with special aids such as a wheelchair or walker. Health professionals evaluate an ill or disabled person's ability to handle activities of daily living in assessing a need for home health care, homemaker support, and other possible aids that will enable the person to maintain an independent life.

Activity deprivation   An inability to fulfill the natural urge for physical activity, such as moving about. Bodily activity is a natural function in all animals, including humans. A person who is deprived of this function because of an illness or disability may experience a great deal of frustration and emotional stress.

Acuity   A measure of clearness or sharpness of perception. *Visual acuity* is the ability to distinguish clearly the shape and details of objects, as measured by identifying objects such as letters of the alphabet from a distance of twenty feet (six meters) or reading fine print from a distance of about sixteen inches. Other types of acuity include *auditory acuity* (sound), *tactile acuity* (touch), and *gustatory acuity* (taste).

Acute   Occurring suddenly with severe symptoms, such as a sharp pain, and usually with a short course.

Acute abdomen   Any disorder within the abdomen that begins with sudden, severe pain. The cause may be determined by a number of different factors, such as the precise location of the pain, whether it is dull or sharp, constant or intermittent, increasing or decreasing, and any activity that alters the pain, such as lying down, bending over, or walking about. Other symptoms, such as changes in bowel movements, also may be significant. *See also* **Abdominal pain.**

Acute allergic reaction   A severe, sudden reaction to contact with a substance to which the person has developed a special sensitivity. The reaction may include increased irritability, breathing difficulty, a bluish skin coloration due to oxygen deficiency, muscle spasms, convulsions, shock, loss of consciousness, and death. Substances likely to cause an acute allergic reaction include allergens such as dusts, plant pollens, venom of wasps or other stinging insects, penicillin, animal serums, and certain chemicals, such as the sulfites sometimes used as food additives. Usually, an acute allergic reaction is an immune response of the body to an antigen (allergen) the body tissues have encountered previously.

The immune system, which protects the body against invasion by foreign substances such as bacteria and viruses, prepares defenses against the substance after the first encounter. Future exposure of the person to the same allergen can trigger the acute reaction, sometimes called **anaphylactic shock**, as the immune system's defenses attack the foreign substance. Acute allergic reaction can be a medical emergency requiring artificial respiration, oxygen, and potent steroids and other drugs to maintain life. *See also* **Immune deficiency.**

Acute respiratory distress   A breathing emergency that may develop during a respiratory disease such as pneumonia, as a result of accidentally inhaling a foreign object, or from many other causes. It is characterized by rapid breathing, shortness of breath, and grunting sounds that accompany expirations. The disorder often follows an illness or injury that involves the chest. It is sometimes associated with asthma or emphysema, but it may also develop in a person with no history of a lung disease. Immediate professional medical care is needed to prevent complications or permanent lung damage. Without treatment, the condition may be fatal. Also called "adult respiratory distress syndrome" and "shock lung."

Adams-Stokes syndrome   A condition of sudden "blackouts" or fainting spells that is caused by a type of incomplete heart block. The person may suddenly lose consciousness when the normal rhythm of the heartbeat is temporarily interrupted. The heartbeat interruption can be caused by failure of one of the lower chambers (ventricles) of the heart to contract or as a result of a short burst of fibrillation (an extremely rapid series of irregular contractions that does not actually pump any blood through the arteries). An attack may occur with or without any earlier feeling of dizziness and regardless of body position. The period of unconsciousness can last from ten to thirty seconds and may or may not be accompanied by convulsions. The person may be pale or bluish and will have no pulse while unconscious.

Consciousness returns when the heart resumes its normal rhythm spontaneously and blood flows again through the arteries. These episodes can occur several times in one day or, in some cases, be separated by many months. However, unless the underlying condition is treated at an early stage, any future attack is likely to be fatal. *See also* **Fibrillation, Heart block.**

Adaptation The ability to make appropriate responses to changing situations by modifying or adjusting one's own behavior. The ability of the body to adapt enables a person to recover from physical or mental stresses and establish a new level of functioning. With age, adaptability may decrease, affecting one's ability to recover and return to a prestress level of functioning as rapidly as a young person.

Addison's disease A partial or complete failure of the functions of the cortex of the adrenal glands and of their production of vital hormones, including glucocorticoids, mineralcorticoids, and male sex hormones. Symptoms include feelings of weakness, fatigue, and lethargy, abdominal pain, diarrhea, nausea, vomiting, and weight loss. The patient has a craving for salt. Other symptoms include reduced hair growth and mottled skin pigmentation, sometimes with very dark freckles appearing in the region from the shoulders to the forehead. The person may experience a high fever, behavioral changes, a lowered resistance to other diseases, and a high sensitivity to stress.

Causes may include a tumor, infection, or hemorrhage in the adrenal gland, but in many cases there is no identifiable cause other than unexplained atrophy of the gland. In addition to the use of hormone replacement drugs and diet changes, therapy includes avoidance of exposure to stressful situations. *See also* **Adrenal gland.**

Adenocarcinoma A cancer of a gland. The cancer is further identified by the type of gland or tissue involved, e.g., *adenocystic carcinoma* identifies a cancer formed by cells around a cyst that usually contains mucus. Adenocarcinomas can develop in the salivary glands, glands of the breast, the large intestine, the endometrial lining of the uterus, or the vestibular glands of the vulva.

Adenoma A noncancerous tumor that may develop in the tissues of a gland. An adenoma may cause the gland to secrete an excessive amount of hormone. An *acidiophilic adenoma* of the pituitary gland is a cause of gigantism and acromegaly, the result of overproduction of pituitary growth hormone. An adenoma of the pancreas may be a cause of **hypoglycemia** because of overproduction of insulin.

Adenopathy An overgrowth or other abnormality of a gland. The term is commonly used to describe enlarged lymph nodes or glands that are usually associated with other disorders, such as **Hodgkin's disease**.

ADH An abbreviation for *antidiuretic hormone,* produced by the hypothalamus. It suppresses the secretion of urine.

Adie's pupil syndrome A neurological disorder involving the reflexes of the eye and marked by abnormal accommodation by the pupil. In near vision, the pupil of the affected eye dilates and contracts more slowly than the normal pupil of the other eye. The affected pupil also fails to react normally to direct and indirect light. Various other reflexes in the body, including the Babinski (knee-jerk) reflex, may also be abnormal in a person affected by the Adie's pupil syndrome. *See also* **Accommodation, Babinski reflex.**

Adrenal cortex The outer portion of the adrenal gland and the part that produces the steroid hormones (androgen, mineralcorticoid, and glucocorticoid) that are essential for normal body functioning. A deficiency of the hormones due to a disorder of the adrenal cortex results in the symptoms of **Addison's disease**.

Adrenal crisis A condition of shock, coma, or severe prostration accompanied by low blood pressure and severe pains in the abdomen, back, or legs, which is caused by a deficiency of adrenal cortex hormones. It can be triggered by a stressful event, such as injury, acute infection, surgery, or excessive loss of body salt because of sweating in a hot environment. The patient may have a severe loss of body fluid with kidney failure and collapse of the blood circulation in the extremities. Because the condition is similar to Addison's disease, the treatment is essentially the same; in some cases the person has been treated for Addison's disease or has shown some of the same symptoms. The outlook for arrest of adrenal crisis is good if treatment is started early. *See also* **Addison's disease.**

Adrenalectomy The surgical removal of a part or all of one or both adrenal glands. If both glands are removed, it is necessary to take a maintenance dose of adrenal steroid hormones for the rest of one's life. An adrenalectomy may be performed to remove a tumor or to control the growth of certain breast cancers or cancer of the prostate gland.

Adrenal gland A small gland located on the top of each kidney that secretes a number of hormones crucial to life. It consists of two separate parts, an outer *cortex* and an inner *medulla.* The cortex secretes hormones (androgen, glucocorticoid, and mineralcorticoid) when it is stimulated by ACTH hormone released by the pituitary gland. The hormones of the cortex control carbohydrate metabolism, mineral balance, and the reproductive processes of the body. The adrenal medulla secretes epinephrine (adrenalin), norepinephrine (noradrenalin), and dopamine hormones in response to stimulation by the sympathetic nervous system. The hormones produced by the medulla, also called catecholamines, influence blood pressure, heartbeat, dilation or constriction of blood vessels, and relaxation of the bronchial muscles. *See also* **Sympathetic nervous system.**

Adrenal virilism   The development of the secondary sexual characteristics of the male in a female as a result of overproduction of androgenic hormones by the adrenal cortex, particularly after the menopause when normal production of female sex hormones declines. The effects also can be due to an ovarian tumor. The virilism may be manifested by enlarged genitalia, male distribution of body hair, male balding pattern, deepening of the voice, diminished breast size, and cessation of menses. Men also may be affected by increased androgen secretion, but the effects are more noticeable in a woman. Treatment may include surgery or medications, or both. If an adrenal tumor is the cause, other adrenal hormone abnormalities, such as **Cushing's syndrome**, also can occur. Also called "adrenogenital syndrome." *See also* **Achard-Thiers syndrome.**

Adrenergic blocking drugs   Agents that inhibit certain actions of the **sympathetic nervous system** that are normally stimulated by epinephrine and norepinephrine, hormones secreted by the adrenal medulla. Adrenergic blocking agents are sometimes classified as "alpha blockers" or "beta blockers," depending upon which part of the nervous system (alpha or beta fibers) is affected by a particular drug. Examples of adrenergic blocking drugs are timolol, used to treat glaucoma, and propranolol, a heart medication.

Adrenomegaly   An enlargement of the adrenal gland.

Adult celiac disease   An inability to tolerate foods that contain gluten, a protein found in cereal grains such as wheat, rye, barley, and oats. Symptoms may range from abdominal discomfort and distention to bone pain, diarrhea, fluid accumulation, and numbness or tingling sensations in the arms or legs. There also may be weight loss, anemia, and skin disorders, which may actually be due to or aggravated by loss of essential nutrients as a result of the condition. The precise cause is the presence in gluten of a substance, gliadin, that acts in the body as an antigen, or foreign substance, that triggers the formation of antibodies much the same as an infection does. The antibody reaction results in damage to the lining of the digestive tract. Adult celiac disease is similar to the celiac sprue of infancy, but the condition may not appear for the first time until the person is in his or her forties or fifties.

Adult onset diabetes *See* **Diabetes mellitus.**

Adult rickets *See* **Osteomalacia.**

Adult sensorineural lesion A loss of hearing that results from organic damage to the tissues of the auditory system located between the inner ear and the area of the brain where nerve impulse messages are translated into sounds. The lesion is usually in the cochlea of the inner ear or in the eighth cranial nerve (the auditory nerve), which carries the nerve impulses from the inner ear to the brain. Causes may be a tumor of the auditory nerve, prolonged exposure to loud noise, a viral infection, adverse effects of drugs, or **Ménière's disease**.

Adverse drug reaction Any physical or mental disorder that results from the use of a medication. Among the more common reactions to drugs are skin eruptions, nausea, blood pressure changes, dizziness, allergic reactions, and heart palpitations. Numerous drugs are associated with impotence. Some drugs also interact with other medications or with certain foods to produce adverse effects; one class of drugs, the **monoamine oxidase inhibitors** prescribed for certain psychological conditions, can interact with wines, aged cheeses, and certain other foods to cause severe hypertension (high blood pressure).

Aftercare Outpatient and rehabilitation services provided for patients who have been discharged from a hospital that promote the restoration of health and to ensure against a relapse.

Age critique A French term, literally translated as "critical age," used to describe the menopausal years.

Age de retour A French term for senility, literally translated as "age of return" (to childhood).

Age spots Discolored areas of the skin that are associated with the aging process. The blemishes, which may be flat or slightly raised, usually appear on skin surfaces that are exposed to sunlight. About 40 percent of people over the age of fifty can expect to develop these skin lesions, which are of several different types. **Seborrheic keratoses** are one-half- to one-inch-wide raised brown or black growths that appear on the epidermis, or surface layer of the skin.

Melanodermas are smooth, flat brown patches that usually occur on the face or on the back of the hand. Melanodermas formed by melanocytes, or tan-producing cells, are also known as "liver spots" because of their coloration; they have no relation to the liver. *Cherry angiomas* appear on the skin as small, bright red bumps. They are caused by clusters of small blood vessels under the skin. Blood vessels also give rise to larger purple blotches in the skin, usually in areas exposed to sunlight.

Ageusia   A loss of the sense of taste. Causes may be organic, as when taste buds atrophy, or the result of an injury or disease. *Central ageusia* is a form of the disorder caused by a lesion in the taste centers of the brain. The cause of *conduction ageusia* is a lesion in the nerves leading from the taste buds.

Agnosia   A loss of the ability to recognize objects, grasp the meaning of words, or interpret sensations. Agnosia is often a sign of organic brain damage, but it also may be due to depression or some other psychological disorder. In one form of the disorder, the person experiences "word blindness" and becomes unable to copy printed material but is able to write spontaneously. The patient also may be unable to read material that has just been read aloud by another person. This condition has been traced to a lesion in nerve fibers that connect the left and right sides of the brain.

AIDS   An abbreviation for acquired immune deficiency syndrome, a viral infection caused by an organism identified in the U.S. in 1983 as a human T-cell leukemia-lymphoma virus (HTLV). In France and certain other countries, the same virus is known as a lymphadenopathy virus (LAV). The virus is generally transmitted by sexual or other intimate contact with an infected person, through the use of contaminated hypodermic needles by drug abusers, or through exchange of infected body fluids, such as from a blood transfusion. The disorder is characterized by swollen lymph nodes (lymphadenopathy) and often by a respiratory infection (pneumocystis carinii pneumonia) and a form of skin cancer (Kaposi's sarcoma). Pneumocystis carinii pneumonia is a lung infection in which lung tissue becomes filled with air or gas-filled cysts. Kaposi's sarcoma causes purple or brown plaques or nodules to appear on the skin of the legs and feet; the disease then migrates into the digestive tract, with a loss of blood that is often a fatal complication.

AIDS is usually detected by a medical test called an enzyme-linked immunosorbent assay (ELISA), which identifies the presence of antibodies to the virus. Antibodies indicate the person has been exposed to AIDS and may carry the virus, but it does not necessarily mean the individual has the disease, which is usually fatal. The body is normally protected against viral and other infections by white blood cells called killer T lymphocytes. The AIDS virus first destroys these protective white cells, eliminating the body's first line of disease resistance and its natural immunity to infections. Although AIDS is often identified as a health problem affecting mainly the young, a survey of AIDS patients in the New York City area found the average age was 38.5 years; some AIDS patients with Kaposi's sarcoma were in their sixties.

Airway obstruction   Any condition in which a person has difficulty in breathing because a foreign object or other obstruction in the respiratory tract has reduced the normal amount of airflow to the lungs. If the disorder is minor, as in a respiratory tract infection such as the common cold, the person is usually able to breathe, although breathing is abnormal, with mild coughing and, sometimes, wheezing. The condition can often be corrected with bronchodilating drugs and by improving the atmosphere by increasing the humidity and eliminating irritants in the environment. If the obstruction is serious, as in choking on food, the person may be unable to speak, may grasp the throat, gasp, and become unconscious. The condition is a life-threatening emergency that requires immediate action to clear the airway, using the **Heimlich maneuver** or other means. If first aid measures fail, the victim should be removed as quickly as possible to a hospital emergency room or a doctor's office where oxygen may be given and, if necessary, a tracheotomy performed. *See also* **Chronic obstructive pulmonary diseases (COPD)**.

Akathisia   A type of restlessness marked by an inability to remain seated for any length of time. It may be caused by a brain disease. It is also sometimes seen in persons suffering from **parkinsonism**, when the effect is attributed to a reaction to phenothiazine tranquilizers. The restlessness also may be expressed by compulsive moving, twisting, or changing positions in a bed or chair, shifting from one foot to another, or pacing about. In cases associated with brain disease, the person may move the limbs more or less continuously in bicycle fashion.

Akinesia   Any of several abnormal conditions marked by a loss or lack of control of muscles that allow voluntary control of the arms, legs, and other body segments. Causes may be exposure to a toxic substance in the environment, such as in lead poisoning; the use of medications that affect the nervous system; a loss of muscle power due to disuse; **parkinsonism**, or an avoidance of any movement that may be painful.

Alcoholism   The chronic use of and dependence on alcohol. The condition may be characterized by a daily need for alcohol in order to function; a tendency to increase consumption; excessive drinking when alone; uncontrolled behavior; periodic binges, benders, or blackouts; impaired social and economic functioning; and severe withdrawal symptoms. Physical effects include cirrhosis of the liver, the fourth major cause of death (after heart disease, cancer, and stroke) among Americans over the age of forty-five; brain damage; damage to the nervous system; and cardiomyopathy (heart muscle disease). Complications may include auditory hallucinations, paralysis, numbness, weakness, loss of reflexes, and impairment of the memory and intellect. Also called "alcohol dependence."

Algodystrophy   A type of wasting of the muscles of the hand. There is localized pain, tenderness, and a loss of bone calcium and muscle tissue. The condition may begin in the hand or in the shoulder and eventually involve the entire limb. It may be accompanied by contracture (inability to straighten the fingers), swelling, fluid accumulation, and bluish (cyanotic) coloring of the skin. The condition may be associated with heart disease, stroke, injury, surgery, or an infection, particularly **shingles**.

Alloesthesia   A referred feeling of pain or other sensation that is felt or perceived on the same or opposite side of the body but not in the place stimulated.

Alkaline-ash diets   Diets that result in production of less acid urine. Foods that tend to increase the alkalinity, thereby reducing the acidity, of urine are milk, cream, buttermilk, almonds, chestnuts, coconuts, vegetables (except for lentils and corn), and fruits, with the exception of cranberries, prunes, and plums. Regardless of the acidity of these foods when eaten, they yield an alkaline "ash" when metabolized. When it is necessary to increase the acidity of the urine, alkaline-residue foods are restricted in the diet.

Alkalosis   An abnormal condition in which there is an excess of alkalinity, or base, in the blood and other body tissues. The disorder may result from a loss or deficiency of acid constituents in body tissues or fluids. Common causes include vomiting, which results in a loss of gastric acid from the stomach, and the use of certain medications, such as antacid stomach remedies or diuretics, that deplete the body's stores of potassium. Symptoms include muscle twitching, weakness, confusion, and irritability. In an effort to compensate, the body attempts to increase the carbonic acid level in the blood through slow and shallow breathing.

Allergen   Any substance that produces an allergic reaction in a person. It is frequently, but not always, a protein or an **antigen**. Examples include plant pollens, certain food products, bacteria, viruses, animal dander, house dust, antibiotics, and fungi. Allergens may not affect all persons to the same degree; thus, for some individuals, strawberries are an allergen, but most people suffer no ill effects from eating them.

Allergy   A hypersensitivity to a particular substance (allergen) in the environment, manifested by a wide variety of physiological reactions. Allergies represent the activity of the body's immune system, which identifies the substance as an allergen (antigen). The allergen is recognized as "foreign" or "nonself," that is, composed of material that is different from the body's own tissue. The immune system attacks and attempts to destroy the foreign substance; it is the reaction of the immune system to the invasion of the body by the allergen that produces the symptoms of an allergy, which may include itching, swelling, skin eruptions, bronchial spasms, blood pressure changes, runny nose, watering eyes, or contractions of digestive tract muscles.

The precise symptoms depend in part upon the area of the body that encounters the allergen, so that poison ivy may cause only a skin reaction, while a wheat allergen produces a digestive tract reaction. Some of the effects are caused by chemicals, such as **histamine**, released by body cells damaged in the conflict between the immune system and the allergen. While many allergies result in relatively mild reactions of itching and watery eyes, some particularly sensitive individuals may experience life-threatening **anaphylactic shock**, with respiratory distress and circulatory collapse, as an allergic reaction to a foreign substance such as a venomous insect sting. People who seem to have more than their fair share of allergies are called "atopic." They are usually afflicted from childhood with various allergies, including hay fever, asthma, eczema, and food sensitivities. Atopy is usually an inherited trait. However, some allergic reactions may appear for the first time in middle age or later in life, depending upon such factors as when the individual develops a sensitivity to a particular antigen.

Alopecia   A partial or complete loss of hair. The condition may be due to aging, inherited factors, a hormonal disorder, a skin disease, or a drug reaction. Certain anticancer drugs cause a loss of hair. *Alopecia areata* is a loss of hair in well-circumscribed patches on the head or other parts of the body. In men, the beard is often the site of alopecia areata. This kind of hair loss tends to develop in those who do not have a skin disorder or other disease that might account for the problem. In a variation of the disorder, *alopecia universalis,* all body hair may fall out. As in cases of alopecia areata, the condition is often temporary. Hair growth may return after a few months, even without treatment. But alopecia also may recur. *Scarring alopecia* is a form of the disorder in which original hair growth is lost due to scar formation, as from burns, injury, X-ray atrophy of the skin tissues, or deep fungal or bacterial infections. Hair rarely, if ever, regrows in the scarred areas. *Male-pattern baldness* is technically a form of alopecia that is linked to heredity and male hormones. *See also* **Baldness.**

Alpha alcoholism A mild form of alcoholism, marked by a psychological rather than a physical dependence on alcohol. The person may use alcohol excessively in order to relieve physical or psychological pain but does not lose control and is still able to abstain. Also called "problem drinking."

Alpha-adrenergic blocker Drugs that prevent the transmission of impulses along certain "alpha" nerve fiber pathways of the sympathetic nervous system. The activity is similar to that of **beta-adrenergic blockers**, except that alpha rather than "beta" nerve units are affected.

Alveolus Any small hollow area of the body. The term is most often applied to the myriad tiny air sacs that give the lungs their spongelike texture. The alveoli of the lungs are air pockets that are clustered like a bunch of grapes at the end of terminal bronchioles; their thin membrane walls contain capillaries that allow circulating blood to absorb oxygen and release carbon dioxide during respiration. A tooth socket is also an alveolus.

Alzheimer's disease A form of dementia, or irreversible brain dysfunction, marked by structural changes in the brain tissue and associated mental and behavioral alterations, usually ending in death. Alzheimer's disease is sometimes classified as "presenile dementia" because the symptoms, usually beginning with memory loss, first appear between the ages of forty and sixty, much earlier than the senile dementia associated with very old individuals. The brain undergoes a loss of cells from the cerebral cortex and other areas; the deep grooves normally present among the convolutions of the brain's surface become wider, and the ventricles, or normal hollow spaces within the brain, become larger. On autopsy, microscopic examination of brain tissue shows lesions called "senile plaques" and tangles of nerve fibers. Symptoms include memory loss, a gradual loss of judgment, failure to recognize or identify persons or objects, and loss of the ability to perform certain tasks, particularly if they are complex.

A patient in the early stages of the disease may be able to perform simple errands, such as going to a store to buy one or two things; but if asked to go to several different stores, he or she may become confused and return empty-handed. A typical early Alzheimer's disease patient may be aware of memory difficulties and write notes to help refresh the memory, then forget the purpose of a note or where it was put. Alzheimer's disease patients tend to become hyperactive, or even agitated. As the disease progresses, victims lose their ability to understand words (aphasia) and the ability to perform purposeful activities (apraxia), such as dressing.

Eventually, they may perform acts that can endanger themselves and others, as when handling machinery or tools. An Alzheimer's disease patient may step out of a moving vehicle, forgetting it is in motion. Deterioration of the brain and its functions is progressive, and the disease, which is generally fatal, may run its course over a span of several years. *See also* **Aphasia, Apraxia, Memory loss, Pick's disease.**

Amaurosis   The sudden partial or complete loss of vision, usually in one eye, in the absence of any organic abnormality. One form of the disease, *amaurosis fugax,* is usually attributed to a deficiency in blood flow to the eye. Other possible causes may include nutritional deficiencies, as evidenced by the discovery after World War II that American prisoners of war in the Far East experienced amaurosis as a symptom of beriberi or pellagra, diseases caused by a lack of the B vitamins thiamine or niacin.

Ambulatory   Pertaining to a person who is not bedridden and is able to walk and be up and about, even though he or she may be ill or injured. The term is sometimes applied to outpatients or to hospital patients who do not require overnight care.

Ambulatory schizophrenia   A mild form of schizophrenia that usually does not require hospitalization. The person may appear to be normal but tends to respond to questions with vague and irrelevant answers. Asked a direct question, the person may begin an answer that is only slightly irrelevant at the start but progressively wanders off the subject.

The patient also may appear to be somewhat eccentric and may show a tendency to wander about aimlessly.

Amenorrhea The absence of menstruation. Amenorrhea is considered a symptom rather than a disorder and is usually divided into two main categories, *primary amenorrhea,* which identifies the failure of a woman to begin menstruating by the time she is eighteen years old, and *secondary amenorrhea,* the cessation of menstruation for at least six months in a woman who has previously menstruated. Absence of menstruation after the menopause is *physiologic amenorrhea* and is a normal condition.

More than a dozen causes have been found for secondary amenorrhea, including crash diets, anorexia, loss of appetite, obesity, depression and other psychological problems, the use of certain medications, including oral contraceptives and tranquilizers, and a number of hormonal disorders. Emotional upsets frequently lead to disruption of normal hormonal functions. Some professional athletes experience amenorrhea that is due to physiological effects of an extremely strenuous training regimen. Diseases that disrupt nutrition and metabolism may also alter normal hormonal activity. *See also* **Menopause.**

Amnesia A partial or complete loss of memory, which can be due to organic brain disease or injury, alcoholism, an epileptic seizure, senile dementia, or an unconscious repression of a memory that may be painful. *Anterograde amnesia* is a loss of memory for events that follow a physical or mental disturbance, such as a blow to the head. *Retrograde amnesia* is a loss of memory for events that occurred before a physical or mental trauma, as in reported cases of persons who assume a new identity after a car crash or a similar accident that "erases" all memory of a life before the mishap. *See also* **Alzheimer's disease, Memory loss.**

Amusia An inability to recognize melodies (a form of **agnosia**) after suffering a stroke or other injury that affects the parietal lobe of the brain.

Amyloidosis A disease in which a waxy starchlike protein substance, amyloid, accumulates in the tissues in amounts that may impair the normal functions of certain organs. Two major forms of amyloidosis are recognized: (1) *primary amyloidosis,* in which amyloid "tumors" develop in the respiratory tract and other organs, and (2) *secondary amyloidosis,* which accompanies an infectious or inflammatory disease, such as **tuberculosis, bronchiectasis, osteomyelitis,** or **rheumatoid ar-**

thritis. When the skin is involved, waxy, translucent papules may appear on the face, lips, ears, and upper chest. The tongue, liver, spleen, and lymph glands can become enlarged. The patient experiences weight loss, fluid accumulation, joint and muscle pain, and purpura (the presence of hemorrhages in the skin). Treatment and outcome depend upon the underlying cause, particularly in cases of secondary amyloidosis, and the organ systems involved.

Amyotrophic lateral sclerosis (ALS) A degenerative nerve disease involving the nerve tracts running from the brain through the spinal cord. As the motor neurons, which innervate the skeletal muscles, degenerate, there is gradual atrophy of the hands, arms, and legs. The disease usually begins in middle age and gradually spreads to most of the body. In most cases, it proves fatal within five years. There is no known cure. It also is known as "Lou Gehrig's disease." Gehrig, a New York Yankees baseball star, died of ALS in 1941, and publicity about the case stimulated general interest in the causes and treatment of the disease. *See also* **Aran-Duchenne disease.**

Anaclisis A condition of extreme emotional and sometimes physical dependence on other people for the satisfaction of basic needs. While normal in infants and young children, the condition in adults is regarded as abnormal. Some individuals consciously or unconsciously select for emotional and physical dependence one who resembles a parent or other significant person who was an important source of comfort in the individual's childhood.

Anacusis A medical term for total loss of hearing.

Anaerobic Pertaining to the absence of air or oxygen, as with those bacteria causing gangrene and botulism that thrive without oxygen. The term also is used to describe physical exercises that require very little muscular exertion, so that increased air intake to inhale additional oxygen is not needed.

Anaphia A loss of or decrease in the sense of touch. The cause can be a lesion in the brain or in a nerve fiber in the spinal cord. A brain lesion, such as one resulting from a stroke, usually results in a loss of the sense of touch on the opposite (contralateral) side of the body. Thus, a loss of the sense of touch on the left side of the body may be due to a lesion on the right side of the brain. If a spinal nerve is involved, the lesion is likely to affect the same (ipsilateral) side.

Anaphylactic shock   An extreme allergic, or hypersensitivity, reaction. It results from contact with an antigen (allergen)—a substance the body's tissues identify as "foreign"—the body has encountered previously, and it causes an overwhelming release of histamine and other body chemicals that affect smooth muscle cells. Symptoms may include intensely itchy skin eruptions, with **wheals** and flares (areas of redness caused by dilated blood vessels beneath the skin), bronchospasm, and, in severe cases, circulatory collapse and shock. Fluid may escape into the alveoli of the lungs, obstructing the flow of oxygen into the bloodstream. The severity of the reaction depends upon such individual factors as the amount or duration of exposure to the antigen causing the sensitivity, the amount and distribution of antibodies produced to fight the antigen, and the amount of antigen causing the current reaction.

Common causes of anaphylactic shock include insect stings, penicillin injections, and vaccines derived from animal serum. An anaphylactic reaction can be a true medical emergency, requiring administration of epinephrine and other potent drugs, resuscitation, and immediate hospitalization.

Anarthria   The loss of the ability to articulate, or to speak properly. The disorder is often due to a disease affecting the neuromuscular tissues.

Anasarca   A medical term for generalized **edema,** or an excessive amount of fluid accumulation in the body.

Anastomosis   The surgical joining of two blood vessels or other tubular body passageways. Anastomoses are commonly performed to allow blood flow to bypass an **aneurysm** or blocked artery or to join two sections of intestine, nerves, fallopian tubes, or ureters.

Androgen   Any of the male sex hormones or related chemical substances stimulating the development of masculine sexual characteristics. Examples are **androsterone** and **testosterone.**

Androsterone   A relatively weak male sex hormone (androgen) that is associated with the growth and development of such masculine sexual characteristics as the genitalia, pubic hair, and deepening of the voice.

Anemia   A general term for any of more than two dozen types of abnormal conditions in which there is a deficiency of red blood cells or insufficient hemoglobin (iron) content in the red blood cells. Anemia itself is a symptom rather than a disease. Some of the milder effects of anemia include feelings of weakness, drowsiness, easy fatigability, difficulty in maintaining balance, ringing in the ears, spots before the eyes, and abnormal behavior. The seriousness of anemia lies in the crucial role of *hemoglobin,* the red coloring matter of red blood cells, in holding oxygen molecules in the red blood cells for delivery throughout the body. When there are not enough red blood cells or the cells do not contain enough hemoglobin to function normally, the tissues of the body experience oxygen starvation (hypoxia). An example of one subtle but serious effect of anemia is the extra effort the heart must exert in order to deliver the reduced amount of oxygen throughout the body; this extra effort may be enough to trigger an attack of **angina pectoris**, congestive heart failure, or shock. An enlarged spleen, amenorrhea, and digestive complaints can be signs of anemia. Anemia can be caused by blood loss; a deficiency of iron, copper, folic acid, vitamin C, or vitamin B_{12} in the diet; infections that destroy red blood cells; enzyme deficiencies; and diseases that interfere with normal hemoglobin manufacture.

Aneurysm   A dilatation or outward bulging in the wall of a blood vessel, usually an artery. An aneurysm usually occurs at a point of weakness in the wall of a blood vessel. The weakness may be aggravated by other health conditions, such as arteriosclerosis, which can cause calcification of an artery wall or high blood pressure. The weakness also can be caused by an infectious disease; thus an untreated syphilis infection can lead to development of an **aortic aneurysm**.

An aneurysm can occur in nearly any part of the body and may rupture, creating an emergency situation. A ruptured aneurysm in a blood vessel in the brain is a common cause of stroke. The risk of an aneurysm generally increases with age, is often associated with arteriosclerosis, and is most likely to develop in the brain, the abdomen, or the legs. An aneurysm in the chest area often causes breathing difficulty, coughing, pain, hoarseness, or swallowing difficulty.

A variation is a **dissecting aneurysm**, in which blood infiltrates between the layers of an artery wall, causing a separation of the layers. A dissecting aneurysm produces a sharp, crushing, or tearing pain that is associated with the part of the body in which it is located. In the chest, the pain may be mistaken for a heart attack. A dissecting aneurysm above the heart may produce a referred pain in the neck. A low back pain can be a sign of an aneurysm in the abdomen. An aneurysm in an arm or leg is usually marked by pain, tenderness, and swelling. It may feel like a cyst. Aneurysms frequently cause pulses to disappear or become unequal in different parts of the body or cause differences in blood pressure between the right and left sides of the body. Absence of a pulse is a diagnostic sign of an aneurysm. Nearly all aneurysms require hospitalization and surgical care to correct or bypass the defect, as well as medical treatment for contributing conditions such as high blood pressure.

Angina pectoris A generally painful sensation in the chest, commonly beneath the breastbone (sternum), that is caused by an oxygen deficiency in the heart muscle. The sensation may range from a vague aching feeling to a severe, crushing pain. The pain may radiate along the left arm as far as the fingers, to the back of the chest, or into the throat and jaw. The pain may also be experienced in the right arm. The discomfort may continue for a period of from one to ten minutes. It is increased by physical exertion and relieved by rest.

The amount of exertion that triggers an attack of angina may vary from one day to the next, but exertion following a meal often produces angina symptoms. Cold weather tends to exacerbate the condition, so that exertion that can be tolerated in warm weather or in a warm room is likely to result in painful symptoms when repeated in a cold environment. There is commonly a time lag between exertion and the onset of angina symptoms, and between the start of symptoms and the relief from pain after the person has ceased physical activity or has taken a prescribed medication. Pain that begins at the same time as physical exertion probably is not a symptom of angina and may suggest a problem involving the skeletal muscles.

In some variations, angina may occur during rest or sleep, particularly if the environment is cold. Angina that occurs during rest also can be due to the shifting due to gravity of fluid from the legs or arms to the chest when the person is in a reclining posture. The symptoms also may be associated with hypoglycemia, emotional upset, or a heart rhythm disorder, such as fibrillation. In most cases, other than pain, there are no physical signs during an attack; in others an abnormal heart rhythm can be detected. Rest, warmth, and nitroglycerin tablets are such reliable methods of reducing the symptoms of angina pectoris that they are used in the diagnosis of the disorder.

While the symptoms of angina also can be caused by many other diseases or disorders, several factors help distinguish angina from the other possible causes. They include the fact that angina pain lasts only a few minutes and usually occurs following a lag period after exertion. *See also* **Myocardial infarction, Valsalva maneuver.**

Angioedema A hypersensitivity disorder, resulting in an allergic skin reaction. The skin lesions are usually larger fluid-filled wheals than are seen in cases of hives or similar reactions to drugs, insect bites, or foods containing **antigens**. Angioedema may be acute or chronic and may be progressive and recurrent. One form is hereditary. Unexplained angioedema may be due to an allergen in the diet, such as a food dye or other additive, or a reaction to a medication.

Angiography An X-ray technique for visualizing the inside of the heart and its associated blood vessels after injection of a radiopaque dye. The method is used in the diagnosis of a wide variety of heart disorders in those who are not allergic to the dye, which contains iodine.

Angioma A small colored skin tumor composed primarily of blood or lymph vessels. A bright red angioma, called a *cherry angioma,* may appear on the chest, arms, face, or abdomen. Nearly every person over the age of forty has at least a few cherry angiomas, and they tend to increase in number as one grows older. However, the angiomas also tend to fade and atrophy in later years. The blue papules that develop in the veins of the scrotum after the age of fifty are also angiomas. These scrotal angiomas may vary from red to a very dark shade of blue and are filled with blood from veins. An angioma comprised of blood vessels is sometimes identified as a *hemangioma,* while an angioma formed from lymph vessels may be called a *lymphangioma.*

Anorexia A lack or loss of appetite as a result of illness. It is a common symptom of gastrointestinal distress. Anorexia may also be a side effect of some medicines or medical procedures.

Anosmia A loss of the sense of smell. The cause may be a nasal swelling or obstruction, atrophy or destruction of the nerve cells in the membrane lining the nasal cavities, or loss of the organs of the sense of smell or the nerve fibers that carry messages from the olfactory organs to the brain because of a head injury, infection, or tumor. The condition may be general, or it may be confined only to certain odors.

Anosognosia The denial or inability to acknowledge that one has a disease or disability. The condition often develops in those with poor vision, hearing loss, disfigurement or loss of a limb, or paralysis. The person may actually be unaware of the physical limitations, or the disorder may be a way of denying reality. The patient may attempt to conceal a disability as by, for example, raising the right arm when asked to raise a paralyzed left arm or by always making turns to the right when his left field of vision has been lost.

Anoxia The total or relative lack of oxygen. The term may be used to refer to an organ or body part that is deprived of oxygen by a circulatory defect, an inadequate supply of oxygen to the lungs, or an anemic condition in which the blood is unable to transport enough oxygen to meet the demand of tissues throughout the body.

Antacids Drugs or dietary substances that absorb, buffer, or neutralize hydrochloric acid in the stomach. There are two types of antacids: *absorbable,* such as sodium bicarbonate and calcium carbonate, which are usually taken for short-term relief, and *nonabsorbable,* such as aluminum hydroxide and magnesium hydroxide, which are weakly alkaline salts that help neutralize the acidity. Each type can produce certain adverse effects if used to excess. Abuse of sodium bicarbonate or calcium carbonate can lead to **alkalosis**; excessive use of aluminum hydroxide can cause constipation, and magnesium hydroxide can cause diarrhea.

Anthracosis An occupational disease of the lungs caused by the inhalation of coal dust. In most cases, the coal dust forms patches around the bronchioles, resulting in their becoming dilated, a type of emphysema. Coal miners who have spent at least ten years working underground are most seriously affected. The coal dust stimulates a fibrous growth in their lung tissues, with destruction of the blood vessel beds in the lungs. Breathing and the ability to continue work become impaired. The condition may be complicated by **silicosis**, depending upon the amount of silica in the coal dust. There is no specific treatment. Also called "black lung disease," "coal miner's pneumoconiosis." *See also* **Silicosis.**

Antiadrenergic Pertaining to drugs or other agents that block or interfere with the transmission of impulses along fibers of the alpha and beta adrenergic pathways of the **sympathetic nervous system**. Examples include substances that block the action of an adrenal gland hormone (norepinephrine) that influences circulation in the extremities and blood pressure, and the **beta blockers** that reduce the rate and force of heart contractions for those with heart disease. *See also* **Alpha-adrenergic blockers, Beta-adrenergic blockers.**

Antiarrhythmics Drugs or other agents that help correct an abnormal heart rhythm. Examples of antiarrhythmic drugs include *digitalis,* prescribed for the treatment of atrial fibrillation; *propranolol,* used for irregular heartbeats; *atropine,* administered for abnormally slow heartbeats; and various sedatives, prescribed for abnormally rapid heart-beats. *See also* **Arrhythmias.**

Antibiotics A family of medications that destroy microorganisms, particularly bacteria, or that interfere with their development or ability to reproduce. Since the introduction of penicillin, the first antibiotic, in the 1940s, many antibiotics have been developed for the treatment of specific kinds of infections. Antibiotics are also employed against a wide variety of diseases caused by fungi, protozoa, Rickettsias, and other organisms in addition to bacteria. However, antibiotics are not effective against viruses, and taking an antibiotic for a viral infection like the common cold is not only useless but increases the risk of developing a sensitivity to the drug, experiencing adverse side effects, or contributing to the production of a strain of bacteria that is resistant to antibiotics.

Some antibiotics, like penicillin, work by preventing germs from building their cell walls; others, such as the tetracyclines, prevent germs from building the protein molecules they need for their normal life functions. Both effects kill bacteria. Certain antibiotics are classified as *bacteriostatic;* they prevent a bacterium from multiplying but do not kill it. It is for this reason that doctors prescribe a specific course of treatment with bacteriostatic antibiotics. If the medication is discontinued too soon, the bacteria can resume multiplying, and symptoms of the infection will return.

Antibody A specialized protein molecule (immunoglobulin) produced by the body to resist infection. There are five basic types of antibodies, each type with a somewhat different function. One type specializes in protecting body surfaces against invading microorganisms; another kind appears to be involved in allergic reactions to milk, penicillin, and other substances in certain sensitive individuals. Antibodies are produced in the lymphatic system. Many specific antibodies may exist, each one adapted to resist a particular allergen or foreign substance that may invade the body. *See also* **Allergy.**

Anticholinergic A drug or other agent that interferes with the transmission of impulses by fibers of the **autonomic nervous system**. Anticholinergic drugs are used to treat symptoms of parkinsonism, to dilate the pupils of the eyes, and to control spasms of the gastrointestinal tract.

Anticoagulant A drug that prevents or slows coagulation (clotting) of the blood. Anticoagulant drugs work by interfering with one or more of the stages involved in the formation of blood clots. *See also* **Blood clotting.**

Anticonvulsant　A drug that prevents epileptic or other kinds of seizures or convulsions. Most anticonvulsant drugs work by reducing the excitability of certain nerve cells in the brain or by preventing an excessive flow of nerve impulses in the affected brain cell areas.

Antidepressant drug　A medication that prevents or relieves psychological depression. Some antidepressant drugs are stimulants; others are believed to work by increasing the amount of epinephrine or related hormones in the central nervous system. *See also* **Bipolar disorders, Depression.**

Antidiuretic　Pertaining to the suppression of urine formation. An antiduretic hormone (ADH) is secreted by the pituitary gland to prevent the release of too much water from the kidneys during urine formation, thereby allowing the body to conserve water for blood volume or to keep salt (sodium) in the body tissues dissolved, among other reasons. Certain drugs, such as nicotine, stimulate production of ADH, while other substances, like alcohol, retard ADH production, increasing urine formation.

Antigen　Any substance that causes the body's immune system to produce and release antibodies whose purpose is to destroy the substance. An antigen is usually a protein that is not normally a part of the body's own system of tissues and therefore is regarded as a "foreign" substance to be rejected. The body's immune system is generally able to identify a molecule as being a part of its own family of chemicals, or "self," or a substance that is "non-self," or foreign. An antigen may be a fungus or bacterium, a toxic industrial chemical, the poison in a bee sting, or a skin graft from another person.

The antibody reaction to the antigen is the cause of inflammatory symptoms associated with infections or allergic reactions, such as itching, redness, pain, or swelling, usually at the site of contact. Occasionally, the body's immune system makes a mistake, identifies some of its own tissues as antigens, and attacks itself. *See also* **Autoimmune disease.**

Antihistamine　A drug that reduces the effects of histamine, a natural body substance with irritating effects that is released from injured tissue cells. Histamine causes many symptoms associated with hay fever, mosquito bites, and other allergic reactions. Antihistamines may produce mild adverse effects such as drowsiness, dry mouth, or constipation.

Antihypertensive Any drug or other agent that reduces high blood pressure. Various antihypertensives work in different ways. Some are diuretics that reduce blood pressure by decreasing blood volume through excretion of water; others dilate arteries directly; and some dilate arteries indirectly by blocking nerve impulses that would otherwise constrict blood vessels. *See also* **Hypertension.**

Anti-inflammatory Any drug or substance that reduces the symptoms of inflammation caused by injury or disease. Examples include such over-the-counter remedies as aspirin and ibuprofen. There also are numerous anti-inflammatory drugs that require a doctor's prescription. Most anti-inflammatory drugs appear to suppress the body's production of prostaglandins, potent natural substances that in tiny amounts cause symptoms of pain, redness, swelling, and heat in the affected body area.

Antilipidemic Pertaining to a drug or other agent, including special diets, that reduces the proportion of fats (lipids) in the blood. Antilipidemics are prescribed for people with high blood **cholesterol** levels or who may be threatened with the cardiovascular effects of **atherosclerosis**. Most antilipidemic drugs stimulate the excretion of cholesterol or triglycerides associated with atherosclerosis. They also may cause excess fats in the diet to form chemical compounds or complexes with bile acids that cannot be absorbed into the bloodstream from the intestinal tract.

Antilipidemic diets are designed to lower blood levels of cholesterol and triglycerides by eliminating food items such as egg yolks, organ meats, and animal fats, which are rich sources of lipids.

Antineoplastic Any drug or other agent that can control or destroy cancer cells. Most antineoplastics attack cancer cells in a manner similar to the way many antibiotics damage or destroy bacteria—by interfering with one of the several steps involved in cell reproduction. Because cancer cells are generally more prolific than normal tissue cells, they divide more frequently and thus are more vulnerable to chemicals that block the formation of substances needed for new cancer cells. The antineoplastic chemical also destroys normal tissue cells as they reproduce, but fewer normal cells are destroyed because they divide less frequently. Because some normal cells are damaged, most antineoplastic agents can have serious adverse effects.

Antiparkinsonian Pertaining to drugs or techniques used to treat **parkinsonism**. Most agents used to treat parkinsonism are substances designed to compensate for an imbalance in neurotransmitter chemicals in the brain. One type causes an increase in the availability of a neurotransmitter (dopamine) that is present in insufficient amounts in parkinsonism patients. Another basic type is an **anticholinergic** that blocks the activity of a different neurotransmitter (acetylcholine) that may be overly abundant in these patients. Nondrug measures include surgical procedures that destroy a part of the brain tissue by alcohol injection, freezing, cautery (burning), or cutting.

Antipyretic Any drug or technique that reduces fever. Commonly used over-the-counter antipyretic drugs are acetaminophen and aspirin. Other methods include an alcohol sponge bath and cooling blankets. An antipyretic drug does not necessarily work in the treatment of an inflammation, and may not offer relief from pain unless, like aspirin, it also acts as an analgesic. Fever is often, but not always, a symptom of an infection. *See also* **Anti-inflammatory.**

Antitoxin A preparation of **antibodies** used to prevent or control a specific disease. An antitoxin does not kill bacteria; it neutralizes the toxin, or poison, produced by the bacteria. Widely available antitoxins include those for botulism, diphtheria, and tetanus. The antibodies are derived from the blood serum of horses that have developed immunity to the infection. Antitoxins are administered by injection and are used with caution because many persons can experience an allergic reaction to the animal serum.

Antitussive Any drug that suppresses coughing by acting on the body's cough reflex. Antitussives should not be given to persons with a productive cough (one that yields sputum) because coughing is helpful in clearing secretions that otherwise would obstruct the upper respiratory tract. Most antitussives are a combination of medications and may also contain a painkiller, alcohol, an antihistamine, and/or an expectorant (a drug that aids in the removal of mucus secretions from the breathing passages) in a syrup form. Although antitussives formerly were prepared with narcotics, such as codeine, the opiate component is now generally replaced by synthetic drugs that are not addictive.

Anton's syndrome A denial (a form of **anosognosia**) by a person with partial or total blindness that there is a loss of vision, despite medical evidence to the contrary. The patient may contrive excuses for an inability to see, insisting, for example, that the examining room is not properly lighted.

Anuria   A failure to produce a normal amount of urine or the inability to urinate. Technically, anuria is measured by a urine output of less than 100 ml (a little less than four ounces) per day; an output of less than 500 ml per day is classified as *oliguria.* Normal adults excrete between 700 ml and 2,000 ml of urine daily. Anuria may be caused by any of several conditions, including an obstruction in the ureters or urethra, kidney impairment or failure, or a drop in blood pressure below the level needed for filtration pressure in the kidneys. Anuria or oliguria often develops unnoticed as a complication of another medical condition, such as burns, serious injury, heat prostration, surgery, heart attack, poisoning, or infection. Untreated, the disorder can progress rapidly to **uremia**, acute renal failure, and death. Among the symptoms of anuria are heart rhythm irregularities, extreme muscle weakness, and numbness due to an accumulation of potassium that cannot be excreted. Although acute urinary retention is usually painful, anuria or oliguria may be painless.

The patient may not have a sensation of fullness in the bladder, and the only physical sign may be a swelling in the lower abdomen. Pain associated with the bladder or the function of urination usually indicates the presence of a bacterial infection causing inflammation, whereas anuria is generally the result of kidney failure. Treatment may require catheterization, dialysis, medications to stimulate excretion of potassium through the bowel, a low-protein diet, and careful management of fluid intake and excretion.

Anxiety   A feeling of apprehension, uneasiness, dread, or agitation as a response to a vague or unknown threat or danger. The response is usually traced to a sense of insecurity or unconscious emotional conflicts. Although anxiety is sometimes distinguished from fear, which is a response to a clear and present danger rather than an undefined threat, the physiological reactions are the same. Anxiety causes muscle tension, an increased rate of breathing, and a faster heartbeat as the body prepares to fight or run from the danger.

Some mild anxiety occurs in most people at one time or another, but when anxiety is severe or persistent, so that it interferes with the normal activities of daily life, the condition is pathological. In some cases of anxiety neurosis, a person may experience an acute attack of anxiety marked by feelings of panic or terror that interfere with rational thinking. Rapid heartbeat may progress to an abnormally fast heartbeat accompanied by palpitations and irregular beats. Rapid breathing may lead to hyperventilation, resulting in **alkalosis**. A tense feeling in the stomach may increase to nausea and diarrhea. Muscle tenseness can become exaggerated in the form of trembling, stiffness, numbness, and weakness. The condition also may be marked by profuse sweating and a fainting sensation.

Anxiety attacks usually are brief, some lasting only a few minutes, but they often tend to recur. Somewhat more common is chronic anxiety, in which symptoms are less severe as compared to those of acute attacks but may persist for weeks or months. These symptoms include fatigue, headaches, insomnia, and feelings of uncertainty about the future. Treatment can include **minor tranquilizers**, **antidepressants**, and/or psychotherapy. Because of their calming effect, **beta-adrenergic blockers** are prescribed for some anxiety cases.

Anxiolytics   Drugs that are prescribed to relieve the symptoms of anxiety. They usually are **sedatives** or **minor tranquilizers**.

Aortic aneurysm   A ballooning (dilatation) of the wall of the aorta, the main artery carrying blood from the heart. The aorta arches upward from the left side of the heart, with branches extending from the top of the arch to the head and upper part of the chest, before it loops downward through the abdomen as far as the pelvis, where it divides into two main trunks, one continuing into each leg. The aneurysm is usually caused by **atherosclerosis** or **hypertension**, or both. The aorta may have been weakened previously by a congenital defect or a disease.

An aortic aneurysm in the abdominal area causes pain in the area of the defect, the pain frequently radiating toward the lower back. An aneurysm of the aorta in the chest area may cause pain near the breastbone, the pain radiating to the left shoulder or left side of the neck. The symptoms may mimic those of a heart attack. If the swollen part of the aorta compresses a nerve to the larynx or a bronchial tube, the symptoms may also include hoarseness and a brassy cough. An aortic aneurysm in the abdomen may become enlarged to a diameter of two inches and press against the spinal column, producing excruciating pain in the back.

Because an aortic aneurysm usually contains calcium deposits, its diagnosis can be confirmed by X-ray. Ultrasound is also used to locate and determine the size of an aortic aneurysm. As there is always a great risk that an aneurysm will eventually rupture or leak blood, the presence of the defect is a medical emergency. Small aortic aneurysms may be treated with drugs that relieve pain and reduce pressure on the weak part of the wall of the aorta. Large and dissecting aneurysms are usually corrected by surgery in which a flexible plastic tube is inserted to replace the weakened section of the aorta. *See also* **Aneurysm.**

Aortic-arch syndrome   A condition in which one or more branches of the aorta become blocked near the point in the chest where it emerges from the heart. The obstruction may be due to **atherosclerosis** or a mechanical defect, such as a constriction. Depending upon the branch artery and the degree of alteration in normal blood flow, the brain may be affected. If the carotid artery in the neck is involved, the person may faint after turning the head to one side. Other symptoms can include fainting spells, temporary blindness, partial paralysis, seizures resembling epilepsy, memory failure, or language difficulties, such as loss of ability to understand words.

Some disorders are progressive if the blockage is not remedied; for example, temporary blindness can increase to total loss of vision. In some cases, the circulatory system may compensate for the obstruction by diverting blood to the affected area through other blood-vessel routes. Surgery may be required to repair a blocked artery or to graft a bypass around the blockage, depending upon the site, the severity of the disorder, and the general health of the patient.

Aortic stenosis   A heart defect in which there is a narrowing or constriction of the aortic valve obstructing the normal flow of blood from the left ventricle of the heart to the main artery of the body. Although the cause often is congenital or due to rheumatic fever, aortic stenosis can also develop in middle age or later in persons without an earlier medical history of heart disorders. In such cases, it is a result of calcium deposits that interfere with the aortic valve function, reducing the heart's output of blood and causing pulmonary congestion.

Symptoms include a faint pulse, **angina pectoris**, breathlessness, fatigue, and loss of exercise endurance. As the condition progresses, physical exertion may cause the person to lose consciousness because blood flow to the brain is impaired. The condition is corrected by surgery to replace the calcified heart valve with an artificial valve.

Apareunia   An inability for any reason to perform sexual intercourse. *See also* **Dyspareunia, Impotence.**

Aphasia   A loss or impairment of the ability to understand or use language, whether written or spoken. The disorder is usually due to an injury or disease affecting a particular part of the brain. Spoken words are processed in a different part of the brain than visual, or written, words, and the specific form of aphasia generally depends upon which brain area may have been isolated by a stroke, tumor, or injury. The cause may be a defect in the sensory portion of the nervous system that interferes with the normal input of sight or sound impulses. The disorder may also be due to a lesion in the brain area in which nervous system impulses are translated into meaningful messages, or a failure of the motor nerves involved in the formation or expression of words.

Aphemia The loss of the ability to speak, which may be due to an emotional disorder or to a brain lesion. The term is sometimes applied to situations in which a person becomes afraid to speak or simply refuses to speak.

Aphoria A condition of physical weakness that is not improved through exerise.

Aphrasia A form of **aphasia** in which a person is able to speak or understand single words but is unable to communicate with words arranged in phrases or sentences.

Apnea The cessation of normal breathing. The term is usually applied to *sleep apnea,* which is marked by a temporary absence of spontaneous breathing and is a fairly common condition among middle-aged and older persons, particularly men. Though chest movements of respiration may continue during sleep apnea, there is no air flow into or out of the nose. Sleep apnea occurs most often in overweight persons whose upper airways (trachea and bronchi) are abnormally narrow. The person may experience choking sensations or awaken suddenly, gasping. Similar sleep apnea effects sometimes occur in persons of normal weight who have an obstruction in their breathing passages. Other causes include brainstem lesions due to a tumor or nervous system infections.

Apraxia A loss of the ability to perform purposeful acts or to manipulate objects. The person afflicted with apraxia may be unable to dress himself or to use tools. The patient may be able to identify an object and describe it yet be unable to demonstrate its use. The condition is the result of damage to that part of the brain involved with memory for certain learned skills. Apraxia occurs in many different forms. Some patients can perform a task with the left hand but not with the right hand; others may perform a different movement than requested, such as brushing the hair when asked to brush the teeth. The precise aberration depends upon the area of the brain that may have been damaged.

Aran-Duchenne disease   A form of **amyotrophic lateral sclerosis** that involves the cells of the spinal cord and progresses at a much slower rate than ALS. Whereas ALS usually leads to death within five years after the onset of symptoms, the Aran-Duchenne patient may survive as long as twenty-five years. The first symptoms usually are muscle-wasting and weakness in the hands. These effects gradually move up the arms, then involve the legs and the rest of the body.

Arcuate scotoma   A functional defect in vision, characterized by an arc-shaped physiologic "blind spot" that develops in the visual field of a glaucoma patient. It is caused by damage to the nerve fibers of the retina. In some patients, the arc extends into a circle, becoming a ring scotoma. The condition is irreversible. *See also* **Glaucoma.**

Arcus senilis   A ring-shaped deposit of white fat that develops at the outer edge of the cornea. This degenerative eye condition generally appears in persons over the age of sixty. A similar opaque circle, identified as *arcus juvenilis,* may develop in the corneas of younger persons, including those of middle age, particularly in individuals with a high level of blood lipids.

Arrhythmia   Any variation from the normal human heart rate of 72 to 78 contractions per minute. Abnormal heart rhythms include premature beats, beats grouped in pairs, missing or dropped beats, **fibrillation,** and atrial **flutter,** a condition in which heart muscle contractions are so rapid that no blood is actually moved by the heart. The normal rhythm of the heart is established by a cluster of hundreds of cells, called pacemaker cells, in the sinoatrial (SA) node. The SA node is located at the junction of the superior vena cava, the second largest vein of the body, and the wall of the right atrium of the heart.

This node (or knot) of specialized heart tissue generates electrical signals at a normally rhythmic rate of about 75 times a minute, and each discharge of the SA node triggers a contraction of the atria (the upper reservoirlike chambers of the heart), followed immediately by a contraction of the ventricles (the lower pumping chambers). The signal from the SA node is carried by systems of fibers that are buried in the heart muscle. The signal system contains another node, the atrioventricular (AV) node, and Purkinje fibers, which are capable of generating heart contraction signals if the SA pacemaker cells miss a beat.

Arrhythmias result from stimulation by hormones, **autonomic nervous system** signals, emotions, illnesses, exercise, and various medications or other substances, including caffeine, nicotine, and marijuana.

Any heart rate of more than 100 beats per minute in an adult is classified as **tachycardia**. An adult heart rate of less than 60 beats per minute is termed **bradycardia** and is also considered abnormal, even though many hospital patients have been found to have resting heart rates of less than 60 beats per minute. Heart rates of less than 60 beats per minute also may be normal for healthy young individuals and trained athletes.

The heart rate also is slower in older persons, who have fewer pacemaker cells in their SA nodes. Some heart arrhythmias are accompanied by symptoms, such as abnormal pulse rates and feelings of palpitations or "skipped beats." Bradycardia can cause a reduced flow of oxygen-rich blood to the brain, resulting in loss of consciousness, convulsions, and death. A beat so rapid that the heart is unable to move blood into the arteries can have the same effect. Feelings of weakness, dizziness, and faintness are common symptoms of heart arrhythmias. However, most arrhythmias require interpretation by a doctor equipped with a stethoscope and an electrocardiogram.

Arterial insufficiency   A condition in which blood flow through the arteries to the arms or legs is diminished by obstructive diseases, including **atherosclerosis**, or by injury or a defect in the artery wall, such as a **fistula** or **aneurysm**. Symptoms may include a pale or mottled skin, indicating inadequate blood flow to the area; a sharp, cramping pain when the arm or leg is exercised; a loss of body hair in the affected area; an absent or weak pulse in the limb; and a feeling of less than normal temperature in the arm or leg.

Treatment may include drugs to dilate the arteries, moderate exercises, a low-fat diet, and elimination of tobacco, because nicotine tends to constrict arteries and reduce blood flow.

Arteriosclerosis   A general term used to identify any disorder characterized by a thickening and hardening of the walls of the arteries. Contributing factors may include accumulations of fibrous tissue, deposits of calcium or other minerals, fatty deposits, or a combination of these that narrow the lumen, or opening, through the blood vessel. When the primary cause is an accumulation of fatty deposits, the condition is called **atherosclerosis**. Arteriosclerosis is often associated with aging and with high blood pressure, kidney disease, and diabetes.

Arteriosclerosis usually produces no symptoms in the early stages, and it is only after damage to the arteries interferes with blood distribution to an organ system or body area that the person becomes aware of the condition. At that point, symptoms may include changes in skin color and temperature, headache, dizziness, and cramping pains in the legs after walking. Untreated, the condition progresses to complete obstruction of vital arteries, resulting in hypertension, stroke, heart attack, kidney failure, and reduced blood circulation in the arms and legs. The condition is usually complicated by diabetes and obesity.

Therapy includes diet changes to reduce the intake of foods rich in animal fats, elimination of cigarette smoking, which causes further constriction of blood vessels, and treatment of the specific medical complications.

Arteritis An inflammation of an artery. Blood vessel inflammations have been classified according to the portion of the artery (inner layer or outer coat) or association of the condition with another disease, such as **rheumatoid arthritis**. *See also* **Temporal arteritis.**

Arthralgia Pain in a joint.

Arthritis A large group of disorders that have in common chronic nonspecific inflammation of the joints, particularly of the legs and arms, usually leading to progressive impairment and sometimes destruction of the joints and surrounding tissues. *See also* **Rheumatoid arthritis, Gout, Psoriasis, Spondylosis, and Osteoarthritis.**

Arthropathy A general term for any inflammation of a joint, which may occur with or without pain. A common form of the disorder, *neurogenic arthropathy,* is particularly serious because it develops without painful symptoms, so that injuries, even small fractures, and accumulations of mineral deposits in the joint may go unnoticed. Among the few clues that abnormal changes are occurring in the joint are the visible evidence that the joint has become unusually large and that the increased size is hard because of new bone formation. Other kinds of arthropathy include *inflammatory arthropathy* and *Jaccoud arthropathy,* a form of the disease that sometimes follows an attack of rheumatic fever.

Arthroplasty The reconstruction of a joint by surgery. The procedure is used to repair or replace a joint that has degenerated as a result of rheumatoid arthritis or osteoarthritis, or to restore mobility to a joint. The operation may involve reshaping of the remaining bone and surrounding tissue or the addition of metal or plastic parts, or both.

Arthroscopy A method of examining the interior of a joint by inserting an instrument with a lens and light source into the joint through a small incision. Arthroscopy also permits removal of small tissue samples for biopsy as well as the removal of deposits, bone or cartilage fragments, or other debris.

Asbestosis   A lung disease, or **pneumoconiosis**, caused by the inhalation of asbestos dust, resulting in fibrosis (an overgrowth of thick fibrous tissue) in the lungs. This decreases the breathing capacity by reducing the elastic quality of lung tissue while also interfering with the absorption of oxygen through the walls of the alveoli, the tiny air sacs that give lungs their spongy appearance. Because asbestos fibers are often microscopic in size, they can be inhaled as deeply into the lungs as the air that carries them. Some inhaled fibers of asbestos become encased in the lung within a deposit of protein, calcium, and iron salts called "asbestos bodies." It is believed the coating is the result of the attempt of the body's immune system to isolate the asbestos fibers and prevent them from irritating the alveoli. Asbestos fibers also inflame the walls of the capillaries that carry blood to and from the alveoli. The condition is not reversible; avoiding further exposure to asbestos does not stop the disease process once it becomes established.

Symptoms of asbestosis include cough, breathlessness, and wheezing, especially when physical exertion is required. The precise symptoms vary somewhat with the type of asbestos one has inhaled, and effects develop gradually over a long period of exposure, usually through working with asbestos or asbestos products. As the condition progresses and not enough oxygen gets into the bloodstream, the patient's skin coloring develops a bluish tint (cyanosis). The condition is aggravated by cigarette smoking, which also increases the risk of lung cancer in asbestosis patients. There is no specific treatment for asbestosis, and therapy is usually directed to relief of the symptoms.

Ascites   An accumulation of fluid within the abdominal cavity. The condition used to be called abdominal dropsy. It is frequently a symptom of a serious disease, such as **cirrhosis, congestive heart failure**, kidney failure, inflammation of the pancreas, or a thyroid gland insufficiency. Ascites due to kidney failure usually is the result of retention by the kidney of sodium (salt) that would normally be excreted. When the body retains sodium, it also retains the water required to keep the salt dissolved. When congestive heart failure is a cause, the process is similar, because changes in blood circulation to the kidney result in sodium retention and fluid accumulation.

The abdomen of a person with ascites may contain so much fluid that the sides of the abdomen bulge outward when the person lies in supine (on the back) position, and tapping the skin on one side of the abdomen may trigger a wavelike motion that moves to the opposite side, an action that can sometimes be seen as a rippling under the skin. Treatment consists of a low-salt diet and, in some cases, diuretic drugs ("water pills") to increase fluid loss through urination.

Asherman syndrome   A form of secondary **amenorrhea** that may develop in an otherwise normal woman as a result of adhesions (scar tissue) in the endometrium (lining of the uterus) that block the flow of menstrual fluid. These adhesions can be caused by inflammation resulting from an infection or from a dilatation and curettage (D&C) procedure. Treatment involves a D&C to remove the adhesions and the insertion of a device that allows healing of the endometrium without formation of new adhesions.

Aspermia   A failure of the male reproductive system to ejaculate semen. The condition is not a sign of infertility but may be due to a defect in the part of the nervous system that controls ejaculation, or the result of a structural abnormality in the bladder neck. Aspermia often develops following bladder surgery.

Astasia   An inability to stand. The person may suddenly develop a feeling of "rubber legs" and fall to the ground. *Astasia-abasia* is a variation of the condition in which the person is unable to either stand or walk normally. Astasia or abasia may be either psychogenic (an emotional effect) or the result of a lesion in central nervous system tissues in a part of the brain that manages body functions over which the person has no direct control. If the person has control of the legs when lying down, astasia is regarded as a psychological rather than a physical, or organic, disorder. The diagnosis is also based on the situation in which an attack occurs; an attack of psychogenic astasia usually occurs only when an audience is present and the fall to the ground is managed so there is little risk of injury.

Astereognosis   A loss of the ability to recognize familiar objects through the sense of touch. The person may also be unable to identify a geometric shape, such as a cube, if it is placed in the patient's hands while the patient's eyes are closed. The condition is associated with a disease or injury affecting the parietal lobes of the brain.

Asterixis   A diagnostic symptom of **Wilson's disease** and other metabolic disorders affecting the central nervous system, in which the wrists develop a "flapping tremor" when the arms are extended, palms down, and fingers spread. The fingers or the hand may tremble in a waving motion. In some cases, the arms will start an involuntary flapping motion like the wings of a bird flying. The tremor also can be detected by asking the patient to squeeze two of the examiner's fingers. Although the patient tries to squeeze, the examiner will feel the patient's fingers alternately clenching and unclenching. Asterixis may also be a sign of **alcoholism, uremia,** or respiratory **acidosis.**

Asthenia   A condition of chronic severe weakness or debility, usually resulting from a muscular or central nervous system disease. The person may feel a complete loss of strength, accompanied by breathlessness, muscular pain, faintness, and heart palpitations. There may also be a loss of appetite, constipation, and low body temperature. Women may experience secondary **amenorrhea.** Specific causes include a pituitary gland disorder and depression.

Asthma   A respiratory disorder marked by spasmodic wheezing and gasping due to a narrowing of the bronchial tubes leading to the lungs. Bronchial tubes swell, become inflamed, and produce a thick mucus that causes these effects. Asthma involves a complex alteration in breathing capacity, causing more air to be inhaled than exhaled during an attack, so that the lungs eventually become overly inflated.

When common **allergens** such as household dust, molds, pollen, or animal dander cause an attack, the allergic reaction is classified as *extrinsic asthma.* If factors such as infections or emotions cause an attack, the disorder is called *intrinsic asthma.* Between attacks, the patient may appear to be in normal health. A wide variety of irritants can trigger an asthma attack in a person who is susceptible. For some individuals, an asthma attack can be triggered by a change in atmospheric pressure, cold air, or the smell of gasoline or paint. Different individuals vary in their symptoms and the severity of their attacks. The typical asthma attack usually begins with an unproductive cough that leads to breathing difficulty. The person may have to rise to a sitting or standing position and bend forward to breathe as the coughing and wheezing attack progresses. The labored breathing often is accompanied by profuse sweating, and the wheezing sounds may be loud enough to be heard across the room.

Asthma that begins after the age of forty is usually more difficult to diagnose than when the onset occurs earlier in life. Older patients rarely show the relationship between asthma and an allergy that is a common clue in diagnosing the disease in younger persons. Asthma attacks in older adults are more likely to be caused by exercise, exposure to cold air, viral infections, air pollutants, emotional factors, and the use of certain drugs, such as aspirin and **beta-adrenergic blockers.** Asthma in older adults also is likely to be complicated by other respiratory disorders, including reduced breathing capacity, and related diseases, such as congestive heart failure. Several types of medications, including drugs to relax smooth muscles, are prescribed for the treatment of asthma.

Astigmatism   A visual disorder caused by a cornea that is not perfectly curved. Because of defects in the curvature, light rays entering the eye are bent unequally so they do not produce a sharply focused image on the retina at the back of the eye. Some of the light rays may be focused in front of the retina, others behind it. The distorted effect has been described as similar to the reflection produced by an amusement park mirror. The condition is corrected by eyeglasses or contact lenses that compensate for the corneal defect, enabling the viewer to focus correctly.

Asymptomatic   An absence of symptoms, in which a person experiences none of the symptoms normally associated with an existing disease or injury. *Asymptomatic diabetes* is a term sometimes applied to the condition in which a person may have abnormally high blood sugar levels without exhibiting actual symptoms of the disease. Glaucoma, hypertension, arteriosclerosis, and osteoarthritis, also may be diagnosed on the basis of clinical signs and laboratory findings before the patient experiences symptoms of the diseases.

Asystole   The absence of heartbeats. The term is often used in cardiac arrest to identify a condition in which the ventricles of the heart are not contracting, as distinguished from **fibrillation** or other **arrhythmias** in which heart contractions continue although they may be inadequate or ineffective.

Ataxia   A loss of the ability to coordinate movements, due to effects of drugs, disease, or injury involving the neuromuscular system. Ataxia can take various forms. A person with *cerebellar ataxia* often has difficulty in turning on his feet and may lurch or sway while walking, holding his arms extended for balance. When ataxia is caused by damage to one side of the cerebellum (the part of the brain that controls voluntary muscle movements), the person may tend to veer to the affected side and walk along a zigzag course in an effort to keep from bumping into objects in his path.

Truncal ataxia (affecting posture of the trunk) may be characterized by an inability to stand or walk normally or to coordinate muscles even while seated or reclining. Ataxia patients often have difficulty in maintaining their balance when standing with their feet together and they walk with the legs unusually far apart. The symptoms are frequently more pronounced in darkness or when the patient is tested with the eyes closed, and are similar to those of multiple sclerosis. *See also* **Astasia.**

Atheroma   An accumulation of fatty material, as an atheromatous **plaque** on the wall of an artery. The term is also used to identify a sebaceous cyst that evolves from an enlarged oil gland in the skin.

Atherosclerosis   An abnormal condition of the arteries marked by **atheromas** that accumulate on the inner walls, narrowing the lumen, or opening, through the affected artery and thus reducing the blood flow through it. Atherosclerosis is a contributing factor in heart disease, stroke, and kidney failure because it tends to occur in the arteries of the heart, the brain, and the kidneys. If the frequently silent and symptom-less buildup of atheromas eventually blocks the flow of blood to the heart or brain, the result is a heart attack or a stroke.

Atherosclerosis also may develop in arteries of other body areas. For example, it causes the leg cramps of **intermittent claudication** when the narrowed arteries restrict blood supply to the calf muscles. The first fatty streaks of atherosclerosis may begin in childhood, but symptoms of obstructed blood flow due to fatty accumulation on the walls of the arteries generally do not appear until after the age of forty-five. (In diabetes mellitus and certain other conditions, the first symptoms may be noted at an earlier age.) A common symptom of atheroslerosis in any part of the body is likely to be a pain produced by **ischemia**, or oxygen starvation in tissues that are deprived of their usual supply of oxygen-enriched red blood cells. In the example of intermittent claudication, ischemia in the leg may send early warning signals in the form of cramping pains that in the beginning may be noticed only when walking. There may be pallor or coldness of the skin, local hair loss, skin ulcerations, or signs of gangrene.

These symptoms signal that atherosclerosis is gradually shutting down circulation to the legs; it is assumed that when atherosclerosis affects the legs it is likely that other parts of the body also are beginning to feel the effects of the disease, even though the effects in vital internal organs may not give as much advance warning.

Atony   A loss of normal muscle tone that can occur in both smooth muscle and skeletal muscle. Atonic skeletal muscle may be character-ized by flaccidity and a loss of muscle tension. Atonic smooth muscle can be a serious condition in which certain normal body functions are impaired, as when atonic constipation results from loss of muscle tone in the digestive tract.

Atopognosia   A loss of the ability to locate the source of a stimulus, such as the pressure of a finger on the body. The cause is usually a lesion in the part of the brain that allows one to attach meanings to sensations or to the personal concept of one's body and its parts.

Atrophy   A decrease in size or function of a body part, such as a muscle or an organ. The wasting away of tissue may occur as a result of disease or a lack of use. Other causes of atrophy include malnutrition and hormonal changes. Various structures atrophy with aging. For example, a decline in the production of the hormone estrogen may cause an atrophic vagina, marked by a decrease in elasticity and in vaginal secretions, resulting in difficulty in intercourse and a need for hormonal or other therapy. Also, chronic gastritis may occur with advancing age as a result of a reduction in the thickness of the gastric wall and a diminished number of glands producing necessary secretions.

Autoimmune disease   Any of a group of diseases in which an abnormality in the functioning of the immune system causes the body to produce antibodies against itself, resulting in tissue injury. Autoimmune diseases tend to be more common in later life, when the immune system seems to lose its ability to distinguish between substances that are "self" and "nonself" and rejects the body's own cells as "foreign" matter. At the same time, the immune system may fail to recognize and destroy cancer cells. Examples of autoimmune disease include **systemic lupus erythematosus** and **rheumatoid arthritis**. *See also* **Antibody, Antigen.**

Autonomic nervous system   The part of the nervous system that is associated with the involuntary or automatic functions of the body, such as breathing, digestion, heartbeat, blood pressure, and most reflexes. The autonomic nervous system is divided into the *sympathetic* and *parasympathetic* systems. Autonomic nervous system functions are generally coordinated with those of the central nervous system and the peripheral nervous system.

Autotopagnosia   A disorder marked by a failure to recognize or relate to parts of one's own body. It is one of a number of functional anatomical disorders that may occur because of a lesion in a localized part of the brain, usually on the right side. In most cases, the patient ignores or disclaims a part of the body, usually on the left side. He or she may neglect to wash the left hand, shave the left side of the face, or wear a shoe or stocking on the left foot, or claim the left arm is not actually an arm but some other object.

Avascular   Pertaining to an insufficient supply of blood to a particular area of tissue. The reduced flow may be due to **atherosclerosis**, blockage by a blood clot, or an interruption of normal flow during surgery or to reduce bleeding, as when pressure or a tourniquet is applied to control a hemorrhage. The term is also used to describe a part of the body that lacks blood vessels.

Avitaminosis   Any vitamin deficiency disease. The cause may be a lack of a particular vitamin in the diet, a failure of the digestive tract to absorb the vitamin, or an inability of the body to utilize the vitamin because of another disorder. The term is generally accompanied by the identity of the vitamin, as "avitaminosis C."

AV nicking   A blood vessel abnormality found in the retina of the eye of some individuals afflicted with a circulatory disorder such as arteriosclerosis or hypertension. A vein that crosses an artery is compressed by the artery, resulting in a "nicked" or constricted appearance when examined by an ophthalmologist. The condition is generally without symptoms but is a common diagnostic sign that the person is afflicted with a cardiovascular disease.

Azoospermia   An absence of spermatozoa in the semen. The disorder may be caused by an obstruction somewhere along the seminal tract, a disease or injury involving the testicles, or a vasectomy. The person is sterile, but the condition does not result in impotence.

Azotemia   An abnormal condition in which the blood contains an excessive quantity of nitrogen products as a result of the kidney's failure to excrete these substances. Uncorrected, azotemia progresses to the more serious condition of **uremia**.

B

Babinski reflex   A basic medical test for certain central nervous system disorders. A blunt instrument is used to stroke a path along the sole of a bare foot from the heel to the ball of the foot, swerving at the ball of the foot toward the great toe. If the complete reflex is present, the great toe will flex upward, the toes will fan, the ankle will flex upward, and, if the patient is lying down, there will also be noticeable flexion of the knee and hip. Each of these responses represents a specific nerve pathway from the brain. The absence of one or more of the reflexes is a clue to the type and location of a lesion in the brain cells that control muscle movements. Also called "Babinski's sign."

Babinski's syndrome   A condition in which a person with partial paralysis, usually on one side of the body, denies or ignores the existence of the defect. As part of the denial, the person may make plans to participate in athletic events or other strenuous activities, despite medical evidence of the disability.

Bacille Calmette-Guérin (BCG)   The name of a strain of modified tubercle bacilli germs sometimes used to vaccinate against tuberculosis in regions where the disease is prevalent. BCG also is used in the treatment of certain kinds of cancer because it can stimulate improvement of the person's immune system, thereby increasing the body's resistance to diseases in general.

Backache   Any pain in any of the areas along or on either side of the spinal column, from the base of the neck to the pelvic region. Although disorders in the chest region, such as **angina pectoris,** may be a cause of upper back pain, most backaches are experienced in the lower lumbar or sacral regions, near the level of the pelvis. Though pain or discomfort also can be caused by many other factors, ranging from tumors of a bone or nerve to heavy metal poisoning to prostate gland disorders in men, the most common causes of backache are strains and sprains of the muscles and related tissues of the lumbar region.

The lumbar region is represented by the first five vertebrae above the sacrum (a spade-shaped bone formed by the fusion of five sacral vertebrae that is joined at the back by the two hipbones). The lumbar vertebrae are designed to support a greater share of the body's weight than vertebrae farther up the spinal column and are more massive, but they have smaller openings for the nerves that connect the spinal cord (the main trunk line of the nervous system that extends from the base of the brain to the tailbone). Lumbar vertebrae have back-to-front flexibility that permits the body to bend at the waist, but the vertebrae are less flexible about twisting movements. Straightening the back from a bending position requires great muscle power. Bending at the waist increases the strain on the spinal column more than sixfold and at the same time compresses the front half of the cartilage disks separating the vertebrae in the lumbar region.

An older person is more likely to feel low back pain than a younger individual after exertion involving the lumbar muscles and ligaments. Studies show that both men and women reach a peak of ability to flex the lumbar spine between the ages of twenty-five and twenty-eight. Ten years later, about 15 to 20 percent of ability to withstand tension and torsion of the lumbar spine has been lost, and after the age of fifty, about 35 percent has been lost. Back pain also can result from tumors, injuries, or substances that can accumulate in the spinal canal, through which the spinal cord passes in the spinal column. A pea-size tumor pressing on the spinal cord or one of its nerve roots can be the cause of excruciating pain, which is relieved only by surgery.

Osteoporosis, a degenerative bone disease commonly associated with the postmenopausal period of a woman's life, can result in a loss of bone mass in the vertebrae. This diminished bone density is often followed by compression fractures (collapse of a weakened vertebrae by the crushing weight of the body above it). A compression fracture may pinch a nerve root trapped in what was previously an opening between vertebrae. Softening of a vertebral bone may also allow a tough cartilage disk that normally serves as a cushion between vertebrae to push inside a weak vertebral bone, causing a spinal column collapse.

In a different kind of degenerative disorder, **osteoarthritis,** it is the cartilage disk that breaks down, so that cushioning between vertebrae is lost while sharp bone spurs grow from the edges of the affected vertebrae. Still another common cause of back pain is the so-called slipped disk, a condition more accurately identified as a **herniated disk**. The disk does not actually "slip," it develops gradually enlarging cracks and tears as a result of repeated compression and tension on the cartilage. Eventually, the disk expands or spreads (herniates) into the neighboring spinal canal, pinching a spinal nerve. The pain that results seems to radiate along the route of the sciatic nerve, producing symptoms of the disorder often called **sciatica**. The effect may also be experienced as a loss of feeling, or numbness, or tingling in the area served by the compressed nerve.

Rheumatoid arthritis and weight gain during pregnancy can lead to low back pain in women; although men are not immune to rheumatoid arthritis, women are much more prone than men to the effects of the disease on the lower back. The condition is often complicated by a loss of muscle tone. Among additional causes of low back pain are infections, blood circulation disorders, birth defects, psychoneurotic disturbances in which anxiety causes tension of the back muscles, which leads to pain, and transitional vertebrae, an abnormal condition in which spinal flexibility is lost because the bottom lumbar vertebra becomes fused with the sacrum.

A few simple tests can provide clues as to the cause of a backache. For example, the pain of a herniated disk can be diminished by lying down. But if there is pain in one leg, and the person lying down lifts the unaffected leg without bending the knee, the pain is likely to increase in the other leg if a herniated disk is involved. If a tumor is the cause, lying down may increase the pain. Sciatica pain usually begins in the buttock, then radiates to the thigh, and may spread down the leg as far as the toes. Coughing or sneezing usually aggravates the pain of sciatica. If the person is unable to lie flat without flexing the knees and hips to relieve the pain, the cause may be lumbosacral strain.

Treatment often includes bed rest on a hard surface, such as a mattress supported by a bed board, sedatives, gentle massage, warm baths, and heating pads. For serious cases, therapy can be an injection of a local anesthetic, a corset or back brace, or surgery. *See also* **Lordosis, Spinal fusion, Spondylosis.**

Bacteremia   The presence of bacteria in the bloodstream. The condition, which is potentially serious, may be temporary or continuous, often developing after surgery, childbirth, or procedures in which urinary catheters or intravenous devices have been used. Bacteremia occurs among drug abusers who inject themselves with contaminated hypodermic needles. Symptoms include a fever that may be intermittent, with periodic high points or "spikes," chills, nausea, vomiting, diarrhea, and skin eruptions that range from small blisters to tiny hemorrhages in or under the skin. If untreated, the condition can progress to septic shock, with circulatory collapse, kidney failure, and, eventually, death. Treatment may involve surgery to drain an abscess or remove infected tissue or the use of antibiotics, or both, depending upon the specific cause.

Bacterial endocarditis   A bacterial infection of the heart muscle (endocardium) or heart valves, or both. The disease is usually classified as either *acute bacterial endocarditis (ABE)* or *subacute bacterial endocarditis (SBE),* depending mainly on the type of bacteria involved. ABE usually is caused by strains of pneumococcal or staphylococcal bacteria, while the causative organism in SBE is a strain of streptococcus. ABE is often due to the use of infected needles by drug abusers, while SBE commonly occurs as a complication of a dental procedure, when bacteria enter the bloodstream through a tooth socket. Heart valves are rarely affected by SBE but may be susceptible in cases of ABE.

Symptoms include a fever that may be irregular or sustained at around 102° F, chills, joint pain (arthralgia), and general discomfort. Because the symptoms mimic those of many other diseases, heart involvement may not be discovered until after heart valve damage or other effects have been diagnosed. Complications include kidney impairment, tiny hemorrhages under the skin and in the eyes, and tender nodules that appear at the fingertips. The infection is treated with antibiotics.

Bacteriuria   The presence of bacteria in the urine. It is a diagnostic sign of a urinary tract infection, a common but potentially dangerous condition. Many kinds of bacteria can cause a urinary tract infection, and specific treatment depends upon laboratory identification of the organism responsible for the infection.

Balanitis   An inflammation of the glans penis. The cause frequently is a sexually transmitted disease, but it may also be the result of a drug reaction, dermatitis, or a fungal infection. The inflammation may be due to the use of self-administered cleansing or other agents, or it may develop without a specific cause. The condition is characterized by tenderness, irritation, and a discharge. There may also be superficial ulceration that erodes the surface of the glans and the prepuce, and swelling can result in constriction of the foreskin. Patients with diabetes appear to be at greater than average risk of developing balanitis. Technically, the condition is identified as *balanoposthisis* in men who have not been circumcised.

Baldness A popular term for hair loss or **alopecia** commonly applied to the male-pattern diffuse hair loss, which is affected by heredity, age, and sex hormones. Women with a relatively high level of male sex hormones may develop a female-pattern baldness after the age of fifty. In both the male and female hair-loss patterns, the hair loss begins at the top of the scalp. Baldness in women is almost always self-limited and never becomes complete. In men, the pattern is one in which the hair loss extends back on both sides from the forehead. It forms an "M" shape that eventually merges with the hair loss that started at the peak of the scalp. In general, the earlier balding begins, the more extensive the hair loss. The gene for baldness is transmitted from grandfather to grandson, with the mother (the daughter of the grandfather) being the carrier to her son.

Ballet's disease A disorder associated with **hyperthyroidism** and characterized by a loss of movements of the eye and its pupil. All other **autonomic nervous system** functions remain normal.

Ballismus A neurological condition marked by "flinging" movements of the arms or legs. It is caused by a lesion in the subthalamic area of the brain. The flailing movements may be limited to one side of the body or to only one arm or leg. The patient may move about the room with dancelike gliding and twisting steps, while making irregular movements of the arms and head. The movements may be so violent as to exhaust the patient or result in injury when they lead to falls.

Bancroft's sign A medical test for an inflammation or clot formation in a vein (**thrombophlebitis**) in the legs. Pain increases when the calf muscle is pushed forward against the shinbone (tibia).

Baragnosis A loss of the ability to estimate the weights of objects that can be held in the hand. The condition is due to a disease or injury affecting a localized area of the brain.

Barbiturate poisoning An abnormal condition caused by taking an excessive dose of a barbiturate sedative. The person usually shows depressed breathing, a bluish skin coloration due to a lack of oxygen in the blood, signs of confusion or disorientation, and headache. Barbiturate poisoning is an emergency condition that requires professional medical care and possible hospitalization. In severe cases, the person may lapse into a coma and have respiratory failure.

Bariatrics A medical specialty that focuses on the prevention and treatment of obesity and diseases related to excessive body weight.

Bartholinitis An inflammation of one or both Bartholin glands, small mucus-secreting glands located in the vestibule (near the opening) of the vagina. The condition may be marked by tenderness or a mass in the vaginal wall. Inflammation may produce a red spot containing pus at the opening of a duct from the gland. It is a common source of **vaginitis** symptoms. A mild infection may respond to hot-water soaks and antibiotics. A severe infection may require surgery to prevent development of a **fistula**.

Basilar artery A short but important artery formed by the junction of two vertebral arteries at the base of the skull. It has numerous branches extending to the inner ear and various parts of the brain. A wide range of symptoms including swallowing difficulty, loss of vision, dizziness, numbness, depression, weakness on one side of the body, and speech difficulties may be caused by any disorder that reduces the blood flow through the basilar artery.

Beck operation Either of two basic surgical procedures for providing collateral circulation (secondary or accessory pathways for blood flow) to the heart muscle when the lumen of the coronary arteries has been narrowed by **atherosclerosis**. By improving the blood supply to the heart muscle, the workload of the heart is reduced, providing relief from the pain of **angina pectoris**.
  The Beck I procedure involves applying an irritant substance to the membrane surrounding the heart in order to stimulate improved circulation. The Beck II operation consists of the grafting of a vein to the aorta and using it as a passage for freshly oxygenated blood to the coronary arteries that nourish the heart muscle. In both types of operations, the coronary sinus, a wide vein that drains blood from the coronary veins, is partially closed by the surgeon. This increases the pressure of blood in the heart's own circulation and improves blood flow to the heart muscle.

Beck's syndrome An abnormal condition caused by an obstruction to the blood flow in the anterior spinal artery, one of the branches of the vertebral artery supplying blood to the brain. Symptoms may include either pain or a loss of the ability to feel pain, weakness, cramps, loss of hearing, and loss of temperature sensations.

Bedsores   Ulcerlike lesions that develop on the skin of patients who are bedridden or confined to a wheelchair. They are caused by continuous pressure of the body against the bedding or chair. This prolonged pressure cuts off the normal blood supply of oxygen to the affected tissues, particularly in areas over bony prominences, such as the base of the spine, the elbows, heels, inner knees, hips, shoulder blades, and ear rims. Older persons, especially those who are obese and suffering from injury or disease, are most likely to develop bedsores. Bedsores are controlled by keeping the skin and bedding dry, repositioning the person every two hours to vary the pressure on the body, and making periodic checks of pressure areas where the sores tend to develop.

Protective methods include sprinkling a thin layer of cornstarch on body areas that show perspiration and placing sheepskins, air mattresses, or foam cushions under the body. Bedsores that are neglected can progress to ulcers that invade tissues deep beneath the skin, requiring surgical treatment and sometimes threatening the life of the patient. Because poor nutrition contributes to bedsores, patients should be given high-protein meals with adequate vitamins and minerals. *Also called* "decubitus ulcer."

Bell's palsy   Paralysis of the facial nerve. The precise cause is unknown but the inflammation producing the symptoms of weakness or paralysis of facial muscles is believed to be due to an infection by a strain of herpes virus, the same type of virus that causes cold sores. Inflammation and swelling of the infected facial nerve may lead to compression of the nerve as it passes through a narrow opening in the temporal bone of the skull; there may also be obstruction of normal blood flow to the nerve, which can suffer permanent damage. The condition usually affects only one side of the face. Symptoms include pain, weakness of the facial muscle, and loss of ability to blink or to close the eyelid on the affected side of the face. The paralysis results in a flat, expressionless appearance on the affected side.

An attack of Bell's palsy often begins with a pain behind the ear and swelling along the path of the nerve. The attack frequently follows exposure to cold temperatures. Because Bell's palsy involves the entire face on one side, doctors generally can assume that the cause is not an injury or disease of the brain, such as a stroke, which usually results in weakness or paralysis only in the area below the eye. Treatment may include steroid medications, physical therapy to prevent contractures of the facial muscles, patching and medication to protect the eye that cannot be closed, and surgery, if necessary. The outcome depends upon a number of individual factors, mainly involving the degree of nerve damage. Complete recovery within a few months can be expected in most cases of partial paralysis.

Benign neoplasm A medical term used to describe a noncancerous tumor. The word "neoplasm" means new tissue or new growth and "benign" suggests a harmless or innocent condition. However, a noncancerous tumor often requires treatment, either for cosmetic reasons or because it may produce harmful pressure on neighboring tissues if it is allowed to continue its growth.

Benign prostatic hypertrophy (BPH) An enlargement of the prostate gland, a condition that commonly affects men after the age of fifty. The overgrowth of tissue that encircles the urethra obstructs the flow of urine from the bladder. The man may experience increased urinary frequency and urgency and a need to urinate during the night, because the obstruction prevents complete emptying of the bladder. Initial symptoms may include hesitation in the start of urine flow and a smaller than usual stream. In some cases, there may be urinary incontinence, dribbling, or urinary retention. As the condition progresses, the bladder becomes greatly dilated, and urinary retention increases. Prolonged urinary retention can lead to **azotemia** and kidney failure. A further complication is the buildup of pressure in the bladder, causing urine to flow back through the ureters and into the kidneys.

The exact cause of the disorder is unknown but the risk of BPH increases with age until 80 percent of men who have lived into their eighties have experienced symptoms of prostatic hypertrophy. Fewer than 20 percent of all men suffer symptoms or obstruction that is severe enough to require surgical treatment. When surgery is required, the preferred procedure is called *transurethral resection,* which requires no incision. A lighted instrument is inserted through the urethra, and small bits of the tissue overgrowth are snipped away and flushed through the urethra. In most cases, sexual potency is not affected by surgery to correct benign prostatic hypertrophy. Also called "benign prostatic hyperplasia."

Beriberi A term for the condition resulting from a deficiency of thiamine (vitamin B_1) in the diet or from failure of the body to absorb the vitamin from food or to utilize what is absorbed, as in cases of liver disease or chronic diarrhea. The condition is marked by an enlarged heart, degeneration of the peripheral nerves, particularly in the legs, and brain disorders resulting from reduced blood flow to the brain. Recovery requires increased daily intake of thiamine and treatment of specific secondary effects, such as fluid accumulation. Persons with fever, hyperthyroidism, or who consume greater than average amounts of alcohol require more thiamine than is available in the typical American diet.

Beriberi heart disease A form of congestive heart failure and lung congestion that is associated with a nutritional deficiency of thiamine, or vitamin B_1. Symptoms include **edema** (swelling due to an accumulation of body fluids), breathing difficulty, fatigue, irritability, and possible skin disorders. Treatment for uncomplicated cases is based on bed rest and an increased intake of thiamine. A contributing factor in the cause of beriberi heart disease is excessive consumption of alcoholic beverages, which increases the body's need for vitamin B_1.

Berry aneurysm A congenital defect of the circulatory system serving the brain, marked by a small saclike dilatation where there is a weakness in an artery or the absence of part of the artery wall. Rupture of a berry aneurysm is a common cause of stroke in later life.

Berylliosis An occupational disease caused by exposure to beryllium compounds or products in the workplace. Beryllium is used in hardening of metal alloys, in chemical plants, and in the manufacture of electrical and electronic products. Inhalation of dusts or fumes of beryllium results in breathing difficulty, coughing, weight loss, and changes in the tissue structure of the lungs. There may be a lag of between ten and twenty years between exposure to beryllium dust and the appearance of berylliosis symptoms. Untreated, the disease can lead to loss of respiratory function and death from heart disease. Treatment is directed toward relief of the symptoms, which may be completely reversible in acute exposure cases. Medications are also usually effective in reducing the symptoms of chronic berylliosis when treatments are started in the early stages of the disease.

Beta-adrenergic Pertaining to a portion of the **sympathetic nervous system** that contains beta-type adrenergic nerve fibers, as distinguished from alpha-adrenergic fibers. The beta nerve fibers provide a specific set of nerve impulse pathways that affect certain body functions, such as the rate and force of heart contractions. Drugs that are administered to reduce or inhibit beta-adrenergic nerve functions are called **antiadrenergics**, "beta-adrenergic blocking agents," or "beta blockers."

Beta alcoholism   A form of alcohol abuse in which excessive drinking has begun to cause physical damage to the liver, kidneys, or nervous system, though the person is neither physically nor psychologically dependent upon alcohol.

Beta blocker   *See* **Beta-adrenergic.**

Bielchowsky's disease   An eye-movement disorder marked by the loss of ability to coordinate movement of the eyes in up and down directions due to a nervous system defect. In a variation of the condition, there is limited movement inward by the eye that is on the same side of the body as a brainstem lesion, while the eye on the other side shows outward, jerking movements.

Bile   A bitter, greenish fluid secreted by the liver and stored in the gallbladder to be released into the intestines when fatty foods are eaten. Bile salts, an important substance in bile, act as a detergent in the intestine, breaking up the large fat globules.

Biliary cirrhosis   An inflammation of the liver involving obstruction of the flow of bile through the ductules of the liver. The cause is unknown, and there is no specific treatment. Symptoms include an enlarged and tender liver, itching sensations, jaundice, and the appearance of yellowish plaques (xanthomas) on the skin, usually around the eyelids and other areas of the face. There also may be pain in the fingers and toes and bone softening or **osteoporosis**.

Although the disease can affect anyone at nearly any stage of life, women in their middle years are most likely to develop the condition. It is not unusual for biliary cirrhosis to occur at the same time as another disease, such as thyroiditis or **rheumatoid arthritis**. Treatment may include drugs to control itching, vitamin supplements, and other supplements as needed, such as calcium tablets to replace bone loss of calcium as a result of the disorder.

Binswanger's disease   A neurologic condition that begins after middle age and is apparently caused by **arteriosclerosis** and loss of the myelin covering of the white matter of the brain. It is characterized by memory impairment, progressive loss of vision, paranoia, speech disorders, and hallucinations.

Biopsy   The removal of a sample of tissue or fluid for microscopic examination or other methods to determine the presence or course of a disease. The sample is often obtained by needle suction, but other procedures, including surgery, may be used.

Bipolar disorder   A psychological disturbance in which there are alternating periods of mania and depression. One phase is usually predominant at any time, although elements of both phases may occur simultaneously. Causes of the disorder are complex and may involve biological, psychological, social, and cultural factors. The manic and depressive episodes may alternate every few days in some individuals, while in others the manic or depressive phase may represent the major characteristic.

During the manic phase, the patient may exhibit an elevated, expansive, or irritable mood, with talkativeness, restlessness, racing thoughts, inflated self-esteem, and a decreased need for sleep. In the community, a manic episode lasting a week or more may be marked by bad investments, buying sprees, and sexual indiscretions. During a depressive phase, the patient may display a mood of unhappiness, hopelessness, and a loss of interest in usually pleasurable activities. Other symptoms can include appetite and weight gains or losses, decreased sexual drive, insomnia or excessive sleep, indecision, guilt feelings, and an obsession with thoughts concerning death. A major depressive episode may end in a suicide attempt.

Bipolar disorders generally begin before the age of forty but reach a peak in the three decades after forty, with depressive episodes becoming increasingly common as aging advances. Patients in depressive episodes are usually treated with **monoamine oxidase inhibitors** or **tricyclic antidepressant** drugs, while manic patients are likely to receive lithium carbonate or **major tranquilizers**. The precise drug and its dosage for a particular patient depend upon the individual response and the person's tolerance for a drug's side effects.

Manic patients given lithium often develop tremors and other neurologic symptoms, requiring the administration of **beta-adrenergic** drugs to counter the effects of lithium. Psychotherapy is provided to supplement the medications. The outlook for recovery of a bipolar disorder patient depends upon a number of individual factors, including compliance with the recommended therapy and acceptance of the patient by the family and others in the community. Bipolar disorder was formerly called **Manic-depressive illness**.

Black lung disease   *See* **Anthracosis**.

Bladder cancer   A malignant tumor in the bladder, which may originate there, often as a consequence of exposure to a cancer-causing chemical in the environment; but the tumor may also result from the spread of a primary cancer in another part of the body, such as the intestine or prostate gland, or from a parasitic infection. Chemicals that are known or suspected causes of bladder cancer include aniline dyes, compounds used in the rubber industry, and, possibly, chemical compounds produced by tobacco. Initial symptoms include a burning sensation when urinating, increased frequency of urination, difficulty in urinating, and the presence of blood or pus in the urine.

When pain is a symptom, it indicates that the cancer has invaded the wall of the bladder. The pain is most noticeable during distention of the bladder, as it stretches while filling with urine. The patient, therefore, finds that emptying the bladder helps relieve the pain and as a result is likely to urinate more often. The specific treatment depends upon the type of cancer cells involved and the degree of tissue destruction by the tumor, and may include surgery, radiation, or chemotherapy, or a combination of techniques.

Blepharospasm An involuntary contraction of the muscle of the eyelid, marked by twitching, blinking, or lid squeezing. Specific causes of blepharospasm can be an irritation of the eye, as from a corneal tumor, or a disorder involving the trigeminal nerve of the face (**trigeminal neuralgia**). Spasms of the eyelid muscle usually increase in the presence of bright light, and intolerance to light (photophobia) nearly always accompanies blepharospasm as a symptom. A tremor of the eyelids is also seen in **parkinsonism**, certain forms of epilepsy, a muscle disorder called myokimia, and other abnormal conditions involving the nerves and muscles that affect facial movements, such as facial expressions. Treatment varies according to the specific cause or condition.

Blindness An inability to see or to receive visual stimuli. The most common causes of blindness, not including head or eye injuries, are inoperable **cataracts**, uncontrolled **glaucoma**, **diabetic retinopathy**, **retinitis pigmentosa**, **macular degeneration**, and rubella (German measles). *Cortical blindness* is a total loss of vision due to a lesion in the area of the brain where nerve impulses from the eye are translated into visual images. The eyes and optic nerves may be normal, but the visual "messages" from the eyes cannot be read by the brain. *Flash blindness* and *solar maculopathy* are forms of blindness caused by looking into a bright light. Flash blindness from viewing an intensely bright flash of light is usually temporary but may be permanent if the light is extremely bright, as in watching a nuclear explosion. Solar maculopathy usually involves some degree of damage to the macula, a portion of the retina, from looking into the sun, as during an eclipse.

Night blindness is a temporary lag in the adaptation of the eye to a darkened room or outdoor environment after being in an illuminated area. *Snow blindness* involves a painful irritation of the cornea and conjunctiva of the eye that results from sunlight reflections from the surface of snow; the reflected sunlight causes ultraviolet burns that can be quite serious. The snowblind person usually cannot open the eyes until the symptoms have diminished.

Most forms of blindness that involve destruction of retinal or optic nerve tissues are irreversible although in some cases, such as glaucoma, damage can be arrested in early stages and further destruction of nerve tissues can be controlled by surgery and medications. It is also possible to restore sight in special cases requiring a corneal transplant.

Legal blindness is a reduction in the best eye to a visual acuity of 20/200 or less, with correction. Legal blindness also is a reduction in the visual field of the best eye of 20 or less. Industry guidelines generally follow the legal definitions but the U.S. Social Security Administration defines blindness as corrected visual acuity of 5/200 or less in the better-seeing eye.

Blind spot   A small gap in the visual field that occurs when light rays from an object become focused on the part of the retina that is occupied by the optic disc, an area of the retina where the optic nerve is attached to the eyeball. Everybody has a blind spot. It is a normal phenomenon because there are no visual receptor cells for detecting images in the optic disc.

Bloating   A gastrointestinal disorder marked by a feeling of abdominal distention, indigestion, and gas in the digestive tract. The person usually has episodes of belching. Some causes are air swallowing, carbonated beverages, eating foods that produce excessive gas, or a psychological disturbance. Severe bloating may be a sign of a more serious disorder, such as an intestinal obstruction.

Blood clotting   The process of clot formation. When a blood vessel is damaged, a natural defense mechanism of the body brings into action substances in the blood called coagulation factors and platelets. They form a jellylike mass at the injury site to protect against further bleeding. Disorders such as **arteriosclerosis** and **varicose veins** may roughen the inner wall of a blood vessel and cause a clot to form. A **thrombus** is a blood clot that remains in place where it forms. An **embolus** is one that breaks loose and flows through the blood vessels. There are also clotting disorders that cause bleeding and bruising. *See also* **Embolus, Thrombus.**

Bone cancer A malignant tumor that may invade any bone in the skeletal system, sometimes originating in the bone (primary cancer) but often occurring as a secondary cancer (one that has spread to a bone from a soft-tissue organ in some other part of the body). A *malignant lymphoma* is the most prevalent bone cancer affecting persons after the age of forty, as compared to most primary bone tumors, which first appear in persons before twenty years of age. It may originate in bone as a primary cancer, spread to bone from a soft-tissue organ, or develop more or less simultaneously in more than one part of the body, such as bone and soft tissue.

The main symptoms are pain and swelling, although in some severe cases the bone may be weakened so that it fractures easily. Malignant lymphoma cases usually have a better prognosis than other types of cancer; many respond to radiation and chemotherapy, so that surgery is not required. Bone cancers are often discovered during examination for symptoms of arthritis or bursitis because the symptoms of pain and swelling are similar. Bone cancers are also discovered during treatment of a fracture, as in some cases of malignant lymphoma in which the bone tissue becomes mottled and patchy from cancer damage and breaks easily. X-ray films show the areas of bone destruction.

Secondary bone cancers can develop from cancer cells carried by the bloodstream from soft-tissue cancers in the breast, prostate, lung, kidney, thyroid gland, and other organs. Any bone may become the site of a secondary cancer, although these rarely develop in the forearm or lower leg. It is not unusual for a secondary bone cancer to be discovered before the original soft-tissue primary cancer has been found. Many noncancerous conditions can produce symptoms resembling those of bone tumors. Examples include cystic bone lesions and disorders in which muscle tissue becomes calcified and bonelike.

Borborygmi A medical term for "gut rumbling" noises, or the sounds made by gas moving through the intestines.

Botulism A very serious form of food poisoning caused by an endotoxin, or poison, produced by a bacterium, *Clostridium botulinum.* The toxin may be present in food that was not properly cooked or otherwise prepared so as to destroy the toxin. Botulism is unique as a food poison in that the bacteria themselves do not have to be present to produce symptoms, and the disease may develop without any symptoms of gastrointestinal distress. In fact, the first symptoms of weakness, fatigue, and visual disturbances may not appear until the following day or several days after the contaminated food is eaten.

There may be nausea, vomiting, or diarrhea, but these symptoms occur in fewer than half of all cases. Among the most commonly reported initial symptoms are visual problems, such as difficulty in focusing the eyes, double vision, and loss of the ability of the pupil to change in response to light changes. Respiration becomes irregular, the patient experiences dizziness, headaches, and has difficulty in swallowing as the attack progresses. Treatment includes antitoxins, sedatives, and efforts to maintain breathing, since most fatalities result from pulmonary complications.

Bowleg *See* **Genu varum.**

Bradycardia An abnormally slow heartbeat at a rate of less than 60 per minute. This slow a heartbeat, compared to a normal adult rate of around 75 per minute, may be considered as normal for a conditioned athlete or a vigorous youngster. It also can be common in people with certain illnesses, such as **myxedema,** or in persons who take propranolol or other **beta-adrenergic** drugs. However, in most other people, bradycardia (derived from the Greek words for "slow heart") can be a life-threatening condition, with symptoms of chronic fatigue, dizzy spells, fainting, convulsions, and cerebral ischemia, a medical term for oxygen starvation in the brain cells.

Bradycardia also can develop without any specific symptoms and may be unrecognized until a situation arises in which the body demands a faster heartbeat, as during a burst of physical exertion or an emotional crisis. Causes may range from an injury that results in a **fistula,** or abnormal passage between a vein and an artery, or another disorder, such as **cholestasis,** due to a bile flow obstruction; but the more frequent cause of bradycardia in older individuals is a failure of the sinus node, a cluster of heart pacemaker cells located at the place where the main vein returning blood to the heart enters the right atrium of the heart. The sinus node cells normally generate the impulses that trigger contractions of the heart muscle at a rate of between 60 and 100 beats per minute in most normal adults. (The rate may be lower during sleep and higher during exercise.)

As a person grows older, the sinus node gradually loses some of its pacemaker cells, as blood flow to the sinus node tissues is diminished and the node accumulates fatty and fibrous tissues. This condition is sometimes identified as part of a *sick sinus syndrome.* The condition may include or lead to other heart dysfunctions, such as **sino-atrial block,** sinus arrest, and bradyarrythmia—a heartbeat that is not only slow but irregular. Diagnosis of the cause of bradycardia usually requires extensive evaluation by electrocardiograms, stress-testing, and injections of drugs that produce specific heart reactions. Test results may suggest causes that could include uremia, an underactive thyroid gland, an infectious disease, brain tumor or brain hemorrhage, or overdoses of a drug, such as **digitalis**, a prescribed heart medication.

In many cases, there may be no particular need for treatment of bradycardia, especially if the heart rate is only slightly below 60 beats per minute. However, if the heart rate drops to 40 per minute, the condition may progress to **heart block**, requiring specific therapy. A heart rate of 30 per minute is considered a medical emergency, and a decline in heart rate to 20 per minute could have fatal consequences. Emergency treatment may include administration of atropine or isoproterenol drugs. Long-term therapy is frequently provided by implantation of an electronic pacemaker. *See also* **Tachycardia.**

Bradykinesia Abnormally slow movements, often seen in older persons who have suffered damage to brain cells controlling actions of the muscles. The person may take a few halting steps in walking, as if learning to walk for the first time. Bradykinesia is sometimes a sign of **parkinsonism.**

Brain atrophy Any disorder marked by the degeneration or loss of nerve cells in the brain. The condition may occur in cerebral **arteriosclerosis, Alzheimer's disease, encephalitis, Huntington's disease,** or **Pick's disease.**

Brain scan A technique for diagnosing disorders that may be caused by a brain injury or disease. A radioactive substance is injected into the blood, and a radiation detection device is then used to survey the distribution of radioactivity in the brain tissues. While normal brain tissue will show little if any absorption of radioactive material, an increase in such absorption, and in radioactivity, usually will be detected in areas of abnormal tissues.

Brain stem A part of the brain at the top of the spinal cord where nerves from the spinal cord enter the cerebrum. The brain stem contains segments of the brain identified as the *midbrain, pons,* and *medulla oblongata.* Circulatory disorders in the brain stem may result in temporary episodes of numbness or loss of feeling in the legs or disturbances of sensations in the fingers. A lesion of the brain stem can be the cause of paralysis on either the same side of the body as the lesion or on the opposite side. Other disorders associated with brain stem injury or disease include facial paralysis; **ataxia**; paralysis of the tongue, throat, larynx, or soft palate; and loss of position sense.

Breast cancer   A malignant tumor of the breast. It is one of the most common types of cancer among women. Nearly all breast cancers are carcinomas, a type of cancer that begins with epithelial cells that normally form the external (skin) and internal surfaces (such as lining of organs) of the body. Breast cancers usually begin painlessly or with only a vague feeling of discomfort as the first symptom. The usual initial sign is a lump in the breast. There may be a retracted nipple or bleeding from the nipple, abnormalities in the breast contour or the areola of the nipple, and enlarged lymph glands around the armpit and shoulder on the same side. There may be fluid accumulation under the skin and pitting or dimpling of the skin over the site of the lesion.

One type of breast cancer, called *inflammatory carcinoma,* is characterized by symptoms that resemble an infection. The skin over the breast becomes red, swollen, warm, and painful. It is a rapidly growing cancer that tends to recur even after radical surgery. Another type of breast cancer is **Paget's disease**, which is marked by a tumor that appears to begin in the nipple; as the cancer cells invade the surface of the nipple, an ulcer develops. This cancer often originates so deep within the breast that no lump is detected at first; the cancer cells then spread along the milk ducts to the nipple.

Breast cancer is unusual in young women, and the risk increases after the age of thirty, reaching a peak in the postmenopausal years. A survey of nearly 750 U.S. hospitals found that one-third of all breast cancer patients were over the age of sixty-four. There is also a familial risk factor, with the incidence of breast cancer being higher among daughters and nieces of women afflicted with the disorder. Among other factors, there is evidence of a hormonal role in breast cancer, particularly from the effects of **estrogens** that are produced naturally or are taken as variations of oral contraceptives to ease the symptoms of the menopause.

In postmenopausal women, there may be continued production of estrogens after the ovaries have ceased producing them. **Androgens**, male sex hormones produced by the adrenal glands, are converted by the body's enzymes to estrogens. The rate of conversion of androgens to estrogens increases as women grow older. Estrogens also can be synthesized from body fat, with the result that some obese postmenopausal women may have higher levels of estrogenic activity in their breast tissue than many women still in their reproductive years.

Because of the increased risk of breast cancer among older adult women, **breast self-examination**, supplemented by mammography and other diagnostic techniques, is particularly important. Some authorities recommend that any mass discovered in the breast of a postmenopausal woman should be regarded as cancerous "until proved otherwise." In the United States, treatment of breast cancer usually includes one of several possible surgical procedures to remove the cancer, the precise approach depending upon such factors as the age of the woman, the type of cancer, and its degree of severity. The surgical techniques are (1) *lumpectomy,* in which only the tumor and surrounding tissue are removed; (2) *simple mastectomy,* in which the breast is removed; (3) *modified mastectomy,* involving removal of the breast and nearby lymph nodes; and (4) *radical mastectomy,* in which the breast, nearby lymph nodes, and muscle tissue underlying the breast are removed. After six months following a mastectomy, cosmetic reconstruction of the breast around a plastic implant is a common procedure. Surgery may be supplemented by radiation treatment, chemotherapy, and/or hormone therapy. In some other countries, breast cancer discovered at a very early stage may be treated with radiation therapy rather than surgery.

When breast cancer is discovered and treated before it spreads to the lymph nodes, there is a better than 70 percent chance of the patient surviving more than ten years. A more encouraging statistic is that 90 percent of all women will never be afflicted with breast cancer.

Breast self-examination   A technique in which women examine their own breasts in order to detect signs of lumps or other possible abnormalities or changes. It is recommended that such self-examinations be performed each month. For menstruating women, the examination should be conducted after the end of the menstrual period, when the breasts are less likely to be swollen or tender. For menopausal women, authorities advise that the examination be performed on the same day of each month. Breast self-examination is especially important for women who are at higher than average risk for breast cancer because they are daughters or nieces of women who have had breast cancer, are overweight, or are childless.

The examination should be conducted before a mirror and with good lighting that will help reveal any skin changes, such as puckering, dimpling, scaly skin, nipple discharge, swelling, or signs of redness or other color change. The breasts also should be compared for symmetry or lack of symmetry, such as outward deviation of a nipple, which can be a sign of breast tissue abnormality. From a standing position, the woman should raise her arms over her head, elevating the pectoral tissues (the chest muscles under the breasts), then place the hands firmly on the hips to contract the pectoral muscles. Next, still in a standing position, one arm should be raised while two or three fingers of the opposite hand gently explore the breast for any unusual lump or abnormality.

   This procedure should be repeated on the other side of the body. The examination should also be repeated by the woman while she is lying on her back, with an arm raised beyond the head. While lying down, the breast tissue is spread against the chest muscle, presenting a different view of the breast surfaces. A final step requires that the woman, while standing, lean forward so the breasts hang independently. This will give a view of any unusual lack of symmetry in the breasts. Although one breast may normally appear larger or more elevated than the other, such differences also can be clues to an abnormality caused by cancer deep within the breast.

   In addition to breast self-examination, women over the age of thirty-five should receive regular mammography examinations, which can detect by low-level X-rays signs of abnormalities that would not be observed by feeling the breast for lumps or masses. Most authorities agree that mammography is not needed by most women under the age of thirty-five. Other diagnostic techniques performed under the supervision of a doctor include thermography, a method of detecting breast lumps by temperature differences between a tumor and normal tissue, and Xerography, which requires higher doses of radiation but produces clearer pictures.

Breathing difficulty   Gasping, labored breathing (dyspnea). When caused by strenuous physical exercise, gasping for oxygen is usually normal, but when excessive or prolonged, or occurring at rest, it may indicate a disorder affecting the respiratory system or the amount of oxygen in the circulating blood. Breathing difficulty may be a symptom of a variety of disorders, such as chronic **bronchitis, emphysema, cancer,** and **heart disease.**

Bronchiectasis   A respiratory disorder in which there is dilatation and destruction of the bronchi of the lungs, usually after a severe bronchial infection. The condition also may follow inhalation of a foreign body or be caused by a tumor that obstructs the air passages. Bronchiectasis is characterized by a persistent cough that produces sputum tinged with pus or blood. It may be accompanied by sinusitis and clubbing of the fingers. The disorder can develop at any age but tends to appear in older individuals after a chronic infection marked by coughing that persists for several years. Treatment is usually with antibiotics, and an effort is made to reduce the risk of complications such as lung abscess or pneumonia.

Bronchitis   An acute or chronic inflammation of the mucous membrane lining the trachea and bronchi. It may develop after a common cold or a similar viral infection. Bronchitis also can be caused by inhalation of mineral dusts such as silica or asbestos; industrial fumes such as strong acids or solvents; hydrogen sulfide; sulfur dioxide; smoke from tobacco or other burning materials; or vegetable dusts that may include fungi or other microorganisms. The primary symptom is usually a cough that produces little or no sputum at first. As the disease progresses, the cough yields a viscous sputum that may contain pus. The patient also may experience laryngitis and breathing that resembles asthma. Other symptoms, such as a mild fever, chills, muscle pain, or sore throat, may actually be associated with a respiratory infection accompanying the bronchitis. Treatment usually requires rest, a cough suppressant, aspirin, a generous intake of fluids, steam inhalations, and antibiotics if there is evidence of a complicating bacterial infection.

Bronchogenic carcinoma   Any of several types of lung cancer that originate in the bronchi of the lungs. Nearly 80 percent of the forms of bronchogenic carcinoma are *squamous cell* or *small oat cell* cancers that are associated with cigarette smoking. There also is a higher risk of lung cancers among workers exposed to asbestos, uranium ore, nickel dust, certain organic chemical fumes, and other air contaminants. Some lung cancers also are secondary cancers that have spread (metastasized) from primary sites in other parts of the body, such as the breast, thyroid gland, intestine, bone, kidney, testis, or prostate gland. Symptoms of bronchogenic carcinoma are cough, sometimes accompanied by wheezing and breathlessness, fatigue, a sensation of chest tightness, weight loss, aching joints, and clubbing of the fingers.

As the disease progresses, chest pain increases, the cough usually produces a bloody sputum, and there is fluid accumulation in the lungs as a result of serum leakage from blood vessels. Persistent localized chest pain is often a sign that the cancer has spread into the chest wall. Treatment usually requires surgical removal of the affected lung tissue. The outcome depends upon the type of tumor and the amount of damage it has caused. Only about 25 percent of bronchogenic carcinoma cases can be aided by surgery, and only about 10 percent of the cases that are operable result in survival for an additional five years. Among the more easily operable cases, the five-year survival rate may be as high as 40 percent. Untreated, however, bronchogenic cancer usually proves fatal in about nine months. Radiation is used to supplement surgery, and radiation may be combined with chemotherapy in some cases. *See also* **Lung cancer.**

Bruit   An abnormal sound heard in the body, usually referring to a heart murmur or to the sound made by blood flowing through a restricted or obstructed artery. It is a diagnostic sign detected by a physician's stethoscope.

Bulbar paralysis A form of **amyotrophic lateral sclerosis** in which there is a gradually developing paralysis that affects the lips, tongue, mouth, and throat muscles. Chewing, swallowing, and talking become increasingly difficult. It is caused by disorders involving the nerve cells that are located in the lower brain stem, at the base of the skull, with nerve fibers that extend into the mouth and throat. That portion of the brain stem at the top end of the spinal cord is sometimes called the "bulb," hence the name of the disease. The muscles of the tongue are affected first, and the tongue shrinks in size.

The chewing muscles of the mouth and the muscles of the throat are usually affected next. Eating becomes difficult, as the person loses ability to manipulate the various muscles in the mouth area, and food may enter the nose or throat by mistake. Because of weakness of the throat muscles, coughing is difficult, so that accidentally inhaled food can become a life-threatening event. Solid foods become difficult to eat, and fluid flow cannot be controlled by the throat, so meals are usually limited to soft foods. Weight loss and breathing system complications, often brought on by choking or pneumonia caused by inhaled food, can be fatal.

Bundle branch block A heart abnormality caused by a failure of fibers in the heart muscle to carry the electrical impulses needed to produce contractions of the heart. The system of fibers that carry the heart impulses is called the *bundle of His,* or the *atrioventricular bundle.* The bundle has a right branch and a left branch. A blockage of a branch of the bundle may result in a reduced heart rate, but as other fibers in the heart's electrical conduction system can replace the blocked impulse route, the condition usually is not critical.

Many persons live for years with a bundle branch block and may require no more treatment than implantation of an artificial **pacemaker**. Bundle branch block may be associated with a congenital heart defect or degenerative effects associated with aging, such as **hypertension**, **arteriosclerosis**, or cardiomyopathy. The condition often is detected by a physician examining a patient's routine electrocardiogram. *See also* **Arrhythmias.**

Bunion A lump at the joint of the big toe that may become painful and inflamed. The condition may force the tip of the toe against or under the adjacent toes. It is usually caused by an improperly fitting shoe. When the deformity or pain are severe, surgery may be required.

Burnett's syndrome (milk-alkali syndrome) An abnormal condition that develops in some peptic ulcer patients who consume large amounts of milk, cream, and calcium carbonate antacids. It is marked by excessive blood calcium and by kidney failure, with symptoms of headache, dizziness, confusion, irritability, depression, loss of appetite, nausea, and vomiting. Other effects may be constipation and "acid rebound."

Burning feet syndrome A disorder characterized by a burning sensation in the soles of the feet. The burning feeling is often more severe at night and may be accompanied by increased sweating and exaggerated sensitivity to pain. In some cases, the hands may also be involved, and the corners of the lips may become cracked and sore. The condition may have no apparent cause but often is traced to a deficiency of pantothenic acid, a member of the B vitamin complex. It also is associated with **polyneuritis, uremia,** and **diabetes mellitus**.

Burnout A popular term for a state of emotional and physical exhaustion, usually related to one's job or career. Many persons perform at a high level of competence for many years until physical illness, psychological stress, or other factors leave them feeling depleted of energy and lacking concern for goals that may have seemed very important at an earlier stage of life. The burnout victim often develops a cynical outlook.

Bursitis A painful inflammation of a bursa, a fluid-filled saclike cushion in a joint. The condition may be acute or chronic and marked by tenderness and a loss of ability to move the joint to its full extent. Bursitis occurs most commonly in a shoulder joint, and is often caused by overactivity such as strenuous exercise. Other common sites of bursitis are the knee, elbow, hip, and hand. The condition may also be associated with an infection, gout, arthritis, or a joint injury.

Bursitis attacks usually last from a few days to a few weeks and respond to treatment with painkilling drugs and anti-inflammatory medications. In severe cases, calcium deposits may form inside the bursa and must be removed. Physical therapy with range-of-motion exercises may be needed to prevent muscle atrophy, which can develop if the patient refrains from using the affected joint.

Buttock pain *See* **Sciatica, Weaver's bottom.**

Byssinosis (brown lung disease) A form of occupational asthma that results from long-term inhalation of dust from cotton, flax, soft hemp, or sisal. It affects mainly people who have worked for many years with textiles. The disease may be complicated by the presence of molds and fungi that can collect on fabrics and are also inhaled. Symptoms include wheezing and shortness of breath. Prolonged exposure is often associated with chronic **bronchitis** and **emphysema**. New workers exposed to cotton or textiles usually manifest these symptoms only on the first day after they return to work following a weekend or vacation; the symptoms then subside.

Gradually, the symptoms begin to continue into the second and third day at work and then last through the work week. For some persons, the only long-term effect is wheezing that occurs at night. For others, the condition becomes progressively worse and the person has to quit working or find employment removed from areas of fabric dusts. The precise cause of byssinosis has not been identified, but it is believed to be an **antigen** in plant dusts that triggers constriction of the bronchial tubes. The symptoms are treated with medications that dilate the bronchial passages. Untreated, the disease may lead to emphysema and an irreversible loss of lung function.

C

Cachexia A condition of extreme weakness and wasting of body tissues, usually due to malnutrition, anemia, or circulatory and muscular disorders. The condition is seen sometimes in cases of cancer, tuberculosis, chronic parasite infection such as malaria, pituitary deficiency, heavy-metal poisoning, or emotional distress. The term is generally identified with the specific disease factor, as *pituitary cachexia* or *cancerous cachexia.*

Caffeine poisoning Effects of excessive use of caffeine in beverages, including coffee, tea, or colas, or in medications containing caffeine, such as "stay awake" pills. The symptoms include rapid heartbeat, heart palpitations, increased need to urinate, tremor, nervousness, irritability, and sleeping difficulty. In severe cases, there may be ringing in the ears, nausea and vomiting, and convulsions.

Because most people learn about their own "caffeine limits" in early adulthood, they usually avoid the extra cup of coffee if that will cause discomfort. Actually, caffeine is rapidly metabolized, or broken down, into other substances by the body and excreted, so it is unlikely that most people would suffer serious ill effects from the amount of caffeine in an average cup of coffee. But a form of chronic caffeine poisoning can develop in someone who consumes numerous cups of coffee daily or who gets additional caffeine from tea, colas, chocolate, or caffeine-containing drugs. Acute caffeine poisoning may occur from overdosing on stay-awake tablets or other kinds of relatively pure caffeine.

Calcium The fifth most abundant element in the body. Most of the body's calcium is located in the skeleton, which contains about 2.5

pounds of the mineral. In addition to the need for calcium in healthy bones and teeth, it is required for coagulation of the blood, normal heart function, the transmission of nerve impulses, the integrity of cell membranes, and other body functions. The calcium levels of various body systems are regulated by the parathyroid glands, located next to the thyroid gland in the neck. When the blood or a part of the body other than bone needs more calcium, the parathyroid gland secretes a substance that helps remove some of the calcium stored in the skeleton.

When the body has too much calcium, the excess is usually excreted. A calcium excess (hypercalcemia) can occur as a result of hyperparathyroidism, hyperthyroidism, bone cancer, excessive intake of vitamin D, immobility, or the use of certain diuretic drugs. Mild cases of hypercalcemia may not produce symptoms, but more severe cases can be marked by loss of appetite, constipation, nausea, vomiting, and abdominal pain. The person may also show signs of mental confusion, stupor, delirium, or emotional changes. In some circumstances, such as inadequate fluid intake, excess calcium may contribute to the formation of kidney stones. A mild deficiency of calcium (hypocalcemia) can occur without symptoms. It also may be characterized by blood clotting problems; various nervous and muscular disease conditions; a bone-softening disorder, osteomalacia; or a condition in which bones become fragile and break easily, osteoporosis. When a calcium deficiency is caused by a parathyroid disorder, the condition is marked by tetany, or convulsive muscle cramps. The average adult needs about 800 milligrams of calcium per day, ideally from dietary sources. This is equivalent to the amount of calcium in two and a half glasses of milk or three ounces of cheese daily. Some authorities recommend significantly more than this for postmenopausal women as a precaution against the development of osteoporosis. There are food sources of calcium other than milk, but for those who are able to tolerate dairy products, they represent the easiest way to obtain calcium in the diet.

Calculus A medical term for a stone that forms within an organ, as a kidney stone or gallstone.

Callus An area of thickened skin that can develop on the foot or other body regions as a result of constant pressure or friction over a bony protrusion. Although a callus usually develops on the foot, it may occur elsewhere, such as on the hand; a professional violinist may develop calluses on the jaw and collarbone. Unlike **corns**, which also tend to develop on the feet, calluses usually do not produce symptoms of pain or tenderness.

Calories Units of measurement of the heat energy in food. It is the heat released by the metabolism of food that maintains a person's body temperature. The greater amount of physical work or play, the more heat generated by your body as food energy is converted into muscle energy and "burned." Even if you don't move out of bed, your body burns a certain number of calories every day to maintain body heat and to keep the heart, lungs, and other systems functioning. The brain alone requires about 500 calories a day. To determine how many calories you need each day, a rule of thumb is to multiply your body weight in kilograms (1 kilogram equals 2.2 pounds) by 35, or a little more if you are quite active physically during the day. The amount of energy in various kinds of foods averages about 4 calories per gram for carbohydrates or protein and 9 calories per gram for fat. There are about 30 grams per ounce. One pound of fat contains about 3,600 calories, which is the amount of weight one can gain by miscalculating one's food intake by only 10 calories a day for a year.

Cancer Any malignant tissue cell disease or tumor that is characterized by uncontrolled growth and is usually capable of invading neighboring tissues and spreading through the lymphatic system or bloodstream to distant parts of the body. A noncancerous, or benign, tumor differs in that it usually is enclosed within a membrane or capsule and does not spread to other parts of the body via the blood or lymph. There are numerous specific types of cancers and many possible causes, including viruses, hormones, mechanical irritation, radiation as from X-rays or radioactive substances, the ultraviolet rays of the sun, and various chemicals in the environment that may enter the body through the skin, respiratory system, or digestive tract. For many cancers, the cause is unknown. In some cases, there appear to be genetic or family factors, as in breast cancers that tend to be more likely to afflict the daughter or niece of a woman who has had breast cancer. There is evidence that one kind of colon cancer (familial polyposis), lung cancer, and leukemia also are more likely to occur in close relatives of persons with those diseases.

Although there are more than 100 known types of cancers, they have a few things in common: They originate in normal tissue cells; they divide more rapidly than the normal parent cells from which they start; they tend to spread into neighboring tissues or migrate to other parts of the body. Cancer cells live longer than normal cells; some cancer cells are theoretically "immortal." But cancer cells serve no useful purpose. They destroy the body's immune (disease-resistance) system, cripple vital organs and tissues by the pressure of their rapidly expanding cell mass, block air passages and blood vessels, and disrupt the blood-clotting system, so that a minor injury for a cancer patient can result in hemorrhage. A benign tumor can also have one of the same effects as a malignant (cancerous) tumor in that it can grow to a very large size, destroying neighboring healthy tissue by sheer pressure of its weight.

Many cancers are believed to develop from a disruption of the genetic material in the parent tissue cells from which they start. The genes in most types of tissue cells (hair and nails excepted) seem to have a built-in mechanism for limiting growth of the particular tissue, so that, for example, a leg bone or earlobe does not continue to grow indefinitely after it reaches a certain size and shape. But a virus, carcinogenic chemical, or burst of radiation energy may be able to change the genetic material so that a cell is no longer limited in its ability to produce new daughter cells and can begin wildly reproducing masses of cells, draining the body's stores of nutrients needed for normal tissue growth and repair and resulting in **cachexia**.

Cancers are sometimes classified according to the basic types of tissue cells involved. For example, cancers that develop from epithelial cells, as of the breast, skin, stomach, or uterus, are classified as *carcinomas,* while cancers that arise from bone or muscle tissue are called *sarcomas.* They may be further subdivided according to the rate of growth, involvement of nearby lymph nodes, and other factors. Leukemias are sometimes identified as "cancer of the blood," which is somewhat misleading, in that the disease actually involves the blood-forming part of the bone marrow rather than tumors of blood cells.

Symptoms associated with various types of cancers sometimes help to identify the source, although careful examination is needed to make a precise diagnosis. Blood in the urine, for example, can suggest cancer of the bladder or kidney, but it could also be a symptom of prostate cancer. A final diagnosis may require extensive laboratory tests, X-rays and scanning techniques, examination of a biopsy sample of the suspected tissue, and, in some cases, exploratory surgery. Treatment of cancer usually requires surgical removal of the tumor and surrounding tissues, including lymph nodes that collect cellular fluid from the cancer site. Radiation or chemotherapy, or both, may be used as a followup to surgery in order to destroy any remaining cancer cells. When cancer can be detected at a very early stage, radiation alone may be able to destroy the cancer cells. However, most cancers are insidious growths and are not discovered until they have begun to interfere with some normal function.

Radiation and chemotherapy, like surgery, may result in the loss of a small amount of normal tissue along with the removal or destruction of tumor cells. But experience acquired in recent years and new techniques have enabled doctors who specialize in cancer treatment (oncologists) to target the therapy more accurately to the abnormal cells, with a minimum loss of normal tissues. The injection of radioactive tracers, for example, helps locate cancer cells rather precisely, because their rapid growth rate makes them absorb more of the radioactive chemical.

The prognosis varies according to the type of cancer, its location, whether it has spread (metastasized), and other individual factors. The rate of recovery for a particular form of cancer is often measured in terms of freedom from symptoms after a time period of five or ten years following the start of treatment. The five-year survival rate for patients with cancer of the colon ranges from 90 percent in cases that were detected at an early stage down to 30 percent among patients with cancer cells that had spread to the lymph nodes before treatment was started. The five-year survival rate for some lung cancer patients following surgery is around 40 percent following surgery, while life expectancy without treatment is less than one year. Some of the most remarkable recovery rates have been recorded among patients with leukemias and lymphomas, mainly as a result of recent advances in chemotherapy techniques. Before the use of chemotherapy, for example, the rate of recovery from advanced Hodgkin's disease was only 5 percent; with chemotherapy, the "cure" rate has been increased to 60 percent. And in some cases of Hodgkin's disease, a combination of chemotherapy and radiation has been found to destroy up to 95 percent of the affected tissue within four weeks, although the percentage of patients who remain disease-free after five or ten years is generally less than the number who obtain remission immediately after treatment.

Because of the many forms of cancer and the myriad possible causes, it is unlikely that a single cure or means of prevention for all types of the disease will be found in the near future. The most ancient medical documents show that doctors have been seeking a cure for cancer since the beginning of recorded history. In fact, the discovery of cures for other diseases, leading to greater average longevity, has increased the risk of cancer for many individuals. As a rule of thumb, the chance of developing most kinds of cancer increases with age. One expert has calculated that one's risk of developing a cancer increases by 1 percent for every year of one's age, so that by the age of fifty, for example, the chances of a person developing a cancer are fifty percent. Some cancers may remain dormant for ten to twenty years and often are not discovered until an autopsy is performed on a person who has died of another disease. *See also* specific types of cancers.

Carbohydrates A category of foods that includes sugars, starches, celluloses, and pectins. Except for milk sugar, all carbohydrates are produced in plants from carbon dioxide and water in the environment, using energy from sunlight. When a carbohydrate is metabolized in the body, this energy is released and the waste products, carbon dioxide and water, are released back into the environment. The body usually stores enough carbohydrates for both physical and mental activities to last about twenty-four hours. (The brain alone requires the equivalent of three to five ounces of sugar daily to function normally.)

A human being can theoretically live without carbohydrates if the diet contains enough proteins and fats, because the body can manufacture carbohydrates from molecules of these other foods. In actuality, however, when the diet lacks carbohydrates, the body begins breaking down the fats and proteins in the body tissues to use as its sources of carbohydrates. Thus, carbohydrates are "protein-sparing" foods, because when they are present in the diet, the body is less likely to literally digest its own vital tissues. The basic carbohydrate unit is a glucose molecule, the simplest form of sugar and the primary source of calories —energy—for the body's trillions of cells. Other sugars and starches are essentially complex collections of glucose units. Most vegetables and grains are composed primarily of starches, which are broken down into glucose units during digestion, and cellulose. Human beings lack the special enzyme necessary to break down cellulose into glucose units, as farm animals are able to do, and are therefore unable to digest this rigid fibrous material that forms the cellular walls of vegetables and grains; but the cellulose portion of fruits and vegetables is a valuable part of the diet, providing the well-publicized fiber that aids digestion by providing bulk for the bowel.

Carcinogen Any substance or agent, or combination of substances or agents, capable of causing development of a cancer. Although numerous substances in the environment have been found to cause cancer in laboratory animals, a much smaller number have been identified as specific causes of cancer in humans. These include arsenic, asbestos, benzene, benzidine, chromium and certain chromium compounds, diethylstilbestrol (DES), mustard gas, soot, tars and mineral oils, vinyl chloride, certain estrogens, and cyclophosphamide. It is believed that most carcinogens produce their effect in at least two stages and may involve more than one agent. In experiments with animals, it has been found that one carcinogen may initiate a cancer, but a second substance usually is necessary to expedite the development of a cancer. Thus, although both asbestos and cigarettes have been identified as causes of cancer, the risk of cancer is much higher for an asbestos worker who smokes cigarettes than for a person exposed to only one of these carcinogens.

Carcinoid syndrome   An abnormal condition caused by a cancerous tumor that may develop in the digestive tract, secreting hormones (such as serotonin) and other substances that result in episodes of abdominal cramps with diarrhea, flushed skin, breathing difficulties, and heart disorders. There may also be skin eruptions that resemble those of **pellagra**. The substances secreted by the tumor include **histamine** and **prostaglandins**, chemicals that are commonly associated with inflammation. It is a particularly insidious type of cancer that usually does not produce symptoms until after it has begun to metastasize (spread to other parts of the body). The serotonin causes flushing, marked by areas of skin that are red but can change in rapid succession to pallor or bluish coloration. The skin effects may be seen on the face and neck and, less commonly, on the abdomen. The most effective treatment is surgical removal of the tumor when the symptoms first occur, even though metastasis has started. Carcinoid syndrome is eventually fatal, but treatment based on radiation, chemotherapy, and careful diet management can extend the life of the patient by ten to fifteen years. A special diet ensures an adequate intake of protein and niacin to compensate for the loss of the amino acid tryptophan, which the tumor converts to serotonin.

Carcinoma   *See* **Cancer.**

Cardiac arrest   The absence of heart sounds, pulse, or blood pressure. The most common cause is ventricular **fibrillation,** in which the heart muscle contracts so rapidly that blood is not circulated properly to the rest of the body, followed by cardiac standstill, a condition in which the heart pumps no blood at all. The person may be unconscious, not breathing, and have dilated eye pupils. Cardiac arrest can be triggered by electrical shock, drowning in fresh water, severe hypothermia or low body temperature, or a spasm of the coronary artery supplying the heart muscle. Cardiac arrest is an emergency situation that requires immediate professional medical care. Cardiopulmonary resuscitation, with mouth-to-mouth breathing and artificial respiration, should be started while awaiting arrival of professional medical personnel.

Cardiac arrhythmias   *See* **Arrhythmia.**

Cardiac failure (heart failure, congestive heart failure)   A condition in which the heart fails to move blood through the arteries normally, resulting in lung congestion and circulatory disorders. Cardiac failure can involve either the left or right ventricles, or both (biventricular). Left ventricular heart failure may be caused by hypertension (high blood pressure), a heart valve defect, a disease of the coronary arteries, or other factors. Right ventricular failure often follows left ventricular failure, which adds to the burden on the neighboring heart chamber. Left ventricular cardiac failure is usually marked by feelings of weakness, fatigue or breathlessness that follows exertion or exercise, intolerance to cold temperatures, and, in some cases, muscle pain associated with poor circulation. Other symptoms of the disease include sudden episodes of breathlessness that sometimes interrupt sleep and are accompanied by coughing spells. The breathlessness may resemble asthma, with wheezing and other abnormal breathing sounds, but, unlike asthma, the lungs do not clear when the patient inhales one of the medicated sprays commonly used to treat asthma. The problem is often caused by changes in the heart muscle, particularly in the area of the left ventricle, which becomes stiff and/or weak and cannot pump blood into the arteries as fast as blood returns through the veins to refill the heart chambers. The condition may be aggravated by lying down, because the heart fills with blood at an even faster rate when the body is in a horizontal position. A normal, healthy heart can adapt to the changes in blood flow that occur when lying down or standing up, but the heart that is abnormal may have trouble coping with them.

When the heart failure patient stands, gravity helps restore the normal balance between blood input and output. The person often finds that a sitting or standing position is necessary in order to breathe deeply or comfortably, or that it may be necessary to get out of bed periodically during the night and walk around. The condition may progress to a more severe form, in which the skin becomes bluish due to a lack of oxygen in the blood, and coughing becomes more intense, resulting in blood-tinged sputum. Heart failure may also become a chronic disorder, with fluid accumulation in the legs, enlargement of the liver, and distended jugular veins, which are a sign of increased pressure in the neck veins. The person begins to experience an excessive urge to urinate at night. The bluish coloration of poorly oxygenated blood tints the ears, lips, and nailbeds. Treatment varies with the specific case, but generally includes rest, sedation if necessary, and appropriate medications, such as digitalis, to improve heart muscle tone.

Cardiac hypertrophy (enlarged heart) A condition in which the heart is larger than average, especially the ventricles, which normally possess more myocardial, or heart muscle, tissue. An enlarged heart may be normal for a person who is an athlete or is otherwise very active physically, but it may be a sign of a heart or circulatory disease if the heart enlargement is the result of an effort by the body to compensate for an abnormality. In a case of hypertension, for example, excessive heart muscle may develop in order to force blood into the major arteries against the resistance of constricted smaller blood vessels farther along the circulatory system. Also called "cardiomegaly."

Cardiac murmur (heart murmur) An audible sound of blood flow in the heart. Under normal conditions, blood flow is silent. The cause of a murmur is usually an abnormal opening or obstruction that diverts the flow and creates turbulence that is heard through a stethoscope as a sound identified as a murmur. Doctors can often identify the cause by the quality of a murmur, which may be low-pitched or high-pitched and occur before, during, or after a heart contraction. Some murmurs are heard only after a person exercises; others may be due to an abnormal thickness (viscosity) or thinness of the blood. A cardiac murmur may be a sign of a heart valve defect or other abnormality, depending upon a number of factors such as whether the sound occurs during heart contraction (systole) or relaxation (diastole), or both.

Cardiac neurosis A psychological anxiety disorder associated with a heart condition. The person may not actually have the condition but may suspect that he or she does, or simply be afraid of developing it. In many instances, the anxiety is generated by heart palpitations or chest pains that are due to emotional stress rather than a true heart disorder. Cardiac neurosis can often be traced to an examining physician whose questions, perhaps pertaining to a history of heart disease in the patient's family, may have been misinterpreted by the patient.

Cardiomegaly *See* **Cardiac hypertrophy.**

Cardiospasm *See* **Achalasia.**

Cardiotonic Pertaining to a substance such as digitalis that increases the efficiency of the heart muscle, usually by increasing the strength of the contractions of the heart.

Cardiovascular Pertaining to the heart and blood vessels.

Cardioversion A technique for restoration of the heartbeat that delivers a synchronized electrical shock to the heart through two metal paddles placed on the patient's chest. The equipment, used in the treatment of heart fibrillation and atrial and ventricular arrythmias, is automatically preset to deliver the charge during the interval in which the heart's own natural pacemaker would normally send its electrical impulse to the heart muscle fibers.

Carotid sinus syncope   An abnormal condition in which a person loses consciousness by turning the head or by wearing a tight collar. The loss of consciousness may result directly from pressure on one of the carotid arteries in the neck, thereby cutting off blood flow to the brain, or indirectly by stimulating the vagus nerve, which runs from the brain to the organs below the neck, resulting in **bradycardia** or a sudden drop in blood pressure. The carotid sinus, a dilatation of the carotid artery, is often more sensitive to such stimuli because of certain diseases or the use of alcohol or digitalis. Persons most at risk are those over sixty years of age who have hypertension or a blockage of one of the carotid arteries that carry blood through the neck to the brain.

Carpal tunnel syndrome   A loss of feeling or a numbness or tingling in the forearm, often accompanied by a weakness in the fingers, due to compression of the median nerve, which extends through the arm to the hand. Compression may be caused by any of more than a dozen factors, ranging from obesity to arthritis, that result in entrapment of the nerve in a tunnel composed of flexor tendons in the wrist. Because of the limited space within the tunnel, any inflammation or abnormality that reduces the space further compresses the nerve. *See also* **Acroparesthesia.**

Cataract   A degenerative condition of the lens of the eye, in which a gray-white opaque area develops that clouds the vision. Early symptoms include an increasing difficulty in reading signs at a distance, doing close work such as sewing, or reading printed material with the "good eye" closed. Some persons see "spokes" radiating from light sources. Cataract formation is associated with aging; the chances of developing the disorder increase to around 45 percent in the seventies.

   There are many possible causes of cataracts, all of them leading to a disturbance of the normal metabolism of the tissue cells forming the lens and interfering with the flow of oxygen and nutrients to the cells. The lens tissues atrophy and eventually "ripen" or crystallize. Among the factors causing cataracts are heredity, injury, infections, diseases such as diabetes, exposure to certain toxic substances such as some nitrogen compounds, drugs, infrared radiation, X-rays, microwaves, and radioactive rays and particles. There are many different types of cataracts, which are classified according to their location in the lens, shape, degree of softness or hardness, and rate of atrophy. Treatment is by surgical removal of the affected lens and its replacement by an implanted artificial lens, contact lens, or cataract eyeglasses. When both eyes develop cataracts at the same time, the usual procedure is to treat one eye at a time, starting with the eye in which vision is poorest. The surgery is relatively simple, and restoration of vision begins within a few days after the cataract is removed. The person may need a short while to adjust to vision with the replacement lens, much as one often needs to practice walking, working, and other activities after first being fitted with bifocal eyeglasses.

Catastrophic anxiety   A near-panic condition that may develop in some persons often after they are afflicted with organic brain disease or aphasia and discover they are no longer able to perform simple tasks as before. They experience anxiety, agitation, fear, and helplessness. Feelings of inadequacy and insecurity may be so strong as to produce pallor and profuse sweating.

Catastrophic illness   Any serious illness that requires prolonged hospitalization with extensive medical and nursing care at costs that exceed the amounts allowed by medical and hospitalization insurance policies. The patient may react to the situation in various ways, such as denying the reality of the illness, or expressing suspicion of being cheated by the medical establishment or fear of family financial ruin.

Catatonia   A complex nervous system disorder characterized by muscular rigidity, stupor, and other symptoms that may be either psychological in nature or physical, or both. Catatonia occurs in **schizophrenia** and **bipolar** mental diseases, but the same symptoms also are observed in cases of brain tumors, brain injuries, stroke, and parkinsonism. The stupor may alternate with periods of excitement. The patient can be mute or speak in meaningless words and phrases. In some cases, he or she may respond to questions by repeating the words just spoken (echolalia) or may imitate the movements of others (echopraxia). Typical symptoms of catatonia include plasticity of the arms and legs, which may remain in whatever posture they are placed, or a passive resistance to stretch movements, even when the patient is trying to cooperate.

Catecholamines   A group of hormones, mainly *epinephrine* (adrenalin), *norepinephrine* (noradrenalin), *dopamine,* and *serotonin,* that are produced in the adrenal glands and cells of the central nervous system and play important roles in the transmission of nerve impulses. It is believed by some experts that catecholamines are involved in certain mood disorders, because abnormally low levels of norepinephrine and serotonin are found in the cerebrospinal fluid of persons suffering from depression, and excessively high levels of these hormones are measured in persons in the manic state. Depletion of dopamine in certain brain areas has been linked to **parkinsonism** symptoms, while dopamine's inhibition of prolactin, a female sex hormone, is believed to be a factor in some cases of **amenorrhea.**

Causalgia   A condition of persistent burning pain and extreme sensitivity of the skin, particularly along the arms or legs. The symptoms are caused by an injury to the nerve fibers in the affected part of the body. The pain and the sensitivity of the skin to external stimuli, even including contact with air, can cause the person to favor the limb, often resulting in muscle atrophy from lack of use. The pain is so extreme that it can also cause emotional upsets. Remedies include tranquilizers, injections of anesthetics, and surgical removal of the troublesome nerve fibers.

Celiac disease (celiac sprue)   An inherited digestive system disease in which the lining of the small intestine is damaged by a reaction with gliadin, a substance in the gluten of wheat flour and in varying amounts also in the flours of barley, oats, and rye. In susceptible persons, the gliadin acts as an **antigen,** or foreign body, that reacts with **antibodies** in the cells lining the small intestine. The reaction leads to inflammation and destruction of the lining. Damage to the intestinal lining makes the digestive tract unable to absorb certain essential nutrients, so that some nutritional deficiencies can develop. The primary symptoms are abdominal discomfort, diarrhea, and weight loss. The celiac patient may also experience bone pain, anemia, and skin eruptions, depending upon the extent of damage. Although the disease may be discovered at any age, it is often not diagnosed until a biopsy is performed on the small intestine of a person who has been plagued by digestive problems; the biopsy reveals damage to the intestinal lining caused by the continued eating of foods containing gliadin. The usual treatment is to discontinue eating foods causing the symptoms.

Cell-mediated immunity (cellular immune system)   The part of the body's immune system that depends upon certain white blood cells (T cells) to resist disease. The T cells defend the body against cancer, viral and fungal infections, and some bacteria, and are responsible for delayed hypersensitivity in skin tests for allergies. Cell-mediated immunity is one of the disease-resistance functions of the body that gradually declines with age. This decline is most noticeable after the age of sixty and can be demonstrated by a lack of response to allergy skin tests that would have produced a positive reaction in the same person at an earlier age. There are wide individual variations, however, and some persons lose their cell-mediated immunity at an earlier age, while others retain their disease resistance in later years.

Cellulitis   A common type of acute skin infection, usually characterized by pain, redness, swelling, and localized heat, that tends to spread
through solid tissues; the legs are commonly affected. The person also
may experience chills, fever, headache, and a general feeling of discomfort. Another type of infection, such as dermatitis, frequently precedes
cellulitis. **Erysipelas** is a form of cellulitis that usually involves the face
and scalp and is often caused by a streptococcus infection. Skin that is
dry and atrophied is a frequent target of such infections. Early antibiotic treatment is necessary for streptococcal cellulitis, which was often
a fatal infection in the days before antibiotics.

Central anticholinergic syndrome   An abnormal mental condition
that results from the additive effect of two or more drugs prescribed for
central nervous system problems, such as antidepressants, antiparkin-
son agents, or tranquilizers. The person may develop symptoms of
agitation, anxiety, partial loss of memory, disorientation, and hallucinations. The problem is corrected by discontinuing one or more of the
drugs.

Central venous pressure   The blood pressure in the vena cava, the
major vein of the body, as it enters the right atrium (the right upper
chamber) of the heart with blood collected from smaller veins throughout the body. The central venous pressure can vary considerably with
changes in posture because of a shift in the blood supply. The result may
be a brief fainting spell. For example, when a person suddenly rises
from a reclining to a standing position, much of the blood in the vena
cava is quickly drained away from the heart and into the abdomen and
legs, in response to the pull of gravity. This rapid drop in blood pressure, called orthostatic or postural **hypotension**, can cause dizziness,
fainting, and falls as blood is drained from the brain. In the fit young
adult, a circulatory system mechanism compensates for sudden drop in
blood pressure so well that the blood shift is hardly noticeable. But as
one grows older, this mechanism loses much of its efficiency with the
result that standing suddenly after reclining in bed, in a warm bath, or
a comfortable chair can cause a momentary disruption in normal blood
circulation with, at the minimum, a loss of balance or, more seriously,
a loss of consciousness resulting in a fall. If a person experiences light-
headedness or dizziness while rising to a standing position, serious
injury can be prevented by returning quickly to a sitting or reclining
position or by rising slowly. *See also* **Cardiac failure, Carotid sinus
syncope.**

Cephalgia   *See* **Headache.**

Cerebral aneurysm A dilatation, or ballooning, of a section of one of the arteries supplying blood to the brain. It may be caused by a congenital weakness, infection, injury, tumor, or **arteriosclerosis**. Symptoms of the disorder are drowsiness, headache, confusion, vertigo, facial pain, weakness of facial muscles, ringing in the ears, stiff neck, visual problems, and partial paralysis. The condition is potentially dangerous since about 50 percent of such aneurysms eventually rupture, resulting in a stroke. Treatment requires placing the person in bed with the head raised at a 45° angle to reduce blood flow to the brain, careful monitoring of the blood pressure, and use of appropriate medications. Various surgical techniques may be employed to prevent rupture of the aneurysm, depending upon its location and other factors.

Cerebral hemorrhage A rupture of a blood vessel in the brain. Symptoms vary somewhat with the location of the hemorrhage, the kind of blood vessel involved, and the cause. Most cases of cerebral hemorrhage are the result of the rupture of an artery that has been weakened by **arteriosclerosis**. Other common causes include congenital **cerebral aneurysm** and head injury. In most cases, the main symptom is a sudden severe generalized headache. The person may vomit, then show signs of a loss of normal control of one or more sets of muscles controlled by the brain, the precise effect on the muscles depending on the part of the brain affected. In some cases, there may be visual disorders, swallowing difficulty, neck stiffness, seizures, or coma, again depending upon the part of the brain involved and the extent of the hemorrhage. A cerebral hemorrhage is a life-threatening event requiring immediate hospitalization and the use of potent painkillers, sedatives, and other measures.

Cerebral thrombosis A blood clot that lodges in an artery of the brain, disrupting blood flow, and thereby causing a **stroke**.

Cervical cancer A carcinoma that develops in the cervix ("neck") of the uterus. After breast cancer, it is the most common malignancy of the female reproductive system. It can usually be detected at an early stage, before there are any symptoms, by a Papanicolaou (Pap) smear, a simple test that should be performed annually. Cervical cancer may signal its presence by the appearance of a watery discharge after straining during a bowel movement or following sexual intercourse. Among many factors associated with the increased risk of cervical cancer are early and frequent coitus, multiple sexual partners, repeated childbearing, viral infections, and poor genital hygiene. When detected at an early stage and treated immediately, the cure rate approaches 90 percent. It is usually treated by surgery and radiation. Although cervical cancer is commonly considered a disease of women during their child-bearing years, those over the age of forty are most commonly affected, and cases have been reported in women in their eighties.

Cervical disk syndrome A condition caused by compression or irrita-tion of one of the nerves that extends from the spinal cord in the neck. A sharp, shooting pain radiates from the neck to the fingers on one side of the body and is aggravated by any motion of the neck, including coughing or sneezing. The thumb and fingers may feel a numbness or tingling sensation. Neck muscles on the affected side are rigid. The condition may be due to an injury, a ruptured or "slipped" disk in the neck, a degenerative disease, or even the simple act of stretching the arms. In many cases, an underlying cause may be a spinal deformity or weakened muscles. Mild pain relievers and special exercises help in most cases, and surgery is usually avoided unless these more conserva-tive measures do not suffice.

Change of life *See* **Menopause**.

CHD Abbreviation for **coronary heart disease**.

Chest pain A sensation of distress, discomfort, or agony due to in-flammation or irritation of nerve tissue in the region of the upper trunk, particularly within the rib cage. Diagnosis of chest pain may be compli-cated by the fact that, in the absence of a crushing or penetrating injury, there may be few, if any, other physical clues, and by panic that the symptoms might signal a heart attack. Most cases of chest pain are caused by heart disease, a spinal nerve compression, or psychogenic factors, that is, stimuli that are psychological rather than physical in origin. Any chest pain should be taken seriously, however, because it can actually be a symptom of a heart attack, pneumonia, or another serious medical problem.

Diagnosis usually begins by efforts to localize the source of the pain to a particular area of the chest wall or deeper tissues within the chest. It is also important to know the duration of the pain and the quality of the pain, that is, whether it is dull, sharp, or crushing. Other clues may be found in what movements, such as deep breathing or stretching the arms overhead, increase or relieve the pain.

The pain of acute **myocardial infarction** (heart attack) usually begins suddenly and lasts more than thirty minutes, with a pain that is often described as a burning, aching, choking tightness combined with a feeling of pressure. It usually occurs in people between the ages of forty and seventy, increases with movement or anxiety and is relieved only by a strong painkiller. The chest pain of **angina pectoris** also may begin suddenly, but it lasts only a few minutes, and it also may produce a burning, choking, aching, or squeezing sensation that can radiate to the jaws and neck and down the arms and back. It is worsened by lying down, eating, anger, worry, stress, physical effort, or cold weather but is relieved by rest and doses of nitroglycerin. A **gallbladder** attack may mimic the pain of a heart attack, although the pain may be felt lower in the chest. It is aggravated by eating or lying down but may be relieved by antacids. The pain of **hiatus hernia** may be worsened by lying down or bending over and relieved by walking or sleeping with the head raised higher than the chest. The pain of **pericarditis** also may resemble that of a heart attack, but it may increase with swallowing, deep breathing, or moving the trunk of the body, and it is relieved by sitting up and leaning forward.

Among frequently unsuspected causes of chest pain are disorders of the spinal column, peptic ulcers, and inflammation of the pancreas. Spinal column disorders include compression of a spinal nerve, which may result from collapse of a thoracic (chest) vertebra, as in a case of **osteoporosis**. Pressure or damage to any of the first six spinal nerves, those extending from the part of the spinal column just below the neck, may be experienced as pain in nearly any part of the chest. Injury to the first thoracic spinal nerve can cause pain that radiates from the shoulder to the forearm, mimicking a heart attack. Pain of stomach disorders, such as peptic ulcers or heartburn, or of an inflamed pancreas may be felt in the lower chest rather than in the upper part of the abdomen.

Cheyne-Stokes respiration   An abnormal breathing pattern marked by cycles of slow, shallow breaths that increase in frequency and depth and then gradually slow again until breathing ceases altogether (apnea). After ten to twenty seconds, the cycle begins again with slow, shallow breaths. Cheyne-Stokes breathing generally occurs during sleep and, as with snoring, the person usually is not aware of it. Causes may include the use of powerful sedatives, a brain tumor, head injury, respiratory infection, or congestive heart failure. A possible cause, particularly among older adults, is a decline in the function of the respiratory control center in the brain.

Chill   A sensation of coldness with shivering of the body, sometimes accompanied by pale skin (pallor) and "gooseflesh." Various diseases, such as influenza or pneumonia, may start with a chill. When the chill is symptomatic of a disease, it is usually accompanied by a fever.

Exposure to wet and cold air may also cause a chill from involuntary contraction of the voluntary muscles. With aging, the body's ability to adapt to both high and low temperatures diminishes, and chills may occur more frequently.

Cholecystitis Inflammation of the gallbladder, nearly always associated with the presence of gallstones and usually complicated by an infection. Acute cholecystitis is characterized by a diffuse pain that radiates from the upper right edge of the abdomen to the right shoulder, with fever, nausea, and vomiting. The pain may range from gripping and burning to excruciating. Attacks may last for hours, but when they subside, it may be a sign that the offending gallstone has moved into the small intestine or has perforated the wall of the gallbladder or the cystic duct linking the gallbladder to the intestine, resulting in peritonitis accompanied by a different severe pain. Tenderness is constant. The abdominal muscles become rigid if peritonitis has developed. The usual treatment is surgery early in the attacks if the patient is able to tolerate general anesthesia. The risk of surgery in acute gallbladder disease is much higher for older patients, the risk of mortality being six times higher for those over the age of sixty-five as compared to those under that age. However, the risk of perforation also is higher for older persons, making surgery a preferred choice despite the risk.

In chronic cholecystitis, gallstones are almost always present, and the gallbladder function is usually lost. The patient has gastric distress, pain in the upper right side of the chest, and nausea. Eating often leads to vomiting. The risk of surgery for the chronic form of the disorder is much lower for older patients and is recommended because chronic cholecystitis, if untreated, can progress rapidly to the acute form. Patients with the chronic form of gallbladder inflammation also have an alternative therapy, whereby the gallstones can be dissolved with the help of oral bile acid drugs taken over a period of several months. However, surgical removal of the gallbladder (cholecystectomy) remains the treatment of choice in most cases.

Cholelithiasis Gallstones in the gallbladder. The stones are a mixture of cholesterol, calcium, and other materials in varying concentrations. It is estimated that about 10 percent of the population will develop cholelithiasis during their lifetime. Twice as many women develop gallstones as men, but the percentage of men with cholelithiasis increases in later years. Factors contributing to the presence of gallstones are heredity, obesity, diabetes, disorders involving the small intestine, the use of supplementary estrogen, and consumption of polyunsaturated fatty acids by certain individuals on special diets.

Cholelithiasis may cause bloating, belching, and food intolerance but often does not produce symptoms until a gallstone blocks the cystic duct through which bile flows from the gallbladder to the small intestine, resulting in a condition sometimes called "gallstone colic." *See also* **Cholecystitis.**

Cholesterol   A waxy steroid substance present in many kinds of animal tissue cells, including bile and blood. (It does not occur in plants.) The human body produces its own (endogenous) cholesterol; it is also found in many foods (exogenous). It has a number of important functions in human health, serving as a component of cell membranes, as a water-repellent protective coating in the skin, and as a raw material for the manufacture of vitamin D and human sex hormones. It is involved in the formation of gallstones, and it can accumulate in the arteries where it contributes to the development of **atherosclerosis** in the form of fatty plaques that are deposited on the inner walls of the blood vessels.

   Cholesterol blood levels in human beings are associated with a group of fatty proteins called *lipoproteins.* One type, called *high-density lipoprotein* (**HDL**), helps remove cholesterol from the arteries to the liver to be stored or excreted, while two other forms, *low-density* (**LDL**) and *very-low density lipoproteins (VLDL)* have the effect of keeping cholesterol in the arteries where it may become deposited on the blood vessel linings. A diet high in saturated fats results in higher blood levels of LDL and VLDL and a greater risk of coronary artery disease, while foods rich in polyunsaturated fats, such as olive oil, increase the proportion of HDL. Exercise and weight loss also help increase the ratio of HDL to LDL in the blood. Women have higher HDL levels than men of the same age until the menopause, after which HDL levels for women fall to the levels measured in men.

Chondrocalcinosis   A form of **arthritis** in which calcium deposits accumulate in the joints. It may or may not produce symptoms. The condition, which resembles **gout**, tends to occur in persons over the age of fifty and favors those who already suffer from **osteoarthritis, diabetes mellitus,** or **gout.** Chondrocalcinosis tends to occur in a familial pattern, suggesting a possible hereditary factor. Because the deposits are made of crystalline calcium, the disease is sometimes confused with gout, which is characterized by deposits of uric acid crystals in the joints. When the calcium deposits result in inflammation of a joint, the disorder is called **pseudogout.** The presence of calcium crystals in the joints does not always lead to pseudogout. The disease does not progress to a deforming type of arthritis and responds well to anti-inflammatory medications.

Chorea Brief, rapid, jerking movements of the arms and legs or the facial muscles over which the person has no control. The condition may occur in a number of disorders, including **Huntington's chorea.** A mild form, called *senile chorea,* sometimes occurs in later life, with few if any serious mental symptoms. A variation, *choreoathetosis,* which may affect older adults, is characterized by movements that are slower, less purposeful, and more continuous than those of true chorea. *See also* **Essential tremor.**

Chronic obstructive pulmonary disease (COPD) A term used to describe any of several disorders resulting in a generalized airways obstruction, including **bronchitis, asthma**, and **emphysema**. The major symptom is a breathing difficulty that may be caused by a number of conditions, such as a narrowing of the bronchial tubes, cigarette smoking, and air pollution. The condition is usually free of symptoms early in life, except for a "smoker's cough" and breathing difficulty following physical exertion. As the person grows older, symptoms of coughing, wheezing, susceptibility to respiratory infections, weakness, and weight loss become more prominent and may be disabling.

COPD is sometimes subdivided into categories of *Type A* (emphysematous) and *Type B* (bronchial), based on diagnosis of individual patterns of symptoms. It is usually diagnosed in Type B patients between the ages of forty-five and sixty-five; the condition in Type A cases is usually found between fifty-five and seventy-five. Treatment is directed at relief of the symptoms and prevention of infections, heart failure, or other complications. The prognosis depends largely upon the degree of lung capacity remaining when the disease is diagnosed. COPD is reported to be second only to heart disease as the cause of disability in men over the age of forty.

Cirrhosis A disease marked by formation of fibrous tissue and nodules in the liver. It is relatively common, particularly after the age of forty-five, being exceeded only by heart diseases, cancer, and stroke as a cause of death. There are two major types of cirrhosis. The most common form, *micronodular,* is caused by excessive use of alcohol and is marked by the formation of small nodules in the liver. The second form is *macronodular,* represented by large, irregular nodules and scar tissue, usually caused by a viral hepatitis infection. There are also mixed types of cirrhosis and other forms of the disease. Although cirrhosis is often associated with the consumption of alcohol, a number of medications, such as methotrexate, and industrial chemicals, including polyvinyl chloride, can produce the same effect. The disorder can follow an infection of viral hepatitis or certain bacterial diseases or be due to a birth defect that alters a person's normal metabolism. Cirrhosis usually begins with symptoms of fatigue, loss of appetite, loss of weight, nausea, and abdominal discomfort. Patients also may experience reduced libido. As the disease progresses, the liver becomes enlarged, followed by enlargement of the spleen. Some patients show signs of wasting of muscles, redness of the palms of the hands, loss of normal feelings and other neurological disorders of the hands and feet, testicular atrophy, and development of female-type breasts in men (gynecomastia). Treatment of alcohol-induced cirrhosis consists primarily of abstinence from alcohol, rest, and a protein-rich diet. As liver tissue has some ability to recover from injury, the prognosis is favorable, except for patients with severe complications, such as **ascites, jaundice**, and hepatic coma.

Claudication   A lameness or limping, usually as a result of a circulatory disorder affecting blood flow to the leg muscles. *See also* **Intermittent claudication.**

Climacteric   An alternative term for **menopause**.

Clubbing (drumstick fingers)   A condition that affects the fingers and toes as a symptom of many diseases of the heart, lungs, digestive tract, and circulatory system. The soft tissues and nails are usually enlarged, and in some cases there is an overgrowth of bone tissue as well. The condition has been noted by physicians for thousands of years, although the cause is not well understood; it is believed to be related to a deficiency of oxygen in the blood. Typically, both hands are affected, beginning with the thumb and index fingers; other fingers and toes become involved later. The nails become curved in a bulbous shape and may appear to be floating because of a thickened layer of soft tissue between the bone and the nail. Clubbing is often a sign of **heart disease, cancer, ulcerative colitis, polycythemia**, and **pneumoconiosis**. Clubbing diminishes when the underlying condition is diagnosed and treated.

Cluster headaches (histamine headaches)   Headaches that are brief and severe and occur in attacks that repeat several times a day or week, followed by long periods that are headache-free. The headaches occur on one side of the head, usually around the temple or on the side of the face, sometimes extending to the neck or shoulder. The attacks are severe enough to cause throbbing, tearing of the eye, and flushing of the skin for periods from fifteen to forty-five minutes. These headaches are sometimes called "histamine headaches" because the same effect can be produced by injecting histamine into a carotid artery leading to the brain, although there is no evidence that histamine is a cause of the headaches.

Colic   A severe, intermittent, griping, abdominal pain. It is caused by spasms of smooth muscle tissue, as occur in the passage of gallstones, appendicitis, lead poisoning, or air-swallowing. Colic is further identified by its source, such as *renal colic,* resulting from one or more stones (calculi) in the kidney or ureter, and *biliary colic,* triggered by the passage of gallstones. Other symptoms may include vomiting, fever, and extreme tenderness in the abdomen.

Colorectal cancer   Adenocarcinoma of the large intestine, the colon, and rectum. The disease is common in North America and occurs almost as frequently as lung cancer. It develops mainly after the age of fifty and affects women more often than men. Because the disease is comparatively rare in Asia and Africa, it is believed that a diet high in refined carbohydrates, animal protein, and fat, and low in fiber, may be responsible for this difference in frequency. The risk of developing colorectal cancer is increased in persons who have had **ulcerative colitis, diverticulosis,** familial polyposis, or excessive exposure to asbestos fibers. Cancers of the rectum are marked by bleeding, pain, and a feeling of incomplete bowel evacuation. Other symptoms include a change in bowel habits; the passage of stools with a black, tarry appearance due to the presence of digested blood; and the passage of relatively fresh blood. Tumors in the colon can constrict the passageway, so that stools are flat or pencil-shaped. Tumors in the ascending colon, on the right side of the abdomen, are sometimes large enough to be felt through the abdominal wall; they may cause anemia, nausea, and bowel movements that alternate between constipation and diarrhea. Most colorectal cancers are treated surgically, with chemotherapy and radiation as alternative or supplementary therapies. The prognosis depends on how early the tumor is identified and whether it has invaded the wall of the intestine.

Complaint   An expression of discomfort or pain that results from an ailment or disease. *Chief complaint* is a medical term used to identify the symptom reported by the patient as the reason for seeking medical attention.

Complexion   The texture, color, and appearance of the skin, particularly of the face. As one grows older, there are changes in the complexion because the skin often undergoes a process of atrophy, accompanied by dryness, roughening, and loss of elasticity in underlying as well as surface tissues. The complexion may also become paler because less blood may be circulating in surface vessels.

Concussion A mild injury to the brain caused by a blow or other trauma, sometimes resulting in a brief loss of consciousness. Other symptoms are dizziness, cold sweats, and visual disturbances. When consciousness is regained, there may also be a headache and sometimes amnesia about events immediately before and after the event. Depending on the severity of the concussion, a "post-concussive syndrome" may follow that can linger for weeks, with symptoms such as insomnia, irritability, inability to concentrate, and depression.

Conductive hearing loss *See* **Hearing loss.**

Confabulation The tendency of a person with a faulty memory to fabricate details of past events in order to account for parts that cannot be recalled. The person may come to accept his or her own fabrications as factual. The condition occurs in **senile dementia** and other organic brain disorders.

Congestion The abnormal accumulation of a fluid, such as blood, bile, or mucus, in an organ or body part. The buildup of fluid may occur from various causes. Examples include blood accumulation in the lowest part of an organ or body area, such as the legs, due to the action of gravity (hypostatic congestion), and dilation of the capillaries of the iris as a result of conjunctivitis (global congestion).

Congestive heart failure A disorder in which the heart is unable to pump the volume of blood that is needed to maintain normal body functions. The ineffective pumping action causes difficulty in breathing and retention of salt (sodium) and water by the body, particularly in the lungs, abdomen, and legs. The disorder may follow a heart attack (**myocardial infarction**), with damage to the heart muscle from an interruption in its blood supply. Treatment includes administration of drugs such as digitalis to strengthen heart muscle action, and diuretics to help eliminate excess fluids (edema) from the body.

Constipation Delayed or difficult passing of stools (feces). The normal pattern of bowel movements varies with each individual, ranging from several a day to one every few days. Efficient functioning of the bowels depends to a great extent on the tone (tension) of the abdominal muscles and those of the rectum and anus, which may diminish with age in the ability to contract and relax efficiently. Harder stools may also result when a person does not drink enough liquids. A potential cause of constipation is inadequate fiber, or "roughage," in the diet; the nondigestible substances in whole-grain cereals and vegetables stimulate the walls of the bowel and induce defecation. Dietary fiber also helps speed the passage (transit time) of fecal material through the colon. The symptoms of chronic constipation include headache, listlessness, a feeling of fullness, and digestive disturbances. **Hemorrhoids** may be a complication of chronic constipation. Fecal impaction, a condition in which hardened stool cannot be expelled, may require special treatment with enemas, or physical removal. The use of laxatives or cathartics without medical supervision is not recommended because they contribute to a "lazy bowel" condition in which the colon becomes dependent on the use of such remedies and fails to function without laxative stimulation. *See also* **Laxatives.**

Contracture   The abnormal shortening of a muscle. The condition, which may be disabling, can be caused by injury, lack of exercise of the muscle, or a disease such as **arthritis** or **fibrosis**. Contracture from failure to exercise a muscle is often the result of favoring a limb or other body part after an injury that makes movement painful.

Conversion symptoms   Symptoms that have no dectectable organic cause but apparently arise unconsciously to mask an anxiety or inner conflict. Conversion symptoms may be used to gain attention, sympathy, or control over others. Typical conversion symptoms are tunnel vision, loss of a sensation of taste or smell, paralysis, loss of voice, headache, loss of appetite, and coughing spells, conditions that can also be symptoms of a physical problem.

Coping   The process of dealing with problems in an effort to adapt to or work through or around them. A person's coping strategies may be conscious or unconscious. For example, a person may deny or ignore the symptoms of a developing physical disorder without consciously recognizing this is being done. However, coping can be a positive tactic as well as a negative one, if it is directed toward correcting the source of a problem rather than relieving the discomfort it causes.

Corns   Small, hardened overgrowths of skin tissue that grow on the feet. They are caused by pressure and friction and often become macerated by the moisture of sweat. Corns are sometimes classified as "hard" corns, which develop on bony prominences, as over toe joints, and "soft" corns, which usually occur between toes. They are removed by surgery or the application of chemicals that dissolve the excess skin growth.

Coronary artery disease (CAD)   Any disorder of the arteries supplying the heart muscle that affects the normal flow of blood to them. The disorders include coronary **atherosclerosis**, coronary **embolism**, coronary **arteritis**, dissecting **aneurysm**, and loss of normal muscle and elastic tissue resulting from an infection, such as syphilis. The most frequent problem is coronary atherosclerosis, which has become a leading cause of death in the Western world. The common symptom of all coronary artery diseases is the crushing chest pain experienced in **angina pectoris**. The pain seems to radiate from beneath the breastbone to the left side of the body, from the arm to the jaw, in most cases. The pain is caused by **ischemia**, a form of oxygen starvation of the heart tissues; narrowing or obstruction of the coronary arteries deprives the tissues of oxygen-enriched blood. The pain is usually increased by physical exertion and relieved by a period of rest.

Diet, stress, lack of exercise, and cigarette smoking are among the most significant factors contributing to coronary artery disease, as shown by long-term epidemiology studies. The CAD increase in North America and other Western nations has been linked to a greater per capita consumption of foods rich in saturated fatty acids, leading to abnormally high blood levels of **cholesterol**, atherosclerosis, and obesity. The twentieth-century increase of sedentary occupations and lifestyles has had the effect of escalating these CAD risks in industrialized countries. Related studies show that physical exercise, reduced consumption of saturated fats, and lower body weight result in lower blood cholesterol levels and a reduced risk of CAD. Adding further to the increasing CAD risks over the past fifty years has been the popularity of cigarette smoking, which narrows coronary and other arteries. The gap in the incidence of coronary artery disease between men and women has narrowed in recent years because more women are smoking cigarettes and have taken stressful sedentary jobs. The use of oral contraceptives also is believed to be a factor in the higher incidence of female coronary artery disease cases, particularly as women grow older and lose their premenopausal hormonal "immunity" to CAD. As risk factors are generally additive, the combination of cigarette smoking and the use of oral contraceptives is more dangerous than either of the factors alone.

Untreated, coronary artery disease leads to sudden death or **myocardial infarction** (heart attack). Nearly one-third of patients with unstable angina pectoris symptoms suffer a heart attack within three months.

The prognosis in CAD is affected by such factors as the number of coronary arteries affected (increasing from an annual mortality rate of 3 percent for one artery to up to 10 percent for all three coronary arteries), the age of the patient, a history of previous heart attacks, and the patient's blood pressure. When sudden death occurs in a CAD patient, there is frequently evidence that fatal ventricular fibrillation was triggered by ischemia of the heart muscle.

Treatment is directed toward either increasing the amount of oxygen available to the heart or modifying the heart's activity with drugs so that it can function with less oxygen. Some patients with severe CAD and a minimum of other risk factors may be advised to undergo **coronary bypass** surgery to correct the symptoms.

Coronary bypass An open-heart surgical procedure in which a blood vessel composed of natural or synthetic material is grafted onto a blocked or narrowed coronary artery to provide a new channel through which blood can flow unimpaired to the heart muscle. Surgeons may remove a segment of an artery or vein from another part of the body and use it for the graft, or they may use a piece of plastic tubing. The operation is usually recommended only when obstruction of a coronary artery is severe enough to be life-threatening and other forms of CAD treatment have failed to relieve the symptoms.

Coronary occlusion Any blockage of one of the coronary arteries, usually caused by gradual narrowing of an artery as a result of **atherosclerosis** or a **coronary thrombosis** (blood clot), or both. In a typical case of coronary occlusion, an accumulation of atherosclerotic plaques on the lining of the artery reduces the size of the opening, restricting the flow of blood. Eventually blood flow is reduced to the point of ischemia (oxygen starvation) and necrosis (death) of the heart muscle cells and **myocardial infarction** (heart attack). Occlusion can also be produced by spasms of the artery, also resulting in a diminished or interrupted blood flow. A coronary occlusion is a life-threatening emergency that requires immediate hospitalization and prompt treatment.

Coronary thrombosis A blood clot that forms within one of the coronary arteries, interrupting the flow of blood to the heart muscle. The result is a **myocardial infarction** (heart attack). There is a tendency for a coronary thrombosis to develop in an artery that is already partly occluded by **atherosclerosis**. *See also* **Blood clotting.**

Cor pulmonale (pulmonary heart disease) Enlargement of the right ventricle (lower chamber) of the heart due to a lung disorder. The cause may be any abnormality that obstructs the normal flow of blood from the right ventricle through the vessels of the lung, including chronic **bronchitis, emphysema, chronic obstructive pulmonary disease**, or pulmonary **embolism**. The right ventricle grows larger in order to perform the extra work needed to force the blood through the diseased lung. Cor pulmonale is most likely to affect middle-aged or older men who smoke cigarettes. It is a common complication of **black lung disease, silicosis**, and other occupational diseases affecting the lungs. Symptoms are a chronic cough, wheezing and breathlessness on exertion, weakness, and fatigue. As the disease progresses, the person tends to breathe more rapidly and may need to stand or sit upright in order to avoid breathing difficulties. Veins of the neck become distended, and a rapid heartbeat develops. It is not unusual for persons suffering from cor pulmonale to experience sudden episodes of drowsiness or loss of consciousness, particularly during physical exertion. The acute form of the disease, caused by pulmonary embolism, may be reversible with proper medical care, including diet and drugs. Prognosis is poor for most patients with chronic cor pulmonale if a significant amount of breathing capacity has already been lost at the time the disease is diagnosed. The incidence of cor pulmonale in North America has increased nearly tenfold since the end of World War II.

Cortical blindness　A form of partial or complete blindness caused by an interruption in the flow of blood to the occipital region of the brain, where visual impulses from the eye are translated into images. The condition is often associated with a stroke.

Cortical deafness　A loss of hearing in the absence of any injury or disease of the ears. The cause is usually a brain lesion that disrupts the normal flow of nerve impulses along the auditory pathway between the ear and the part of the cerebral cortex that interprets the impulses. *See also* **Agnosia.**

Cramp　An acutely painful, usually sudden, spasm of a muscle or group of muscles. The condition may be caused by heat, cold, fatigue, or a particular occupation, as in miner's cramp. Some involuntary muscular contractions, such as writer's cramp, are classified as "occupational neuroses" because they tend to occur only when the person is working under stress or against a deadline. Heat cramp is caused by a deficiency of sodium chloride (table salt) and is both prevented and treated by eating foods or drinking fluids containing salt. Calcium is necessary for normal muscle tone, and a lack of it in the diet may result in muscle cramps in physically active adults. Some cramps may be a symptom of a disease, such as chronic kidney failure.

Crepitus A grating sound produced by the friction of facing tissue surfaces rubbing against each other. Crepitus may be heard in cases of **osteoarthritis, rheumatoid arthritis,** and **scleroderma.** Other types of joint noises are creaking, which is produced by bone surfaces of joints rubbing together when there is a loss of cartilage cushioning in the joint, and crackling, which is attributed to gas bubbles in the fluid that normally lubricates a joint.

Creutzfeldt-Jakob disease A slow virus infection of the central nervous system that causes progressive mental deterioration, often with symptoms of psychotic behavior. Muscle wasting and involuntary muscle activity such as spasticity, tremor, and rigidity are other characteristics of the disease. It begins in middle age, and deterioration is noticeable from one week to the next, usually ending in death within a year. It is an uncommon disease, and the method of transmission is uncertain. However, patients have acquired the disease through organ transplantation and through insufficiently sterilized medical instruments previously used in the treatment of patients with Creutzfeldt-Jakob disease.

Crohn's disease A chronic inflammatory bowel disease that generally affects two age categories: those under thirty or over forty. The onset of symptoms for the older group reaches a peak around the age of seventy. The inflammation usually involves the ileum, a portion of the small intestine, but also may spread to the colon and rectum. Symptoms include attacks of diarrhea, severe abdominal pain, loss of appetite, weight loss, chills, fever, and weakness. The patient usually has three or four bowel movements daily, producing semisoft stools. Complications include abscesses and fistulas. Experiments with laboratory animals suggest the disease may be transmitted by a virus or similar microorganism. Treatment includes drugs, diet, and surgery. In some cases, the patient may be fed intravenously to allow the digestive tract to rest and recover from episodes of inflammation.

Cup arthroplasty A surgical procedure for replacement of the head of the femur, the bone of the upper leg, at the hip joint with a metal or plastic substitute that fits into a metal cup inserted into the hipbone. The procedure is performed to relieve pain and increase the range of motion in cases of arthritis, fracture of the head of the femur (upper leg bone), or congenital defect aggravated by **osteoarthritis**. The damaged or diseased bone surfaces are removed, and the replacement parts are shaped to match the original bony joint.

Cyanosis A bluish color visible through the skin and mucous membranes. It is a sign of an insufficiency of oxygen in the blood or of a circulatory disorder. Cyanosis first appears in surface areas of the body, such as the lips, nailbeds, and ears, where coloration is normally pink because of the presence of oxygen-rich blood.

Cyclothymic disorder A form of depression observed in older adults characterized by periods of depression and mania that are not serious enough or which do not last long enough to be considered major episodes of bipolar (manic-depressive) disease. The person may exhibit a loss of interest in most activities, complain of fatigue and sleep disorders, have tearful, pessimistic episodes, and shows signs of social withdrawal. *See also* **Bipolar disorder.**

Cystitis An inflammation of the urinary bladder or the ureters that carry urine from the kidneys to the bladder. The symptoms are low back pain or pain above the pubic area, a feeling of an urgent need to urinate, frequent urination, urinary difficulty, and—especially in women—blood in the urine. Causes can include a bacterial infection (most common), tumor, or a kidney stone. A bacterial infection of the bladder is far more common in women than men and often results from an infection that spreads upward from the urethra; it may be caused by a bacterium acquired during sexual intercourse. In men, the disorder may follow an infection that migrates upward from the urethra, possibly having spread from a prostate gland infection or caused by medical use of a catheter. Treatment includes antibiotics when the cause is a bacterial infection, medication to control bladder muscle spasms, increased fluid intake, and, in certain cases, surgery.

Cystometry A diagnostic technique used to help find the causes and cures of disorders involving the bladder, including incontinence. It involves measurements of the capacity and pressure of the bladder and the condition of the urethral sphincter, the round muscle of the urethra that controls the flow of urine when voiding.

Cytomegalovirus disease (CMV) An infection caused by a virus related to the herpes virus. It may occur without symptoms or be characterized by fever, swollen glands, general feelings of discomfort, enlarged spleen, and, occasionally, a rash, respiratory system effects, and jaundice. CMV can occur at any age, and the risk of infection increases as one grows older. The majority of older adults have had CMV infection, whether or not they recognized it. The disease is particularly dangerous in pregnancy because the virus can be transmitted to the fetus, causing spontaneous abortion, stillbirth, birth defects if the fetus survives, or severe postnatal problems.

D

Dark adaptation   The ability of the eye to adjust to the absence of light when entering a darkened room or going outdoors at night after being in a well-illuminated area. Impaired dark adaptation is associated with glaucoma.

Deafness   *See* **Hearing loss.**

Decalcification   The loss of calcium from the bones and teeth, resulting in **osteoporosis, osteomalacia,** and dental diseases. The causes may be a diet that lacks calcium, poor absorption of calcium from the diet because of a deficiency of vitamin D, a deficiency of the stomach acid that aids in the absorption of calcium from foods in the diet, or an excess of foods rich in fat or oxalic acid, substances that can convert calcium in the digestive tract into forms that the tract cannot absorb. Decalcification can also result from a defect in the parathyroid hormone system, which controls the calcium levels of body tissues. People who are not physically active are also likely to experience some calcium loss because the body tends to maintain only as much bone density as is required by the usual daily level of activity.

Decubitus ulcer   *See* **Bedsores.**

Defecation   The normal physiological process of eliminating solid wastes from the body through the anal opening of the rectum. Defecation itself is a natural function, but the ability to postpone the act is a learned behavior that is controlled in part by the brain. It also requires

99

an intact system of nerves and reflexes, mental awareness, and normally functioning smooth and skeletal muscles. Most people are able to maintain their learned ability to control defecation throughout life, but the complex network of brain cells, nerves, and muscles involved in postponing defecation can be disrupted by a variety of accidents, including stroke, causing fecal incontinence. Other causes of impaired control can include diabetic neuropathy involving the colon, dementia, spinal cord disease, fecal impaction, and laxative overuse. A more common complaint, particularly among older persons, is **constipation**. People who are physically active generally have fewer bowel problems than those who are inactive. *See also* **Constipation.**

Defibrillation   A method of treating **fibrillation** of the heart by administering an electric shock. The technique is used primarily to control ventricular fibrillation but is also applied in certain cases of atrial fibrillation that may not respond well to the administration of digitalis. The shock is given through two electrodes, one placed over the right side of the heart and one near the left armpit or shoulder. The electrical charge is usually a measured amount of direct current electricity. If time permits, the patient is given a sedative or analgesic. **Acidosis** builds up quickly as a complication of ventricular fibrillation, and death or brain damage can occur within a few minutes, so the entire procedure must be done quickly. Medications are given to counteract acidosis and to help restore heart muscle tone after the event.

Deficiency disease   Any physical or mental ailment resulting from the lack of one or more nutritional factors necessary for normal human health. The cause may be a failure to eat foods containing the essential minerals and vitamins, amino acids, and fatty acids; a digestive disorder that prevents absorption of one or more of the essential nutrients from the digestive tract; a failure of the body to manufacture an enzyme needed to help digest a crucial food element; or a disorder in which the body excretes a nutritional factor needed for normal health, as in the excessive excretion of potassium by patients taking certain diuretic medications. Examples of deficiency diseases include **scurvy**, caused by a lack of vitamin C; iron-deficiency **anemia; beriberi**, resulting from a thiamine deficiency; and **pellagra**, caused by a niacin deficiency. More common than overt nutritional deficiencies, particularly among older adults, are subclinical nutritional deficiencies, or borderline health disorders, such as sores that are slow to heal because of a mild deficiency of zinc or vitamin C in the diet. The deficiencies might be detected by laboratory tests but are not severe enough to be disabling.

Degenerative disease   Any disease marked by the deterioration of a body structure or function, such as **osteoarthritis, arteriosclerosis, cancer**, and **dementia**. Degenerative joint disease can affect the neck, spine, hips, knees, and other body areas, causing pain, muscle weakness, neurological disorders, and instability of the joints, making movements unsteady and leading to falls. Dementia is usually the result of degeneration of the brain and is characterized by impairment of intellectual functions, such as loss of memory, comprehension, reasoning, judgment, and discrimination. **Intermittent claudication** and **coronary heart disease** are both caused by atherosclerotic degeneration of the arteries, and **emphysema** is a degenerative disease of the lungs. In addition to their direct effects on a body system, degenerative diseases can also be immobilizing, increasing a person's susceptibility to infections and other disorders associated with physical inactivity. *See also* **Spondylosis.**

Deglutition   *See* **Dysphagia.**

Dehydration   Excessive loss of water from the body tissues, which can be the result of diarrhea, vomiting, fever, or simply a failure to consume enough fluids to balance the body's normal loss of water through breathing, urination, sweating, and defecation. It is often associated with a disruption of the body's **acid-base balance.** Symptoms of dehydration include feelings of confusion and irritability, a flushed, dry skin, coated tongue, and inability to produce a normal amount of urine. The pulse and breathing are usually rapid, the body temperature is often below normal, and the skin may feel cold. Persistent or frequent dehydration can lead to kidney disorders. Persons who take diuretic medications are particularly susceptible to dehydration, as are those who are exposed to extreme hot or cold temperatures, and they must increase their intake of fluid accordingly.

Delirium   An abnormal mental condition marked by confusion, loss of orientation as to time and place, and reactions that are inappropriate to the situation. There also may be hallucinations, delusions, illusions, restlessness, agitation, muttering, and fear that can easily progress to panic. Symptoms of delirium may develop suddenly, over a period of hours, or gradually. A major symptom is a "clouding of consciousness," in which the person appears to be not clearly aware of his environment. There also is a tendency to misinterpret what is seen or heard; the patient typically becomes unable to identify familiar persons. Other symptoms include incoherent speech and sleep disturbances, usually in the form of insomnia and a desire to sleep during the day. Among the causes of delirium are a small **stroke, dehydration, hypoglycemia,** head injury, brain infection, high fever, reaction to a drug or toxic substance such as carbon monoxide gas, or prolonged emotional stress or exhaustion. Symptoms of delirium may also develop in older persons who are compelled to make a sudden disorienting or fear-inducing change in their environments, such as being hospitalized or placed in a nursing home.

Dementia   A generalized term for forms of mental deterioration usually associated with an organic brain disorder. Dementia is often broadly applied to degenerative disorders that affect the "mature mind," after adult speech and other characteristics have been acquired, to distinguish the condition from types of mental deterioration that have their onset in younger persons. **Alzheimer's disease, Pick's disease, Huntington's chorea, Wilson's disease,** and **Creutzfeldt-Jakob disease** are among the dementias that usually start after the age of forty. Regardless of the causes, dementias tend to follow a similar pattern of deterioration, with recently acquired mental faculties being among the first lost. Thus, memory for recent events is lost before memory for earlier events. Abstract thinking ability is lost before concrete thinking. If the person acquired a sizable vocabulary before the onset of symptoms, that part of the intellect may be retained. The person becomes less venturesome in thought and action, relying on old habits and responses rather than trying new ways and ideas; in fact, the challenge of a new situation can trigger symptoms of **delirium.**

As the mental deterioration progresses, the person may exhibit signs of antisocial behavior that was latent but suppressed in earlier adult life, much as a person under the influence of alcohol may be less inhibited in social behavior. About half of all cases of dementia are of the *primary degenerative type,* involving permanent alterations in the number and structure of brain cells, as in Alzheimer's disease. About 25 percent of the cases are of the reversible, treatable type that may respond to certain medications and psychotherapy. The remainder may include cases of dementia associated with the effects of drugs, hormonal disorders, nutritional deficiencies, and other factors, such as *multi-infarct dementia,* caused by a series of strokes that are too small to result in paralysis or other disabling effects and cannot be detected through brain scans.

Superimposed on the organic aspects of dementia may be symptoms of **bipolar disorders,** particularly episodes of depression. Depressive traits may have been present but suppressed in earlier adult life. In other cases, depression may surface as an inversion of the person's earlier personality. When depression is an underlying factor in dementia, the condition may be reversible. The prognosis is also more hopeful when a nutritional deficiency disease, such as **pellagra**, can be found to be the cause of dementia.

Demyelination A degenerative change in certain nerve fibers in which there is loss of the amount of fatty (myelin) insulation that sheaths them. There is some slight demyelination of the central nervous system in all persons after the age of forty and a more serious form of the disorder in certain types of organic brain disease and in persons with some diseases of fat metabolism.

Dental disorders Various problems of the teeth and gums that may occur increasingly with aging. One recent survey found that slightly more than 50 percent of all Americans over the age of sixty-five had lost all of their natural teeth, and 67 percent were toothless in at least one jaw. In addition, in a typical year, 15 percent of all persons over sixty-five are treated for **periodontal disease**, 18 percent are treated for cavities (dental caries), and 40 percent require new dentures or repair of existing dentures or bridgework. Such data are based on patients of a generation that received less preventive and maintenance dental care than those now in their forties. Future generations of older adults should experience fewer dental disorders because of the emphasis on fluoridated public water supplies and improved dental care since World War II. Much of the dental work required by persons over the age of forty now involves treatment of secondary caries, or decay that develops around existing fillings. Also, after the age of forty, the incidence of caries below the gumline increases by 300 to 400 percent, because receding periodontal tissues expose the roots of the teeth.

Dentate nucleus calcification A type of neurological disorder that commonly occurs in older adults and is characterized by mild degrees of loss of control of the skeletal muscles involved in body movements. It is caused by calcium deposits in a portion of the cerebellum, at the base of the brain, called the dentate nucleus. In severe cases, the calcification produces symptoms of **Huntington's chorea** or **Parkinson's disease**. Similar symptoms may be caused by calcium deposits in another area of the brain (the basal ganglia) in older persons. It is usually a progressive disorder.

Denture problems Pain or other disorders caused by pressure on mouth tissues from false teeth (dentures). Symptoms include pain, bleeding gums, or hard pads (dental granulomas) at pressure points. The condition is corrected by a dentist who will modify the dentures so they will not irritate the gums and who will also relieve the symptoms of gingivitis (gum inflammation).

Dependent person   An individual who requires assistance from others for physical care, food, warmth, shelter, protection, or emotional attention, or a combination of these factors. Studies show that in the past two decades, partly because of the increasing proportion of older adults, the ratio of dependent persons has been increasing three times as fast as the general population. One survey found that 17 percent of all Americans over the age of sixty-five were bedridden, homebound, or otherwise limited in mobility, and 40 percent of the same age group needed assistance in some of the **activities of daily living (ADL)**.

Depressed breathing   A breathing pattern characterized by slow, shallow respirations. The condition is usually caused by medications that depress activity of the breathing center located in the medulla portion of the brain.

Depression   A major disturbance of mood, characterized by apathy, withdrawal, loss of self-esteem, and loss of interest or pleasure in most or all of one's usual activities. Depression is the most common psychological disorder in older adults. It is a complex condition that may occur independently of a physical illness or accompany it. There also are varying degrees of depressive symptoms, ranging from feelings of normal bereavement in response to the death of a loved one or concern about income to a severe dysphoric mood with delusions and preoccupation with suicide and death. An older adult may simply appear depressed because of physical changes in the face and posture, or as a reaction to the use of any of dozens of drugs, from alcohol and antipsychotics to steroids and sulfonamides, that can cause symptoms of depression. Many older adults may also appear depressed because of sensory deprivation, in the form of impaired hearing or vision, that has the effect of socially isolating them. In some cases of "masked depression," physical symptoms may be a psychosomatic manifestation of depression in a person who was trained in earlier years to suppress normal expressions of sadness or other emotions.

After middle age, many people begin losing much of what they had acquired earlier in life, including stature in the community or profession, their job, income from other sources, old friends and relatives and other social contacts, as well as such physical assets as mobility, vision, and hearing. A person who has been driving an automobile since the age of sixteen may be deprived of that ability fifty years later because of failing vision or a stroke, with a consequent loss of the sense of autonomy. Some individuals welcome their new dependent role, while others may become severely depressed by the restrictions imposed on them by the routines of medical care personnel or other persons.

Among biological factors that may contribute to depression in older adults may be a genetic predisposition, as there is evidence of this influence based on family histories of patients treated for severe forms of the condition. There are also changes in body chemistry that increase the risk of depression as one grows older. Levels of an important neurotransmitter substance (monoamine oxidase) increase, while concentrations of catecholamines decrease. Catecholamines include natural stimulants, such as epinephrine (adrenalin), that make the heart beat faster and raise the blood pressure. Monoamine oxidase is an enzyme that destroys the body's natural stimulants. Thus, a part of the aging process has the effect of reducing the body's own "uppers" while increasing its natural "downers." In support of this theory is the fact that one of the drugs prescribed for the treatment of depression is a **monoamine oxidase inhibitor (MAOI)**, which inhibits the action of the "downer" enzyme.

Physical illnesses that may contribute to symptoms of depression in older adults include viral and bacterial infections, metabolic disorders, and hormonal problems. Specific illnesses common to older depressed patients are bacterial and viral pneumonias, encephalitis and meningitis, endocarditis, tuberculosis, urinary tract infections, diabetes mellitus, neurosyphilis, dehydration, and acid-base imbalances.

Physical symptoms associated with depression can include weight loss, loss of appetite, fatigue, weakness, anxiety, sleep disturbances, general aches and pains, dizziness, heart palpitations, breathing difficulties, constipation, urinary problems ranging from incontinence to increased frequency, headache, backache, memory problems, and feelings of numbness. Sleep disturbances, particularly insomnia, are common complaints of persons suffering from depression, though true insomnia must be differentiated from the changes in sleeping patterns that normally occur with increasing age. On the other hand, a number of diseases, such as parkinsonism and hyperthyroidism, produce symptoms that are often mistaken for signs of depression. In order to treat depression properly, the doctor must carefully sort out the various possible physical and psychosocial factors that may be the cause of the symptoms.

Treatment of depression often requires correction of the factors causing or contributing to the physical symptoms as well as restoring the mental health of the individual, when possible. The choice of treatment depends upon factors causing the condition and may include antidepressant and/or antipsychotic drugs, electroconvulsive therapy, individual and/or group psychotherapy, and such supportive measures as improving the person's environment, involving family and friends in the treatment process, and encouraging participation in mental and physical activities. Because of side effects and varied individual responses to drugs, the choice of medication may require several weeks of testing of the different alternative drugs and dosages.

Dermatomyositis A disease of the connective tissue marked by symptoms of an itching, eczemalike skin inflammation and weak, tender muscles. There may be swelling of the face and eyelids, and a loss of weight. As muscle tissue is lost, the patient may find movement and performance of simple tasks difficult. Among possible causes are viral infection, reaction to a medication, and an internal cancer. The disease is sometimes classified as a form of **polymyositis** that involves the skin. Treatment is with steroids and other drugs, which may include antacids and mineral supplements for severe cases. The prognosis varies widely, with some patients responding within weeks and other requiring treatment for five years or more, while still others may succumb to a complication involving the heart or lungs.

Detached retina *See* **Retinal detachment.**

Detrusor The name of a group of muscle fibers that surrounds the urinary bladder. Contraction of the detrusor muscle produces pressure for emptying the bladder. An unstable detrusor muscle may contract involuntarily, causing urinary **incontinence. Stroke** or brain damage from other causes can cause a person to lose the ability to prevent detrusor contraction when he or she feels the urge to urinate. This inability results in **uninhibited bladder** and urinary incontinence.

Diabetes mellitus A disorder characterized by inadequate secretion by the pancreas of insulin, a hormone essential for normal carbohydrate metabolism, resulting in excessive levels of blood glucose (blood sugar). The condition is often complicated by disorders of the blood vessels, nervous system, and acid-base balance. Diabetes is a complex metabolic disorder, with five different subtypes of the disease determined by such factors as whether the patient requires insulin injections (insulin-dependent) or can be treated instead with oral drugs (hypoglycemics). A diagnosis of diabetes is based primarily on the ability of the person's body to utilize glucose, the basic chemical building block of carbohydrate molecules, when the pancreas fails to secrete enough insulin. A glucose tolerance test, in which a person fasts for ten to sixteen hours before drinking a glass of glucose dissolved in water, is sometimes helpful in making the diagnosis. Analysis of blood samples taken at thirty-minute intervals after drinking the glucose solution reveals how well the body tolerates the measured dose of glucose. Inadequate insulin secretion results in glucose intolerance. The diagnosis also is based on the various symptoms of diabetes, including excess thirst, excessive urination, abnormal hunger, lethargy, and weight loss. Uncontrolled diabetes also can affect metabolism of proteins and fats, resulting in additional complications.

The incidence of diabetes mellitus rises sharply after middle age. For persons below the age of thirty-nine, the prevalence of diabetes is only 1.5 percent. After the age of forty, the incidence jumps to 8.4 percent, and after sixty to 17 percent. In addition to the figures for the prevalence of diabetes, another 10 percent of the over-sixty age group has been found to have relative insulin insufficiency or impaired glucose tolerance. However, much of the glucose intolerance among older adults is caused by a resistance of the body's tissues to the action of insulin and not by a failure of the pancreas to secrete enough insulin. This condition, sometimes called adult-onset, or non-insulin-dependent, diabetes, is aggravated by obesity and often can be corrected by weight reduction and exercise.

The causes of diabetes mellitus are partly hereditary and partly environmental, including lifestyle influences. Most people who develop diabetes mellitus after the age of forty, and have the adult-onset (non-insulin-dependent) form of the disease that does not require injections of insulin, have a family history of the disorder; the genetic evidence is particularly strong among identical twins. They also tend to be obese and have some degree of **atherosclerosis**. Among the reasons for impaired glucose tolerance and increased blood glucose levels in older adults are reduced physical activity and a normal change in body tissue composition as fat replaces muscle.

Inactive persons with a higher proportion of body fat require less glucose than physically active people with more muscle and less fat. The higher blood glucose levels contribute to a diuretic effect, so that one of the earliest symptoms of diabetes is an urge to urinate more frequently. The increased concentration of glucose in the urine can lead to a yeast infection, **monilial vaginitis** (genital candidiasis), in women.

In addition to optimum weight control and exercise, control of adult-onset diabetes usually requires an individualized diet with no increase in the frequency of feedings, which is the opposite of the dietary regimen for patients with insulin-dependent diabetes. Among other differences, day-to-day consistency of calorie amounts of carbohydrates, fats, and proteins and consistency of timing of meals, factors important in insulin-dependent diabetes, may not be necessary for patients with adult-onset diabetes. The diet usually restricts calorie intake from fats to less than 30 percent of the daily total and maintains carbohydrate intake at between 55 and 60 percent of total daily calories. Patients, including those with impaired glucose tolerance, should have their blood glucose levels checked regularly by a physician. Although "do-it-yourself" test strips are available for measuring blood glucose levels in the urine, many older adults may be unable to interpret the results as accurately as medical technicians.

Diabetic retinopathy A degenerative disease of the blood vessels in the retina of the eye resulting from effects of **diabetes mellitus**. Abnormalities of the cells of blood capillaries of diabetics lead to **aneurysms** of the small vessels, hemorrhages, loss of fluid, and the formation of new tissues in the retina. The condition also results in a clouding of the normally transparent substance filling the eyeball, so that vision is gradually lost. The condition can sometimes be treated with use of a laser beam that seals the leaking blood vessel.

Dialysis A method of removing certain substances from the blood by a process that filters the blood through a semipermeable (semiporous) membrane, allowing certain chemicals to pass through while others remain in the blood. Two basic procedures are employed. *Hemodialysis* utilizes a machine fitted with an artificial membrane. *Peritoneal dialysis,* performed within the body, uses the peritoneum, the membrane that lines the peritoneal cavity of the abdomen. Dialysis is used in the care of persons with severe kidney disorders and in the treatment of life-threatening poisoning by drugs, chemicals, or natural substances. A complication of dialysis is *dialysis dementia,* a neurologic condition of progressive mental deterioration that develops occasionally in patients who have been treated by this technique. The exact cause is unknown, but as it tends to occur more frequently in certain geographical areas, it is believed that a toxic substance in the local water—possibly high levels of aluminum—may be a factor. There is no specific treatment for the disorder, which eventually leads to death. Dialysis also is associated with an increased risk of brain hemorrhages, migraine headaches, muscle cramps, and vitamin deficiencies. These complications can be treated with drugs or, in the case of bleeding in the brain, by surgical drainage.

Diaphragmatic hernia *See* **Hiatus hernia.**

Diastole The phase of the heart contraction cycle when the muscles of the heart chamber are briefly at rest, which is between the end of a contraction and the point at which blood begins to fill the heart chambers for the next contraction. During diastole, the force (pressure) of blood flow from the heart ebbs, to build again as a result of refilling of the heart chambers with blood. Circulation in the coronary arteries peaks during diastole because relaxation of the heart muscle allows the arteries to expand. *See also* **Systole.**

Dilate   To open wider, as when the pupil of the eye becomes enlarged or the bore of a blood vessel is increased.

Diopter   A measure of the refractive power of a lens that is used in prescribing and making corrective lenses for eyeglasses. It is based on the metric system and is equal to the number 1 divided by the focal length of the lens in meters. Thus, a 2.0 diopter eyeglass lens would have a focal length of ½ meter, or about 20 inches, and a person with a prescription for 2.0 diopter eyeglasses would find objects most clearly focused when held at a distance of about 20 inches. As the number of diopters increases, the focal length shortens, so that a 4.0 diopter lens has a focal length of 10 inches, and so on.

Diplopia   Seeing double, a visual abnormality in which a single object appears as two. Diplopia can occur in several ways, with the images in horizontal, vertical, or diagonal relationships to each other. It is a functional defect and can be caused by a failure of coordination of the external eye muscles, a cataract, or an irregular cornea. In crossed diplopia, the image seen with the right eye may appear to the left of the image seen with the left eye, or vice versa.

Disability   The loss of a body part or function that results in an impaired ability to carry on one's activities without assistance. A disabled person may or may not also be handicapped, depending upon his or her ability to cope with an impairment. Thus, blindness is a disability, but it becomes a handicap in situations when help is needed, and paraplegia becomes a handicap when the patient requires assistance in boarding a bus or airplane.

Discectomy   A surgical procedure for removal of a **herniated disk.**

Disengagement   A mental process whereby a person withdraws or disengages from life's activities. The condition may begin to show up in an older adult who prepares for a less active role in life by denying the importance or value of objectives that would inspire or drive a younger person. Disengagement may be manifested by quiet withdrawal or by expressions of anger and bitterness, acting-out behavior, and frantic efforts to restore a feeling and image of youthfulness. How a particular individual disengages may be affected by such factors as cultural values, mode of life, and economic and social conditions.

Disk *See* **Cervical disk syndrome, Herniated disk.**

Dissecting aneurysm An aneurysm that is caused by blood leaking between the layers of muscle in the wall of an artery, forming a column that separates (dissects) these layers. This abnormal condition tends to occur at a place where the lining of the artery is weakened by the death or degeneration of some of the tissue cells. Middle aged or older men with high blood pressure are most commonly affected. Dissecting aneurysms usually involve the aorta, the main artery carrying blood from the heart to all parts of the body. If uncorrected, the dissection or splitting of the layers of the artery continues in a direction away from the heart, involving arteries that branch away from the aorta. In most cases, the aneurysm eventually ruptures. Symptoms are a severe tearing pain that occurs in the area of the aneurysm and follows the path of the dissection as it continues. The pain is nearly always in the abdomen, chest, and back, and may be accompanied by breathing difficulty, loss of consciousness, profuse sweating, and an abnormally rapid heartbeat. Treatment often requires lowering the blood pressure so that surgery can be performed to replace the damaged artery with a length of plastic tubing before a rupture occurs.

Disseminated intravascular coagulation (DIC) A term for any of a variety of blood coagulation disorders, such as infections or illnesses that prevent normal coagulation of the blood.

Disuse phenomena Degenerative changes that occur in the body from lack of use of a body part or system. The phenomena are experienced by persons who are confined or immobilized by disease or injury. The changes may be psychological as well as physical. Psychological changes are sometimes manifested in disorientation and alterations in time sense and memory, similar to those experienced in cases of sensory deprivation. Physical changes often include a breakdown of the skin, contractures, constipation, bone loss, kidney stones, respiratory disorders, and thickening of the blood. Skin tissue changes are caused by body pressure on skin surfaces combined with inadequate airing of the skin surfaces. Contractures result from prolonged holding of an arm, leg, or other body part in a fixed position. Muscle and bone tissue atrophy rapidly when not fully exercised regularly. Loss of abdominal muscle tone contributes to constipation, while bone minerals tend to accumulate in the kidneys. Respiratory disorders evolve from pooling of secretions in one part of the lungs, which remain moist, while other lung surfaces become dry; simultaneously, mucus accumulation fosters the growth of bacteria. Persons who are inactive often tend to drink less fluid than normal, increasing the viscosity of the blood so it is more likely to form clots that can lead to a heart attack or stroke.

Diuretic (water pill) A drug or other agent that stimulates the production and excretion of urine. Diuretics are prescribed in the treatment of such disorders as **hypertension, congestive heart failure**, and **edema**, in which symptoms are relieved by reducing the volume of fluid in the body. Some diuretics can have adverse effects in persons being treated for certain diseases. Thiazide and chlorthalidone diuretics, for example, can produce hyperglycemia, thus aggravating diabetes mellitus, and may also result in an excessive excretion of sodium and potassium. Certain diuretics are capable of modifying blood levels of cholesterol, electrolytes, and uric acid and may deplete body fluid volume, exacerbating the symptoms of gout. They may also interfere with anticoagulant and digitalis drugs taken by heart patients. Diuretics can cause dehydration in older patients who do not drink enough fluids. Several natural substances, such as alcohol and caffeine, also have a diuretic effect.

Diverticulitis ("left-sided appendicitis") An inflammation of a diverticulum in the large intestine, usually caused by an abscess in this "pocket" that has formed in a weakened part of the wall of the colon. Diverticula are comparatively common in persons over the age of fifty and appear to be the result of low-residue diets eaten over many years. Diverticula themselves usually do not produce symptoms; though in some cases there may be occasional rectal bleeding and periods of constipation. Diverticulitis produces pain and tenderness in the lower left side. Other symptoms are nausea, vomiting, fever, and constipation or diarrhea. Because the inflamed segment of colon is near the kidney and bladder, the pain is sometimes mistakenly identified as a disorder of the urinary system. Treatment may include bed rest, antibiotics, and intravenous (IV) feeding while the abscess is healing. Complications include hemorrhage or peritonitis. Surgery to remove the inflamed section of the colon is sometimes indicated.

Diverticulosis The presence of small pouches or sacs (diverticula) formed by the protrusion of the lining of the bowel, particularly the colon, through its muscular wall. There may be a dozen such outpocketings in a person with diverticulosis. The diverticula may be a cause of chronic diarrhea and other bowel diseases, because the sacs become filled with fecal material and bacteria, and interact with food substances such as unabsorbed carbohydrates and fatty acids passing through the digestive tract. The person may be symptomless unless the diverticula become a source of rectal bleeding or inflammation. Treatment may include medications to relieve abdominal distress, local heat application, rest, and a diet that provides adequate bulk, or roughage, for moving fecal material more rapidly through the bowel. Surgery may be required in cases of severe intestinal bleeding. *See also* **Diverticulitis.**

Dizziness   A sensation of a loss of balance while in a sitting or standing position. The person may feel faint, experience nausea, giddiness, and blurred vision, and may feel a sense of swirling motion. If standing or walking, he or she may also feel unsteady and weak in the legs. The person who experiences dizziness should lower the body or be lowered to a safe position in a chair or on the floor or another solid surface. Dizziness is a common cause of falls resulting in serious injuries. Causes of dizziness include **orthostatic hypotension**, or a sudden draining of blood from the head when arising from a lying, sitting, or standing position; a small stroke; central nervous system disease; heart disorders, or an abnormality in the inner ear, where the sense of balance is controlled. The most common cause of dizzy spells is an inner ear, or labyrinthine, disorder. *See also* **Ménière's disease.**

Dopamine   A **catecholamine** neurotransmitter of the sympathetic nervous system that is found in certain areas of the brain and in the blood vessels of some of the skeletal muscles. It is produced within sympathetic system nerve cells by the action of an enzyme on the amino acid tyrosine. There is evidence that some disorders, such as **parkinsonism**, can be caused by a deficiency of dopamine. Drugs that increase the production or use of dopamine by the brain cells are used to treat parkinsonism. Dopamine is also used in the treatment of shock, falling blood pressure, and low heart output, and as a diagnostic aid in triggering the symptoms of central nervous system disease such as **Huntington's chorea.** Abnormally high levels of dopamine have been measured in schizophrenic patients, and the substance has been found to inhibit the release of prolactin hormone while enhancing the release of growth hormone. Dopamine is converted by enzymes into two other catecholamines, epinephrine and norepinephrine. Dopamine generally has a balancing effect on levels of another important neurotransmitter substance, acetylcholine. Factors that increase dopamine activity in the nervous system decrease acetylcholine (cholinergic) types of neurotransmitters, and vice versa. Thus, cholinergic drugs can precipitate symptoms of parkinsonism by reducing dopamine levels, and dopamin-ergic drugs can lower levels of cholinergic substances in the nervous system, causing symptoms of Huntington's chorea or other disorders. Because of this delicate balance, extreme care must be exercised in prescribing medications that can affect the nervous system and result in serious side effects, particularly for older adults whose neurotrans-mitter balance may be easily upset.

Dreaming A series of images that occur spontaneously during sleep. The images may be based on past events or experiences, anticipated future events or experiences, or efforts to solve problems or resolve inner conflicts. One study suggests that while dreams remain individu-alistic in the aging person, aging does affect their content, and the frequency of dreaming diminishes. Various psychiatric theories have been proposed to explain dreaming, and much of the practice of psy-choanalysis involves dream interpretation. Dreaming tends to occur four or five times a night and during specific periods of sleep, which can be identified by rapid eye movements (REM) and recorded with an electroencephalograph that registers brainwaves. The **hallucinations** that occur in the minds of some mentally disturbed persons produce the same kind of brain-wave patterns as dreams.

Dressing apraxia A symptom of certain brain disorders in which persons are unable to dress themselves properly. The subject might, for example, put clothing on the left side of the body, neglecting the right side. The condition is associated with a body image defect, expressed as a failure to recognize parts of one's own body. The same patient may wash or shave only the left side of his face or fail to attach the bow of his eyeglasses over the ear on the right side, which he may disclaim as a part of his body. The brain defect usually involves tissues that inte-grate various functions.

Dribbling A term used to describe spillover of fluid to the outside of the body. Dribbling of saliva from the mouth can be a symptom of **parkinsonism** or an overclosure of the bite of dentures. Dribbling of urine can be a sign of stress incontinence in women or a prostate problem in men. If necessary, urine dribbling can usually be corrected surgically. *See also* **Incontinence.**

Drop attacks Falls that may occur without loss of consciousness. The cause is often a circulatory disorder, such as a constriction of an artery supplying the brain so that the blood supply to a part of the brain is suddenly curtailed. The affected portion of the brain may be a center that controls balance, muscle tone, or nerves that contract the "anti-gravity" muscles of the legs. Drop attacks also may be due to arthritic damage to a knee or hip joint. The attacks occur without warning, and the person usually is not aware of the onset of falling until he finds himself on the ground. Women occasionally experience what are called *cryptogenic drop attacks,* for which no cause can be found. Some drop attacks have occurred in persons who are in unfamiliar surroundings or suffering periods of confusion or disorientation.

Drowsiness   A condition marked by a low level of alertness, because of fatigue, the imminence of sleep, or a disease or injury. A person who is merely resting or drifting into sleep usually has assumed a relatively natural, comfortable position. One who is drowsy because of an acci-dental impairment of consciousness may show an absence of such natu-ral signs as yawning and swallowing. Also, one whose drowsiness is caused by injury or disease may have a slack jaw with the mouth partly open, and the eyelids may be at least partially open. A drowsy person is easily aroused and is able to respond to questions. In the absence of paralysis or numbness, the drowsy person will also react to mildly painful stimuli, such as pinching or the pricking of the skin by a needle. The condition may also be described as *lethargy. See also* **Stupor.**

Drug eruption   A skin disorder that may occur in persons who are particularly sensitive to certain drugs. Eruptions may occur as erosions of the tongue and lips, skin discolorations of the hands and face, and premature graying of the hair. Drugs that may cause skin eruptions include diuretics, tranquilizers, antibiotics, steroid hormones, and anti-malarials. Treatment may include use of emollients, wet compresses, antihistamines, and elimination of the medication.

Drug intoxication   A severe adverse reaction caused by taking over-the-counter, prescription or illegal drugs. The reactions may be caused by an accidental overdose, a drug allergy that has developed from previous use of the drug, or an individual hypersensitivity due to an inherited susceptibility. Symptoms may include abnormal movements of the eyes, abnormally dilated or constricted pupils, drowsiness or stupor, loss of consciousness, low body temperature, flaccid muscles of the jaw and arms, depressed breathing, vomiting, diarrhea, dry skin, rapid heartbeat, and excitability. Fatal toxic drug reactions have re-sulted from such common medications as aspirin and penicillin.

Drug metabolism The chemical interactions between drugs and the affected tissues and other substances present in the body, leading to physiological changes such as reduction of fever, elimination of bacteria, or increased heart muscle tone. Drug effects vary widely among individuals. While older adults are more sensitive to the effects of painkillers and sedatives, and may require lower doses, they are more resistant to **beta adrenergic** blocking drugs. An older adult may require a dose of a particular heart stimulant that is as much as six times the amount of the drug that would produce a similar effect in a younger person.

Factors that affect drug metabolism in older adults include a 12 to 18 percent increase in body fat and a decline of 10 to 15 percent in total body water, resulting in a smaller volume of blood and other body fluids. Other factors influencing drug metabolism in older adults include increased stomach acidity affecting the absorption of drugs, reduced heart output, altered liver function, and reduced kidney activity. Use of alcohol, tobacco, and other medications also may influence the metabolism of a particular drug differently in the body of an older adult.

Dry skin Skin that lacks sufficient moisture or sebum (oil), or both. It may be characterized by itching, roughness, scaling, fissuring, cracking, and cross-hatched patterns caused by scaling. Natural changes in the skin, particularly the reduced production of sebum, is related to a diminished production of androgens (male sex hormones) in older adults. In women, the changes become noticeable after the menopause; men usually begin to feel the effects later in life. This natural drying of skin can be aggravated by cold, dry winds, hot indoor temperatures with low humidity, wool clothing, and excessive bathing with soap and hot water. Uncorrected, the condition can progress to a form of eczema, while scratching can result in skin infections. Treatment includes the use of antihistamines to reduce the itching sensation, the use of mild, superfatted soaps for cleaning the skin, and the application of bath oils and emollients, which are more effective if applied after a bath while the skin is still damp.

Dumping syndrome The rapid emptying of the stomach contents into the small intestine that is an aftereffect of surgery for the treatment of stomach ulcers in which a part of the stomach is removed. When this smaller stomach is nearly filled by a meal, the person may have a sense of distress in the upper abdominal region, without pain, but with a feeling of nausea, weakness, and heart palpitation. The patient may show pallor and sweating. The symptoms diminish after the patient learns to eat smaller meals with a greater frequency, which the abbreviated stomach can accommodate.

Duodenal ulcer A peptic ulcer in the duodenum, the first segment of the small intestine. It is the most common type of peptic ulcer. A duodenal ulcer usually produces a pattern of symptoms that repeats each day. The pain is usually relieved by a meal but returns several hours after eating. A duodenal ulcer also tends to produce pain in the middle of the night but not early in the morning. The symptoms may vanish for a period of time but return, usually in the spring or autumn. The symptoms also return during periods of emotional stress. During periods of remission, the ulcer may heal completely. But half of the "cured" duodenal ulcers recur within two years.

Treatment of duodenal ulcers usually begins with conservative measures, such as eliminating certain food items, particularly pepper and caffeine, from the diet and taking antacids. Ulcers that fail to respond to diet and antacids may be treated with medications, including drugs that inhibit action of nerves controlling stomach acid secretion, that combine with proteins to form a protective coating over the lining of the digestive tract or that lower the level of acidity. Severe cases may require radiation therapy or surgery, especially when an ulcer penetrates the wall of the duodenum, leading to peritonitis. Surgery may be used to sever the vagus nerve fibers that cause an increase in the flow of gastric acid. It may also may be needed to control hemorrhage, a common complication of duodenal ulcers. Hemorrhage treatment also may require blood transfusions, flooding the digestive tract with ice water, and feedings of bland foods, such as milk. *See also* **Peptic ulcer.**

Dupuytren's contracture A hand deformity that tends to develop in some men after the age of forty as a tightening and thickening of the tissues beneath the skin of the palm. It causes the little finger and ring finger to bend toward the palm and to resist efforts to straighten them. The condition usually begins in one hand but eventually involves both. The first sign is the appearance of a small nodule in the palm, near the base of the ring finger, which gradually grows to form a band or plaque of hard tissue. The contracture is usually painless and can be corrected by surgery in the early stages.

Dysarthria A loss of the ability to speak distinctly, usually as a result of a disease or injury affecting the central nervous system. It is a common effect of stroke.

Dysautonomia Abnormal functioning of the autonomic (sympathetic) nervous system, characterized by symptoms of drooling or dry mouth, excessive or diminished sweating, and impotence. The condition occurs in parkinsonism and diabetes and accounts for the loss of voluntary muscle control in **drop attacks, vertigo**, and fainting spells.

Dyschezia A failure of the defecation reflex of the nervous system, resulting in constipation. Causes can include degeneration of the nerve cells that activate the anal sphincter and other muscles of the bowel; travel or change of residence that may disrupt toilet habits; laxative abuse; loss of appetite; and joint or muscle factors, such as arthritis of the hips or loss of coordination that prevent a person from assuming a natural posture of squatting or sitting on a toilet seat.

Dyschromia A medical term for changes in skin pigmentation, such as appearance of liver spots, blood blisters, or cherry angiomas. *See also* **Angioma, Complexion.**

Dysesthesia An unpleasant sensation, as occurs in spinal degeneration when herniation of a vertebral disk results in numbness, or muscle weakness, or impairment of a part of the body supplied by fibers of a compressed nerve root. Dysesthesia may occur suddenly and painlessly.

Dysequilibrium A loss of balance that may occur without the symptoms of **dizziness** or **vertigo**. Dysequilibrium can lead to **falls** or **drop attacks** and can arise from instability of joints due to **arthritis**, interrupted blood flow to a brain center that controls muscles in the legs, or loss of ability to stand or coordinate muscles because of **organic brain disorders**.

Dysgraphia A loss of the ability to perform the hand movements needed for writing or drawing according to spoken instructions. Damage to the link between the sense of hearing and the part of the brain that allows visual imaging of what is to be created interferes with the ability of the person to carry out the task. However, the person may be able to copy someone else's work.

Dyskinesia any involuntary muscular activity, such as a tic, spasm, or seizure. The term is also used to identify a voluntary movement that appears distorted because of a **neuromuscular disorder**.

Dyslexia A loss of the ability to understand written words or numbers due to organic brain damage. Vision and speech ability may be normal. The condition varies with different individuals. Some may be able to read letters but not words, words but not numbers, numbers but not letters or words. The disorder may be complicated by anxiety or other emotional problems.

Dysmenorrhea   Painful menstruation. The condition is usually marked by severe abdominal cramps in the lower front pelvic area. The cramps are often accompanied by headache and backache. The symptoms usually begin just before or at the start of menstrual flow and may last a few hours to a few days. For most women, the condition is mild and brief and requires no particular treatment, but for at least 10 percent of women, dysmenorrhea can be disabling. Symptoms of dysmenorrhea can be aggravated by endometriosis, pelvic inflammation, pelvic tumor, or a displaced uterus.

Dyspareunia   Any condition that causes sexual intercourse to be painful for a woman. For postmenopausal women, the cause may be atrophy of the tissues lining the vagina.

Dyspepsia   *See* **Indigestion.**

Dysphagia   Difficulty in swallowing. Among various causes are a narrowing of the opening in the esophagus, a rigidity of the wall of the esophagus, an obstruction in the esophagus due to inflammation or a tumor, or a goiter. In some cases, the cause can also be a loss of normal coordination or functioning of the nerves and muscles that control the passage of food between the mouth and the stomach.

Dysphasia   A difficulty in speaking or understanding speech. The condition is due to damage in a speech center of the brain. The person may be able to understand or speak individual words but may not be able to communicate with words in an organized meaningful pattern.

Dysphoria   A personality pattern disorder marked by depression, anxiety, restlessness, and discontent.

Dyspnea   *See* **Breathing difficulty.**

Dyspraxia   A loss of the ability to perform functions that require skill in muscle coordination. The cause of the problem is an organic brain disorder rather than a defect in the muscular system.

Dysthymic disorder   A form of depression in which a major symptom is a loss of interest or pleasure in one's usual activities. The patient may appear depressed, but the symptoms are not severe enough to be classified as true depression, and the patient also shows no particular signs of **bipolar disorder**. Also, the depressed moods may occur at intervals separated by months of relatively normal behavior. The dysthymic form of depression is often observed in older persons.

Dystonia   A muscle tone disorder marked by slow involuntary contractions of the muscles of the trunk and limbs. The movements, such as repeated arching of the back, are caused by a disease of the central nervous system.

Dysuria   Difficult or painful urination. The person may experience hesitancy in starting the flow of urine or have to strain to maintain the stream, usually because of a partial obstruction in the urethra or because of a disorder involving the complex nervous system control of the urination process. Causes may be a stone or blood clot in the bladder or urethra, an enlarged prostate in a male, a spinal cord tumor, or cancer of the urethra.

E

Ear fungus An eruption of the skin of the external ear, usually as a result of an allergy or bacterial infection. Symptoms include oozing, redness, crusting, or swellings on external ears. The cause of contact dermatitis or atopic eczema of the ear is often an allergic reaction to the materials used in earrings. Treatment is with medications that are determined by the actual cause of the skin reaction. Although the term ear fungus is commonly used to identify the condition, a true fungus infection is rarely the cause.

Eaton-Lambert syndrome A condition of muscular weakness that is often associated with an underlying cancer. This defect is due to impaired release of acetylcholine neurotransmitter at the nerve ends. The symptoms resemble those of myasthenia gravis. The muscle weakness is usually in the shoulders and pelvis and is often associated with a lung cancer that frequently is not located until after the onset of the symptoms. Unlike true myasthenia gravis, muscle strength can be recovered through exercise. The symptoms diminish if the tumor is removed or destroyed.

Ecchymosis A bruiselike patch of bluish or purple coloration of the skin. It is caused by an accumulation of blood beneath the skin following the rupture of capillaries. Ecchymoses may be caused by mild injury, such as bumping into furniture, and tend to occur more frequently in older adults who have lost some of the subcutaneous fat that normally cushions against contact with an object. The skin of the older adult also may be thinner and thus more translucent, so that bleeding beneath the skin is more visible than in a younger person.

Eccrine gland   A medical term for sweat gland.

Eccrine tumor   A growth in a sweat gland, whether benign or malignant.

Echolalia   A condition in which a person's speech consists only of a repetition of words and phrases uttered by another person. The automatic mimicking also may include a repetition of the other person's movements and gestures. Echolalia may be observed in organic brain diseases, including **Alzheimer's disease** or **Pick's disease**.

Ectropion   An atrophy of eyelid tissue that causes the lid margin to fall outward or away from the eyeball. This exposes the conjunctival membrane that lines the eyelid and part of the eyeball and protects the surface of the cornea, leading to drying, irritation, and redness of the eye, as well as poor tear drainage across the eye surface. The tears may run down the cheek of the patient rather than into the duct that normally drains tears into the nasal cavity. The condition may involve only the lower eyelid or both the upper and lower eyelids. The underlying cause may be paralysis of the facial nerve, but it is often the result of loss of tissue firmness with aging. Treatment may require surgery.

Eczema   A type of dermatitis, or skin inflammation, characterized by itching, redness, swelling, and eruptions that take the form of pimples or blisters that sometimes break, causing the area to "weep." If the condition is not treated, the skin areas can become dark, leathery, thick, crusted, and scaly. Factors causing eczema include heredity, emotional stress, allergy, poor nutrition, hormonal imbalance, or a combination of these factors. Eczema usually forms in the skin folds of the knees, elbows, neck, or face, but during a severe attack it may spread to other skin surfaces. *Atopic eczema* occurs in people who are generally sensitive to more than one kind of allergen and who have a history of hay fever, asthma, or other reactions to dusts, molds, or other environmental irritants.

Edema   An abnormal accumulation of fluid, particularly in spaces between tissues or as in tissues of the legs or in the alveoli (spaces) in the lungs. Edema can be a symptom of a wide range of disorders, from a minor inflammation, injury, or burn to life-threatening congestive heart failure or kidney or liver disease. The underlying disorder may cause leakage of the fluid from capillaries; result in an obstruction of the vessels that normally collect fluid in body spaces; cause disturbances in the body's fluid and acid-base balances; signify or be a reaction to

...fection or a toxic chemical. Edema often begins insidiously and is first noticed as an unexplained gain in body weight; it eventually becomes apparent as puffiness in the face or swellings in the legs.

Pulmonary edema, or fluid in the lungs, causes symptoms, especially shortness of breath, that may interrupt sleep with coughing spells. The coughing, when present, is often coarse and may be accompanied by wheezing and gurgling sounds. The patient may find that getting out of bed and walking around for a few minutes provides some relief so that sleep can be resumed. Edema that is a sign of **congestive heart failure** is usually marked by fluid that leaks in from capillaries and accumulates in the ankles, creating a condition sometimes identified as *pitting edema,* because small pits can be made to appear temporarily in the flesh by poking a finger into the fluid-swollen area. When the person is lying down, the fluid may move into the lower back area.

Allergies to drugs, foods, or other substances, such as poison ivy, may result in edema of the subcutaneous tissues, which is manifested as blisters or hives. A disorder of the kidneys may result in a failure to excrete sodium, causing fluid accumulation. A similar form of edema can result from excessive salting of foods. Treatment of the various types of edema requires correction of the underlying cause.

Effort syndrome A functional disorder with symptoms that resemble those of **angina pectoris** but that are associated with anxiety. The symptoms may include heart palpitations, dizziness, and fatigue. The person also may have cold, moist hands, **breathing difficulty**, and chest pains following a period of exercise, whereas in a true case of angina, the symptoms would more likely occur during exercise. Although effort syndrome is sometimes called "soldier's heart" and is associated with complaints of soldiers in combat, the condition is actually more common among civilians and affects women more frequently than men.

Effusion The escape of fluid from blood vessels, as in **edema,** into the body cavities. The term is usually combined with the part of the body affected. Thus *pleural effusion* refers to fluid seepage into the pleural cavity around the lungs. Effusion into an internal cavity may produce signs and symptoms detected indirectly, as with a stethoscope, but effusion into a joint may be visible, marked by a swelling or bulge in the skin around the joint, and may affect normal movement of the involved limb.

Egoisme à deux Literally "mutual selfishness," a psychiatric term sometimes applied to older married couples who deny the reality of physical or mental decline in each other because they do not want to contemplate the major changes that must eventually be faced. Because day-to-day changes are rarely noticeable, it is possible to foster the denial until the deterioration becomes too obvious to ignore.

Ejaculation   The emission of semen from the penis during orgasm. The semen, containing secretions from the prostate, seminal vesicles, and other sources, is propelled through the urethra by the rhythmic contractions of muscles at the base of the penis. In most men, the force of ejaculation and amount of ejaculate decrease with aging, but the incidence of premature ejaculation also decreases.

Ekbom's syndrome   *See* **Restless legs syndrome.**

Electrocardiogram (ECG or EKG)   A recording of the electrical activity of the heart made on an instrument called an electrocardiograph. It is a noninvasive and painless means of verifying normal heart function and of detecting heart abnormalities. Electrocardiograms are usually included as part of a periodic medical examination. Previous ECG's can be compared with more recent ones to reveal any changes in heart function. An ECG is recorded through a group of electrodes (leads) placed on the chest and, for electrical balance, at points on the arms and legs that are theoretically the same distance from the heart. Electrical impulses generated during contractions and relaxations of various heart muscle fibers produce the patterns recorded on the ECG. Each peak or spike of the trace pattern represents one of the stages of the cardiac cycle, from the spread of the initial electrical impulse originating in the atria (upper chambers) onward through the ventricles (lower chambers).

Electroencephalogram (EEG)   A recording of the electrical activity of the brain, made by attaching electrodes at various points on the scalp. The electroencephalogram translates the electrical activity into brain-wave patterns associated with different mental states, such as deep sleep, dreaming, drowsiness, or alertness. EEG's also provide clues regarding brain tumors, lesions, strokes, or seizures, including the location of brain tissue affected by or causing symptoms of the defect. Because various brain areas have been carefully mapped, partly from studies of effects of specific brain injuries on mental and physical functions, the EEG can be used to help diagnose some central nervous system disorders. For example, in examining a blind person whose eyes appear free of defects, an EEG can be made with electrodes set to register any response by brain tissue in the occipital region of the brain, where visual images are formed, when a light is flashed before the patient's eyes. If the stimulus fails to produce an "evoked potential" (brainwave), the person may have **cortical blindness**. Similar EEG tests can be made in tracing losses of hearing, of the sense of touch in a particular body area, or of other functions.

Electrolyte   A chemical element or compound that becomes an ion, or atom or group of atoms with an electrical charge, when dissolved in water. Most minerals and many proteins and other substances function as electrolytes in the body. Among the most important electrolytes in the human body are sodium, chloride, potassium, and bicarbonate. An excess or deficiency of an electrolyte can produce adverse health effects. While the body attempts to automatically keep the electrolytes in balance, that balance is dependent upon a proper fluid balance, and many factors in turn affect this. Certain diseases, conditions, and medications can upset the body's normal electrolytic balance, producing a wide range of symptoms.

Vomiting and diarrhea are common causes of electrolyte imbalance because they may lead to dehydration and excessive loss of potassium, chloride, and sodium. Alcohol, diuretics, and a low-sodium diet can result in a potassium deficiency, a condition marked by weakness, decrease of normal reflexes, weak pulse, falling blood pressure, and heart rhythm changes. Too much potassium, on the other hand, can produce muscle cramps, nausea, excitability, dizziness, and sensations of numbness. Abnormal kidney function affects sodium (salt) balance. So does high fever, which can double the body's need for water and salt. However, too much sodium can cause irritability, lethargy, weakness, confusion, stupor, and coma. Treatment involves restoration of the normal fluid balance, correction of the underlying cause of the electrolyte imbalance, and adjustment of the intake of foods providing the necessary electrolytes.

Electromyography (EMG)   A system of recording the electrical activity in muscles through electrodes placed in various muscle groups. EMG is used to study the condition of muscles in cases of weakness or fatigability, in which there is no clear cause of an abnormality.

Electrosurgery   A technique of using an electric current to remove senile and seborrheic keratoses, leukoplakia, warts, unwanted hair, and certain moles and hemangiomas from the skin.

Embolic cerebral infarction   A type of stroke produced by an obstruction (embolism) in a brain artery. An embolus often begins in or near the heart area and may be composed of blood platelets, red blood cells, and other solid components of blood, or fragments of atherosclerotic deposits from the lining of arteries, and is carried upward to blood vessels in the brain. The embolus may lodge in a small artery, disrupting blood flow to a large area of brain tissue, or break into smaller pieces to be carried into lesser blood vessels, eventually interrupting blood flow to smaller areas of brain tissue but allowing circulation to be restored to the larger brain area. Approximately 30 percent of brain damage due to strokes involves an embolus.

Embolus   Usually a dislodged **thrombus** or other particulate matter that circulates in the bloodstream. The object may be a bit of tissue, a blood clot, a fat droplet, or even a bubble of air or gas. When the embolus becomes lodged in a blood vessel, circulation to the area of tissue normally nourished by the blood is suddenly deprived of oxygen, causing pain and tissue injury or death. If the embolus blocks the blood flow to the heart muscle, an area of the brain, or the lung, the situation can be life-threatening. When feasible, a surgical incision is made into the blood vessel to remove the embolus. *See also* **Thrombophlebitis.**

Emesis   A medical term for vomiting.

Emmetropia   A condition of normal visual accommodation and eye refraction. Images of distant objects are focused clearly on the retina. When accommodation and refraction are not normal, corrective lenses may be needed. *See also* **Myopia, Presbyopia.**

Emphysema   An irreversible breathing disorder caused by overinflation of the tiny air sacs (alveoli) of the lungs and the destruction of their walls. This gradual destruction of the alveoli reduces the elasticity of the lungs and the amount of oxygen that the blood vessels in the walls of the air sacs absorb with each breath. The lungs are in a constant state of inflation because of the difficulty of exhaling. Common causes of emphysema are cigarette smoking and chronic exposure to air pollutants, particularly dusts and fumes in the workplace. The patient with emphysema tends to pause momentarily between exhaling and inhaling. When breath sounds can be heard, they are decreased. As air becomes trapped in the lungs, the volume of the lungs increases and the chest walls acquire a more or less permanent "barrel-chest" appearance of a person taking a deep breath. The patient experiences breathlessness with less physical exertion than healthy people. Any effort that involves the lungs, even shouting or laughter, may trigger a coughing spell. This may produce a minimal amount of thick, heavy phlegm.

A common medical test for emphysema has the patient attempt to extinguish a lighted match held six inches from his or her open mouth, by taking a deep breath and blowing through the open mouth (without pursing the lips). Fewer than 20 percent of patients with severe emphysema can pass this test. *See also* **Black lung disease, Chronic obstructive pulmonary disease (COPD).**

Empty nest syndrome   A mental state of some older parents characterized mainly by depression and associated with the departure from the family home of their children who have reached maturity and are ready to establish their own homes and families.

Empty sella syndrome   A disorder involving a decrease in size of the pituitary gland, located in that part of the skull called the "sella turcica." The patient, generally a middle-aged woman, may or may not show any signs or symptoms of a hormonal disorder. In most cases, she is overweight, has had several pregnancies, and suffers from hypertension. The primary symptom is headaches and occasionally there are visual difficulties. In some cases, the cause is believed to be a rebound effect of the pituitary gland, which normally becomes enlarged with each pregnancy but may gradually shrink to a much smaller size after the pregnancies.

Encephalitis   Any inflammation of the brain. It may result from a viral or bacterial infection. (Bacterial infections of the cerebrum are also called "cerebritis.") Symptoms for both types of infection are similar and may include headache, fever, stiff neck, nausea, and vomiting. Invasion of the brain tissues by a virus may lead to irreversible damage of at least some brain tissue. Either type of brain infection can be fatal if not treated quickly and effectively. Because of the similarity of symptoms in bacterial and viral infections, diagnosis may be difficult. Except for one form of viral encephalitis, when the cause is herpes simplex Type I, there is no specific treatment. Herpes simplex encephalitis can be treated with a viricide. Most bacterial infections of the central nervous system respond to treatment with antibiotics.

Encephalopathy   Any alteration of the normal structure and function of brain tissues, usually caused by injury, disease, poisoning, or degenerative conditions. Encephalopathies also can result from metabolic or nutritional disorders. Changes in the brain and peripheral nerves of older adults may be the result of a lack of certain B vitamins. Some older adults also may exhibit signs of encephalopathies due to effects of medications or combinations of medications that alter functions of the brain or peripheral nerves. Hepatic (liver) encephalopathy results when ammonia or other metabolic waste products enter the brain and cause symptoms that range from euphoria, restlessness, and confusion to stupor, drowsiness, tremors, slurred speech, and loss of consciousness. Treatment depends upon the cause of the encephalopathy and can include diet changes, drugs, and use of substances called "chelating agents," which bind poisons in the tissues so they can be excreted easily.

Endocarditis An inflammation of the lining of the chambers of the heart and the heart valves, usually caused by a bacterial infection. Symptoms of the disease include chills, profuse sweating, loss of appetite and loss of weight, joint pains, fever, pallor, and small hemorrhages under the skin and nails. The disease is insidious because the symptoms are often misleading, suggesting many disorders that do not involve the heart. Endocarditis may result from a bacterial infection acquired during dental work, when bacteria in the mouth accidentally enter the bloodstream. Persons with prior heart damage as well as previous heart valve infections are particularly susceptible. Endocarditis may be complicated by the formation of an embolus from cellular debris and bacterial colonies growing on the heart valves. Endocarditis is also frequently complicated by kidney involvement leading to glomerular nephritis. Treatment is with antibiotics. Endocarditis is especially dangerous for older adults since they have a death rate from this disorder that is nearly double that of younger patients.

Endometrial cancer (uterine cancer) A malignancy, usually adenocarcinoma, of the endometrium, or lining of the uterus. It is the most common type of cancer of the female reproductive tract and is most frequent in postmenopausal women between fifty and seventy. The cause is not clear, but is believed by some to be related to a relatively excessive production of the female sex hormone estrogen. Estrogen secretion may continue after the menopause because of hormone-secreting ovarian tumors or the conversion of fat deposits to estrogen by male sex hormones (androgens) circulating in the bloodstream. Fat is a source of estrogens, and obesity increases the chances for a woman to develop endometrial cancer. Being ten to twenty pounds overweight doubles a woman's risk for endometrial cancer, and being more than twenty pounds overweight increases the risk by three to ten times. Other risk factors are late menopause and never having given birth. Symptoms of endometrial cancer are vaginal bleeding, which is always abnormal after menopause, as well as low abdominal and low back pain. A "Pap" test does not always reveal cancer in the body of the uterus, because (unlike cancer of the cervix, the neck of the uterus) the cancer cells are not shed in the early stages. Jet washing of the uterus or vacuum curettage is usually required to obtain samples of endometrial cells for cancer tests. Treatment of endometrial cancer is by total **hysterectomy**, often with radiation therapy before and after surgery.

Endometrial hyperplasia An overgrowth of the lining of the uterus caused by continued secretion of the female sex hormone estrogen when it is not modified by the secretion of a second female sex hormone, progesterone. A natural function of estrogen is stimulation of endometrial growth. When estrogen secretion continues during and after the menopause in the absence of progesterone, which is normally produced during the menstrual cycle, the lining of the uterus becomes thick and glandular. Because of the risk that endometrial hyperplasia may progress to **endometrial cancer**, progesterone therapy is sometimes used or a hysterectomy is performed. A symptom of endometrial hyperplasia is abnormal vaginal bleeding after the menopause. If such bleeding occurs, the patient should be examined for possible endometrial cancer.

Entrapment neuropathy An abnormal condition caused by entrapment of a nerve or nerve root under a ligament, as in carpal tunnel syndrome; between two groups of muscles, as in pronator syndrome; or by a bone degeneration, as in root entrapment syndrome. Symptoms may include pain, tingling sensations, loss of muscle strength, or failure of the affected area to respond to stimulation by vibration or pinprick. Contributing factors may be a metabolic disorder, such as diabetes mellitus, or a vitamin deficiency, arthritis, occupational diseases that result from use of vibrating tools, and tumors. Treatment depends upon the underlying cause and may include physical therapy, exercises, surgery, and diet changes.

Epicondylitis (tennis elbow) A painful inflammation of the muscles and other tissues of the forearm near their origin at the elbow joint. It is caused by repeated strain on the forearm, with extension and twisting of the wrist. The strain may be produced by a number of activities, such as turning a screwdriver, as well as playing tennis. Treatment usually involves rest and the use of analgesics, sometimes hydrocortisone injections, and strapping of the forearm.

Epilepsy (seizure disorders) A neurological disorder characterized by recurrent episodes of convulsive seizures, inappropriate behavior, loss of consciousness, and/or sensory phenomena (aura) in the form of strange odors, colored lights, or unusual sounds. There are approximately twenty types of epilepsy, but the seizures commonly follow a pattern of loss of consciousness followed by jerking movements of the arms and legs. The seizures are believed to be triggered by an abnormal electrical discharge from a small area of diseased or injured brain tissue in response to a stimulus that may come from within or outside the brain. The electrical aberration can sometimes be recorded on an **electroencephalogram (EEG)**.

Although cases of epilepsy frequently become established in childhood, an increasing proportion of cases are first diagnosed after the age of fifty. Epilepsy that develops in older adults may be caused by tumor, cerebrovascular disease, stroke, head injury, or brain infection. Tumors account for 10 percent of the seizure disorders in patients over fifty. Cerebrovascular disease and stroke are other common causes; in many cases, seizures begin within a year after a first stroke. Epilepsy attacks in older persons do not always take the form of convulsive seizures; they may be also expressed as spells of dizziness or vertigo. In some cases, the epilepsy attacks may be confused with alcohol withdrawal symptoms or effects of an electrolyte imbalance.

Diagnosis of epilepsy is difficult because of a lack of a reliable diagnostic test; although an EEG may detect a seizure, many epilepsy patients show normal EEG's, and abnormal EEG's may be recorded in the absence of other symptoms. Diagnosis is based primarily on the patient's history of seizures, careful medical examination, and family medical history, particularly evidence of central nervous system injury or infection affecting the individual before or during birth or in early childhood. Treatment is with anticonvulsant drugs.

Epistaxis Bleeding from the nose caused by rupture of the blood vessels in the mucous membrane that lines the nasal cavity. Causes may include injury, infection, irritation of the mucous membrane, and high blood pressure. Although the frequency of nosebleed is highest in childhood and adolescence, epistaxis is often more serious in older adults. It may be accompanied by vertigo, apprehension, respiratory distress, nausea, and even loss of consciousness with significant blood loss. Swabbing the mucous membranes inside the nostrils with petroleum jelly and increasing the humidity of the environment may be helpful in preventing epistaxis.

Epithelioma Any malignant tumor that develops from cells of the epithelium, the layers of tissue forming the skin and mucous membranes. Because it presents a large tissue surface exposed to carcinogenic agents of the environment, epithelium frequently becomes the site of cancers. A common example of an epithelioma is a basal cell skin cancer. It may be caused by excessive exposure to sunlight in susceptible patients. The prognosis is very good for epitheliomas when treatment is started before they reach one inch in diameter. An epithelioma is usually removed by surgery, except when it appears on the face and the patient prefers treatment by radiation so the site will not be marked by a scar.

Epulis   A general term for a tumor or swelling of the gingiva (gums). The term literally means "gum boil," but it may also be used to identify a fibrous tumor (fibroma) of the tooth socket, a pyogenic (pus-forming) cyst, or a small mass of bone-forming tissue. An epulis may be caused by an overgrowth of soft or bony tissue, an infection, or something that irritates the gums.

Erosion   A wearing away of an organ or tissue surface, as a dental erosion characterized by the loss of the enamel layer of a tooth. A skin erosion is limited to the epidermis and usually heals without leaving a scar. An erosion of the skin or mucous membrane is often marked by an ulcer.

Eructation (belching)   The act of bringing up gas or air from the stomach.

Erysipelas   A bacterial infection of the skin and the tissues beneath the skin caused by Group A streptococci. Symptoms include a high fever, chills, general discomfort, and a red, raised, warm, tender area around the face and ears, but any skin surface can be involved. There may be small or large blisters and swelling due to fluid accumulation. It often begins at the site of a skin wound, an area where the skin has been scratched, or as a compliction of ear piercing. Treatment includes bed rest and antibiotics.

Erythrasma   A ringwormlike skin infection that is prevalent in warm, humid climates. It tends to develop in areas of skin folds, as between the toes, in the armpits, and in the anal-genital area, and is marked by light red patches, scaling, fissuring, and maceration of the skin. It affects mainly persons with **diabetes mellitus** and middle-aged, over-weight women. Treatment is with oral antibiotics.

Erythema   Any redness or inflammation of the skin or mucous membranes. It is caused by dilatation of the capillaries in response to an infection, injury, or other stimulus. Erythema of the palms is often a sign of chronic liver disease.

Erythrocyte   A red blood cell.

Erythromelalgia   A disorder of the hands and feet, marked by a burning pain that seems to be activated by a change in skin temperature. There is evidence that the disorder may be hereditary and that it may lead to polycythemia (an excessive red blood cell count). Aspirin and a cool environment provide temporary relief, but the condition is resistant to curative measures.

Esophageal cancer   A carcinoma of the esophagus. It usually does not produce symptoms in the early stages, but as it progresses the patient may begin to experience painful **dysphagia**, regurgitation, loss of appetite, and loss of weight. Suspected causes include reflux of gastric acid from the stomach and excessive use of alcohol and tobacco. Treatment often involves surgical removal of the esophagus and replacement with a tube prosthesis. Radiation may also be used.

Esophagitis   Inflammation of the esophagus, often caused by backflow (reflux) of gastric acid from the stomach, and often associated with **hiatus hernia.**

Essential hypertension   High blood pressure that is not caused by a known or identified disease or condition. The exact cause is unknown, but it is believed to involve the structures or functions of the **autonomic nervous system** and the small arteries. Numerous theories have been offered for the development of the condition, such as obesity, emotional stress, excessive salt intake, or a kidney enzyme defect. Such factors may aggravate an existing condition of hypertension, but the basic cause remains unknown. There is evidence that a susceptibility to essential hypertension may be inherited.

Untreated essential hypertension often leads to premature death or disability from stroke, heart attack, or kidney failure. There is no known cure, but therapeutic measures to control the condition include drugs that reduce blood pressure, dietary restrictions as needed to reduce body weight and sodium intake, physical exercise as recommended by a physician, and avoiding the use of cigarettes. Also called "primary hypertension." *See also* **Hypertension.**

Essential tremor   Involuntary contractions of the hands, head, and face, especially during ordinary movements of the body. Initially the tremors are minute but may become more pronounced as the patient grows older, when the same condition may be identified as "senile tremor." Essential tremor is sometimes confused with **parkinsonism,** which is marked by additional symptoms. It is an inherited condition that may be exacerbated by mental stress, particularly in social situations, as when the patient is unable to hold a teacup on a saucer without the embarrassment of a loud rattling sound. The disorder sometimes partially responds to treatment. Alcohol may help suppress the tremors, but it should not be used as a substitute for prescribed medications.

Estrogen   The primary female sex hormone, produced during the woman's fertile years mainly by the ovaries and, in pregnancy, by the placenta. Small amounts of estrogen also may be produced in the adrenal glands and in the male testes. The purpose of male estrogen, which appears in traces in male urine samples, is unknown. In the female the hormone plays a key role in preparing of the uterus for implantation of a fertilized ovum and in supporting the pregnancy once it is established. As menopause approaches, estrogen production by the ovaries begins to decline; after menopause it is reduced significantly in most women, but it is not entirely absent. Because of the chemical relationships among various male and female sex hormones, it is possible for the body's tissues to convert one hormone to another. It is also possible for the body to create estrogen from fat deposits in the body. Thus, women who are obese may continue producing estrogen after the menopause in amounts approaching estrogen levels of some premenopausal women.

A negative aspect of substantial, continuing estrogen production in postmenopausal women is that it can be a contributing factor in the development of ovarian, uterine (endometrial), vaginal, and vulvar cancers. During the fertile years, the ovaries also secrete a second female hormone, progesterone, which tends to inhibit the role of estrogen as a cancer producer; but progesterone production ceases with the menopause and is no longer present to suppress the estrogen-induced cancers. Some doctors prescribe estrogen therapy for menopausal women who experience "hot flashes" or vaginal atrophy. Because of a wide range of possible adverse effects, including gallbladder disease, vaginal bleeding, uterine cancer, sore breasts, and nausea and vomiting, menopausal patients are usually given the smallest effective dose for a limited period, and the therapy is discontinued if side effects develop. Some authorities explain that the estrogen-replacement drug given menopausal women is actually a substitution of hormones, and it does not truly mimic the natural or physiological estrogen present in the woman's body during her reproductive life.

Exclamation mark hairs   Broken hairs that resemble exclamation marks, being thick near the top and gradually becoming thinner toward the base. They are a symptom of alopecia areata. They occur along the edges of balding spots where the hairs break easily, about one-tenth of an inch above the surface of the scalp.

Exfoliative dermatitis   A skin disorder marked by a generalized eruption and scaling. The widespread eruptions may vary from fine reddish granular scales to large red plaques. There is intense itching and excessive peeling or shedding of the skin. The lymph glands are usually involved. In many cases, the condition develops spontaneously in apparently healthy persons, with no known cause. In other instances, causes may include drug reactions, topical agents, scarlet fever, **leukemia**, and **lymphoma**. Treatment is with various drugs, including antihistamines, with special attention given to the prevention of secondary infections, which may be fatal.

Exophthalamos   An abnormal bulging or protrusion of the eyeball. The condition may involve one or both eyes and may develop as a result of a brain disorder, injury, tumor, or disease, such as **hyperthyroidism**. Treatment depends upon correction of the underlying disorder and protection of the eye from drying, infection, or damage to the cornea.

Exposure deafness   A loss of hearing caused by prolonged exposure to loud sounds, generally noise above the level of 85 decibels, which is around the intensity of sound at a busy street intersection or a small light plane flying overhead. Louder noises, above 105 decibels, which includes the sound of a nearby jet aircraft, can be painful or deafening for some individuals.

Extrapyramidal diseases   A category of disorders that are characterized by involuntary movements of the body or body parts, such as tremors, tics, spasms, and walking irregularities. The term is derived from a group of central nervous system nerve fibers called the extrapyramidal tract (located outside a pyramid-shape nerve tract) of the brain; the nerves control muscle tone, body posture, coordination of muscles, and other functions.

Extremities   The arms and legs, those parts of the body that are separate from the trunk. Also called "limbs."

Extrinsic allergic alveolitis   A respiratory disease with pneumonia symptoms, which is an allergic reaction to dusts containing organic matter, that causes an inflammation of the alveoli, or air sacs, of the lung. The person will have developed an extreme sensitivity to the **allergen** as a result of a previous exposure to it and will have developed

antibodies that are quickly mobilized to fight and reject the **antigen**. The foreign substance is usually protein material present in mold spores, bird excrement, in moldy hay or mushroom compost, wood dust, moldy cheese, wood bark, cork dust, or even an enzyme present in some laundry detergents. The person who has become sensitized to the protein from a previous exposure usually develops influenzalike symptoms several hours later. The symptoms may include chills, fever, headache, cough, breathing difficulty, and a general feeling of discomfort; there may also be a rapid heartbeat, fever, and asthmatic wheezing. In most cases, the symptoms subside within twelve to twenty-four hours, particularly if the individual has been removed from the source of the dust causing the reaction. The best treatment is complete avoidance of exposure to the organic dust causing the reaction. In some cases of very severe reactions, steroids or other drugs may be administered. Repeated exposure to the offending dust can lead to structural changes in the lung tissue, resulting in premature death.

Exudate   A leakage from the blood vessels or tissue cells, usually consisting of fluid containing proteins and fatty substances.

Eyelash sign   A test of the eyelid reflexes of an unconscious person. If the loss of consciousness is due to hysteria or another functional disorder, stroking the eyelashes should result in a movement of the eyelids. If the person is unconscious because of injury or disease of the central nervous system, the eyelid reflex will not occur.

Eye pain   *See* **Glaucoma, Temporal arteritis.**

F

Fabrication   *See* **Confabulation.**

Face-hand test   A test for certain types of brain damage, in which the person's face and the back of his hand are touched at the same instant. If the person is unable to detect the separate touch sensations, it is evidence of certain types of brain damage.

Facial paralysis   *See* **Bell's palsy.**

Faint   *See* **Syncope.**

Falls   An involuntary and sudden collapse or drop from a standing or sitting posture. Falls often are associated with slipping, tripping, or losing one's balance while carrying a load or while standing at a height above ground level, as on a ladder or stool. Among older adults, falls account for approximately 25 percent of all health impairments. As one grows older, the risk of a serious fall increases, so that 70 percent of all fatal injuries from falls occur in persons beyond the age of sixty-five. A large share of falls among older adults is due to an increasing loss of stability in walking. Changes in breathing, bones, joints, muscles, and nerves that coordinate body movements begin to occur in the late thirties. Studies of marathon runners show a rather steady decline in running ability after the age of thirty-five, all due to the natural changes in their anatomy and physiology.

Fractures that result from metabolic bone disorders such as **osteoporosis** and **osteomalacia** are a major factor in falls by older adults. In some cases, spontaneous fracture of a hip weakened by osteoporosis can be the cause of a fall. However, it is now agreed that the fall as an initial event is much more frequently the cause of hip fractures in patients with osteoporosis. Postmenopausal women are at a particular risk because of osteoporosis. Also contributing to the increased risk of falls by older adults is a decline in the sense of balance, so they learn to walk more slowly and cautiously with a wide stance. Women may develop what is known as a "waddling gait," while men acquire a flexed posture and short-step gait. There is increased postural sway in these **gait disorders** of an older person, and the feet are not raised above the ground with each step.

Age-related factors that further contribute to loss of stability in standing and walking include **orthostatic hypotension**, a condition that affects nearly 25 percent of older adults and is marked by a feeling of faintness as blood drains rapidly from the head upon suddenly rising to a sitting or standing position. Other conditions include degenerative joint disease (osteoarthritis), muscle weakness due to disuse, effects of small strokes, foot and leg diseases or deformities, and poor vision. Also contributing to falls by older adults are **drop attacks** in which sudden severe leg weakness of presumed neurological origin causes collapse. Other causes include **syncope**, epileptic seizures, and a wide range of drugs that affect the central nervous system, including alcohol, sedatives, antidepressants, tranquilizers, and hypertension medications. Many of the causes of instability in walking and standing can be treated by physical therapy, medications or changes in medications, surgery, and, in some cases, by dietary changes that promote normal bone maintenance, with emphasis on appropriate intakes of calcium and vitamin D.

Familial   Pertaining to a disorder that tends to occur in members of some families and not others. A familial disease may or may not be hereditary; the fact that members of the family share the same environment can sometimes account for the disorder. The incidence of a familial disease occurring in an affected family is greater than would be expected by chance. *See also* **Hereditary.**

Familial hypercholesterolemia   An inherited disease characterized by extremely high blood levels of cholesterol and a much greater than average risk of developing atherosclerosis and coronary heart disease. Persons who acquire familial hypercholesterolemia have a 16 percent chance of experiencing a heart attack by the age of 40. By the age of sixty, the risk of heart attack increases to 66 percent. The condition can be treated with a strictly controlled diet and medications that lower cholesterol levels in the blood.

Familial tremor *See* **Essential tremor.**

Fanconi's syndrome A kidney disorder marked by the loss through excretion of sugar, amino acids, potassium, phosphorus, bicarbonate, and uric acid in the urine. The disease can be inherited or acquired. It is sometimes inherited along with other hereditary disorders, but symptoms may not appear until the person reaches middle age. The acquired form can be due to exposure to cadmium, copper, lead, mercury, or other toxic chemicals; from the use of outdated tetracyline antibiotics; following a kidney transplant; or as a complication of **amyloidosis** or **multiple myeloma**. There is no specific treatment, and therapy is directed toward control of complications, such as acidosis or potassium deficiency.

Farsightedness *See* **Hyperopia.**

Fasciculations Small twitchings of muscles that are visible through the skin. The twitchings are caused by spontaneous muscle contractions triggered by an irritated nerve and may be associated with degenerative diseases of the spinal cord or brain stem. The condition also occurs in **amyotrophic lateral sclerosis.**

Fat A general term for any of a number of substances composed of fatty acids and glycerin. At normal room temperatures, they vary in consistency from fluids (oils) to solids (greases and tallows). Fats are insoluble in water but are soluble in fat solvents, such as alcohol. They are an important source of body fuel because they contain more than twice as much energy per ounce as pure sugar. The body stores excess calories as fat; one pound of fat represents around 3,600 calories. About 25 percent of the body of an average person is fat, and the proportion is much higher in an obese individual. Besides serving as a source of fuel, fat provides cushioning and insulation for body tissues and is a source of sex hormones. *See also* **Fatty acid.**

Fatigue A feeling of tiredness, weariness, loss of strength, or exhaustion, which may be a natural consequence of physical activity or a symptom of an underlying disorder. Malnutrition can contribute to fatigue if the body lacks the carbohydrates or other nutrients needed as fuel to keep its systems functioning in optimum condition. A respiratory or circulatory system disorder may interfere with the distribution of oxygen and other bloodstream nutrients to the body's tissues. Anemia, marked by a deficiency of hemoglobin that carries oxygen in the blood, can limit the amount of oxygen delivered to the tissue cells as sufficiently as required, and symptoms of fatigue may result.

Certain diseases can result in an accumulation of poisonous substances that interfere with normal body functions. Even in a normal, healthy body, individual tissues, such as muscles and nerve cells, experience fatigue and require brief rest periods in order to accumulate energy or electrical charge before making the next contraction or other response to the activity demands of the body. In addition, a person's mental attitude, such as boredom, anxiety, or frustration, can contribute to feelings of fatigue.

Fatty acid   Any of a group of about forty substances found in plants and animals that have a similar chemical formula, with carbon, hydrogen, and oxygen atoms arranged in the same proportions. Human beings use only seven or eight of the total number of fatty acids, but only three—linoleic, linolenic, and arachidonic acid—are essential for normal health.

Fatty liver   A popular term for an accumulation of fatty acid compounds in the liver, producing symptoms of enlarged liver, abdominal pain and discomfort, jaundice, and loss of appetite. Causes include cirrhosis due to alcohol abuse, toxic chemicals, use of certain medications, and protein-calorie malnutrition, as well as a number of inherited disorders. Fatty liver is generally harmless in itself but is often a symptom of an underlying disease that requires treatment. The problem is usually resolved with treatment of the cause. *See also* **Cirrhosis.**

Febrile   Pertaining to a fever.

Fecal fistula   An abnormal passageway from the colon to the surface of the body. A fecal fistula may develop as a result of injury to the pelvic organs, a tumor, or a complication of **diverticulosis.** An artificial fecal fistula, such as a colostomy, may also be created surgically, as a temporary or permanent measure, to permit diversion of fecal flow away from a segment of the large intestine being treated for a cancer, ulceration, or perforating injury, such as a bullet wound.

Fecal incontinence   *See* **Incontinence.**

Felty's syndrome   A complication of **rhumatoid arthritis** marked by an enlarged spleen and an abnormal decrease of white blood cells, with increased susceptibility to infections. The cause is unknown, and surgical removal of the spleen is helpful in only about half of the cases. *See also* **Hypersplenism.**

Femoral neck fracture A fracture of the neck of the long bone (femur) extending between the hip and the knee. The femoral neck is a portion of the bone that branches at an angle from the direction of the upper leg toward the insertion in the hipbone. Femoral neck fracture is one of the major causes of disability and immobility among older adults. It is often a complication of **osteoporosis.**

Festination A tendency by some persons with neurological disorders to gradually increase their speed while walking, in order to overtake a displaced center of gravity and prevent them from falling forward. The symptom is observed in cases of **parkinsonism.**

Fever Any abnormal increase in body temperature above the accepted normal level of 98.6° Fahrenheit (37° Celsius). Fever is generally a symptom of a disease, although other factors such as exercise or dehydration can cause a higher than normal body temperature in a healthy person. Among the many causes of fever are infections, cancers, severe injuries, and certain medications. A condition called "fever of unknown origin" is one in which the body temperature reaches 101° F (38.3° C) or higher on several occasions, that lasts at least three weeks, and the source of which cannot be diagnosed in one week of hospital observation and tests. In about half of the cases of such fevers, the cause is later found to be an abscess, tuberculosis, hepatitis, endocarditis, temporal arteritis, or a pulmonary embolus. Most older adults experience a mild fever of about 100° F (37.7° C) for two or three days following major surgery. It is not considered as serious unless it persists beyond the third day or goes higher.

Fever blister A cold sore caused by the herpes simplex virus. *See also* **Herpes zoster.**

Fiber A term commonly used to identify the cellulose or lignin fibers that form the cell walls of plants, including fruits and vegetables. Plant fiber is composed of the same types of carbohydrate molecules as sugars and starches, but they cannot be digested by human beings, who lack the digestive juice enzymes of cattle and other animals needed to convert these fiber molecules into smaller units that can be used by the body as energy sources. However, fiber in the diet provides bulk and binds water to provide a mild laxative effect in maintaining normal bowel function and preventing **constipation**. Dietary fiber helps move food waste through the digestive tract and reduces the risk of **diverticulosis**. For several reasons, fiber is also believed to reduce the risk of colon cancer. Studies show that fiber in the diet lowers blood sugar levels of persons with diabetes. A diet containing adequate proportions of fruits and vegetables should provide sufficient fiber for the general health of most people. Excessive use of fiber in meals can have a detrimental effect, because fiber can bind certain minerals and other nutrients so they cannot be absorbed from the digestive tract.

Fibrillation Repeated abnormal contractions of muscle fibers, particularly heart muscle fibers. The term is usually associated with the area of heart muscle tissue involved in order to identify the problem more precisely, such as *atrial fibrillation,* when the upper chambers of the heart are contracting abnormally, or *ventricular fibrillation,* if the problem involves the lower heart chambers. In atrial fibrillation, contractions of the muscles of the atria occur continuously in an irregular, chaotic manner, quite unlike the regular, orderly contractions associated with a normal heartbeat. The rate of contractions in atrial fibrillation have been estimated to range above 300 beats per minute, compared with a normal resting heartbeat of about 72 per minute. In many cases, fibrillation is such that the heartbeat cannot be measured accurately. Common causes of atrial fibrillation in older adults may include **arteriosclerosis, hyperthyroidism,** and **hypertension**. Ventricular fibrillation is also characterized by rapid, irregular, chaotic heart muscle contractions (**arrhythmias**) and often may follow a heart attack (**myocardial infarction**) within minutes. It also may be triggered by electrical shock, drowning, or an overdose of certain medications. In ventricular fibrillation, the ventricles contract so wildly that no blood is moved into or out of the heart. It is treated with **defibrillation**, a type of electrical countershock that can be administered in a hospital or by an emergency medical service. If ventricular fibrillation cannot be controlled, there is no pulse or blood pressure, and the person loses consciousness and dies.

Fibromyositis Any disorder marked by inflammation and tenderness of the muscles and connective tissues, with pain and stiffness. In typical cases, symptoms begin with sudden joint or muscle pain that is aggravated by movement of the afflicted part. There may be muscle spasm, but fever is absent unless the condition is associated with an infectious disease. Rheumatic disorders are sometimes related. Other possible factors can include exposure to cold and dampness or an injury. *See also* **Rheumatism.**

Fibrosing alveolitis   An inflammation of the air sacs (alveoli) of the lungs, marked by breathing difficulty and oxygen deficiency of the tissues. It occurs as a complication of **rheumatoid arthritis** and other disorders of the immune system. It also occurs as a reaction to a number of inhaled allergens. The normally resilient membranes of the air sacs are gradually replaced by stiff fibrous tissues that reduce the ability of the membranes to handle the exchange of inhaled oxygen entering the capillaries in the membrane walls and carbon dioxide released from the capillaries for exhalation. Treatment requires use of bronchodilators, physical therapy, mechanical breathing assistance, and other techniques, depending upon the degree of respiratory failure resulting from the disorder.

Fibrositis   An inflammation of connective tissue, usually marked by pain and stiffness. The condition tends to occur in the neck, shoulder and trunk. The affected area may be painful when arising in the morning but is relieved by mild exercises. In some cases, there are small nodules on the affected muscle, believed to be filled with fat or fluid, or both, and a cause of muscle spasms.

Finger-nose test   A test for a possible neurological disorder. The person is asked to extend the forearm and then to slowly place the tip of the index finger on the nose. The test is done twice, once with the eyes open and again with the eyes closed. An inability to perform the finger-nose test properly with the eyes open may be a sign of a disorder involving nerve tracts of the cerebellum. An inability to perform the test with the eyes closed may suggest a disorder involving the spinal cord, resulting in a loss of the sense of position. If a tremor develops during the test, it may be a sign of disease in the cerebellum.

Fissure   An abnormal cleft or split in the skin or mucous membranes, or a normal groove in a body part. Cracklike fissures can occur at the corners of the mouth and are often caused by a vitamin deficiency. An anal fissure is a painful fissure that extends up into the anal canal.

Fistula   An abnormal opening or channel between an organ and the body surface or between two organs. The condition may be congenital, but it may also be caused by an **abscess**, occur in a disorder such as **ulcerative colitis**, or be a complication of abdominal surgery. An anal fistula may also be an indication of **Crohn's disease**.

Flaccid bladder   A urinary bladder condition in which the normal reflex control of the bladder through the spinal cord has been lost.

Symptoms are overfilling of the bladder, lack of a full bladder sensation, and an inability to urinate voluntarily. The condition often results from injury and requires retraining of the person, who must use the toilet every two hours. The flaccid bladder can be emptied by pressure on the lower abdomen, which overcomes the controlling pressure of the sphincter muscle of the urethra. Medications are available to help start emptying of the bladder and reduce the chance of incomplete emptying, leaving residual urine, which would have to be removed by catheterization.

Flatus *See* **Gas.**

Floater An object that drifts through the eyeball, casting a shadow on the retina that gives the appearance of a spot passing in front of the eye. Sometimes the shadow may appear to be a part of a cobweb or insect. An occasional floater is usually a harmless bit of tissue that may have been in the eye since birth. But the sudden appearance of several floaters may be a sign of a retinal detachment, tumor, blockage of a vein, or other abnormality resulting in a leakage of blood into the interior of the eye, requiring immediate medical treatment to prevent blindness. Floaters tend to occur more often as one grows older.

Fluid balance The balance between fluid intake and the excretion of water through urine, feces, respiration, and sweating. Fluid balance is related to **electrolyte** balance and the body's need to keep the volume and composition of body fluids relatively constant. Fluid intake is often neglected in the older adult who, for various reasons, is more likely than a younger person to suffer dehydration without necessarily feeling thirsty. An increased rate of fluid excretion in older people may not be important if a person has easy access to water and drinks freely of it, but if he or she fails to increase the intake of fluid to compensate for the higher rate of urine excretion, electrolytes become more concentrated in the body tissues, causing various adverse health effects.

Fluid wave A wavelike phenomenon associated with fluid accumulation in the abdomen as a result of **congestive heart failure, cirrhosis** of the liver, and other disorders. When such fluid is present, the wave can be produced if the person lies face up and another person places his hands on either side of the abdomen. When the abdomen is tapped on one side, a wave travels across to the other side, where it may be felt. Fluid in the abdomen also may cause the flanks to bulge on either side when the person is lying face up. The presence of fat in the abdomen of an obese person can interfere with either of the tests. *See also* **Ascites.**

Flush *See* **Hot flashes.**

Flutter A condition of extremely rapid abnormal heart muscle contractions, similar to atrial **fibrillation**, except that the beat is regular. The rate of heartbeat during atrial flutter is about 300 per minute, and the pulse rate is often around 150 per minute. In some cases, atrial flutter is self-limited and ends without treatment. However, because it can also change to atrial fibrillation and heart failure, efforts are made to correct the rhythm abnormality. Flutter tends to occur with **myocardial infarction**, arteriosclerotic heart disease, **rheumatic heart disease**, and inflammatory disorders involving the atria.

Folate (folic acid) A substance that is part of the vitamin B complex and is necessary for the normal production of red blood cells in the bone marrow, among other important functions. People with inflammations, cancers, or anemia may require additional amounts of folate in their diets. Alcohol and certain drugs, particularly those affecting the bone marrow, can interfere with absorption of the vitamin from the digestive tract, even when the diet includes foods rich in folate, such as liver, yeast, whole wheat, and leafy vegetables. Older adults are especially vulnerable to health effects of a folate deficiency.

Folliculitis An inflammation of the hair follicles, the shafts from which hairs grow. Older adults ocasionally are afflicted with a folliculitis of the scalp that produces intense itching. It is caused by a local bacterial infection and usually requires treatment with antibiotics.

Forgetfulness *See* **Memory loss.**

Fremitus Vibration tremors of the chest wall, particularly the vibrations produced when a person speaks. By placing the palm of the hand over the chest while speaking, one can feel the vibrations conducted to the chest wall from the vocal cords. Vocal fremitus is used by an examining physician to check the condition of the lungs. Fremitus is increased near consolidated lung tissue in pneumonia or in inflammation around a lung abcess, but is diminished or absent in the case of pneumothorax, fibrosis, or when fluid in the pleural cavity of the chest obstructs the vibrations.

Friction rub A dry, grating sound heard by an examining physician through a stethoscope placed on the chest. By analyzing the sounds, the condition of various organs and tissues can be studied; some sounds are normal, others are abnormal. A friction rub in the area of the heart that occurs simultaneously with the heartbeat is presumed to be caused by the layers of the pericardium (membranes covering the heart) rubbing together. A sound like that of two pieces of leather rubbed against each other may suggest that the pericardium is inflamed, resulting from the loss of the lubricating fluid that is normally present between the membrane layers.

Frontal lobe degeneration   A condition marked by the loss of normal personality factors, such as social judgment, initiative, purposeful behavior, and tact, which are controlled by the frontal lobes of the brain. The condition may be caused by chronic abuse of alcohol and by brain disorders, such as **Alzheimer's disease** and **Pick's disease**.

Functional age (biological age)   A concept that the age of an individual should be judged by the age level at which he or she functions rather than the age in calendar years. Many people over the age of sixty can perform some mental and physical tasks as well as those who are forty years old or younger. Performance by a chronologically older person at a younger age level in one or several areas does not ensure that the older person can compete with younger individuals in all areas, but it is a more accurate measure of aging than the number of years a person has lived.

G

Gait disorders Abnormalities in the manner or style of walking due to neuromuscular, arthritic, or other changes in the body. As a person grows older, the body's center of gravity tends to shift forward, resulting in altered flexion of the knees in order to maintain balance when walking. The flexed knees give the person an appearance of crouching, with a forward-leaning posture. With aging, there may be increased difficulty in starting or stopping the body movements involved in walking. With the shift in the body's center of gravity, maintaining balance while walking is difficult, so that the older person takes steps more slowly and uses shorter steps in order to prevent falls. Caution in walking may also result from impaired vision or inner ear disturbances that affect the sense of balance. In more serious gait disorders, particularly those complicated by a neuromuscular disorder, the person may walk with a shuffling gait or move forward with lurching motions. Because of starting and stopping difficulties, a sudden change of direction may require that the person pause briefly and make several steplike movements in order to turn the body into the new direction. Abnormal walking patterns also can be the result of reactions to drugs prescribed for heart disorders, anxiety, hypertension, or other problems; such drugs can cause confusion, loss of coordination, and other effects that alter normal gait.

Gallbladder disease Any disorder involving the gallbladder, a small pouch in the upper abdomen that stores bile produced by the liver, releasing it as needed to help digest fatty foods. The bile is released into the small intestine through a series of ducts connecting the organs. The gallbladder and its associated ducts can be the site of cancer; benign (noncancerous) tumors; gallstones; acute or chronic cholecystitis (inflammation) caused by infection or chemical irritation; gangrene following interruption of blood supply to the organ; diverticula; fistulas; and perforation, which can result in peritonitis. The bile in the gallbladder is a a greenish to brown-colored fluid containing a number of solid but dissolved substances. If too much water is lost from the bile while it is in the gallbladder, the solid substances become so concentrated that they form gallstones (cholelithiasis). If the gallstones obstruct the release of bile through the ducts, the person suffers the excruciating pain of a gallbladder attack. The condition affects about 10 percent of men and 20 percent of women in their fifties. Many patients are overweight. The symptoms are pain and tenderness in the upper right side of the abdomen, which often radiates to the right shoulder blade, nausea, and vomiting. The location of the pain is one of the major diagnostic signs. Diagnosis also may be based on visualization of the gallbladder and its ducts by cholestography (X-ray films made after a dye has been swallowed or injected), ultrasound, or radioactive scans; gallstones may not be easily visible if they do not contain an opaque substance, such as calcium. The usual treatment is surgery to remove the gallbladder.

Gallbladder cancer   A cancer of the gallbladder, the body's bile reservoir, usually associated with the presence of gallstones. The disorder rarely occurs before the age of forty, is most common after sixty, and is found mostly in women. The symptoms are weight loss, loss of appetite, nausea, vomiting, jaundice, and increasing pain in the upper right side of the abdomen. Many patients experience pain and dyspepsia for several years before the cancer is discovered. The severe pain may develop only in advanced stages of the disease, and the cause often is not discovered until exploratory surgery is performed. Carcinoma of the bile duct is less common and affects mostly older men, especially those who have been treated previously for ulcerative colitis, gallstones, or parasitic infections by liver flukes. Symptoms include jaundice, pain, and a generalized itching sensation, caused by bile pigments in the skin. Surgery or other treatment depends upon the precise location of the cancer and the stage of its development.

Gas   Air or other gases that accumulate in the digestive tract, resulting in belching, bloating, abdominal pain, and flatus. Gas is generally regarded as a symptom of a minor digestive disorder and is more often a cause of embarrassment than a sign of a disease. Most of the gas in the esophagus, stomach, and duodenum (the first segment of the small intestine) consists of nitrogen and oxygen from swallowed air and carbon dioxide produced by the neutralization of stomach acid and organic acids of foods after they reach the duodenum. Much of the swallowed oxygen that becomes trapped below the stomach is absorbed while the nitrogen is passed on through the intestine, though both gases may be trapped by fluids in the stomach. Most of the gas produced in the intestine consists of carbon dioxide and hydrogen, as well as some methane from the fermentation activity of intestinal bacteria on carbohydrates in the diet. Some complaints of intestinal gas in older adults are possibly due to a deficiency of enzymes needed to help digest carbohydrates in milk, fruits, or vegetables. Dental defects, such as missing teeth or poorly fitted dentures, may result in improper chewing of food and air swallowing. *Also see* **Lactose intolerance.**

Gastritis An inflammation of the mucous membrane lining of the stomach. At one time or another, the condition affects much of the general population but it increases in frequency as one grows older, partly because of a lifetime of accumulated dietary insults to the digestive tract. In a younger person, there is a comparatively constant reproduction of cells in the mucosal lining, so that injured or destroyed cells are rapidly replaced. But in the later adult years, the rate of replacement of cells damaged by alcohol, aspirin, and other chemicals is much slower, leaving a thinner mucous membrane and fewer cells to produce gastric juices needed for digestion. In some cases, there may be a total lack of stomach acid, a condition known as **achlorhydria.**

Gastritis associated with degenerative changes of the aging process is known as *atrophic gastritis.* The prevalence of atrophic gastritis increases with age and is marked by a loss of stomach muscle tissue as well as changes in the mucosal lining, which gradually begins to resemble the lining of the intestine. Two basic types of atrophic gastritis are recognized. One type is often accompanied by achlorhydria and pernicious anemia, due to the lack of a substance (intrinsic factor) produced by cells normally functioning in the mucosal lining of the stomach. Another type of atrophic gastritis is less likely to be marked by achlorhydria and pernicious anemia, but it is far more common and is more likely to produce symptoms of dyspepsia. The risk of stomach cancer also is thought to be higher among persons with the latter type of atrophic gastritis. Treatment may include antacids to relieve dyspepsia, even though there may be no stomach acid to neutralize, and vitamin B_{12} to control anemia. Other forms of gastritis, which may involve bacterial infections or peptic ulcer complications, are treated with surgery and antibiotics.

Gastrointestinal changes with age Alterations in the digestive system, which extends from the mouth to the anus, due to the natural aging processes. Some changes begin with the atrophy of alveolar bone supporting the teeth and recession of the gums, resulting in loosening and loss of teeth and increased difficulty in chewing food. The reduction in saliva secretion affects how well food is digested because the saliva contains an enzyme needed to begin digestion of starches. Swallowing difficulty may increase with decreased action of the muscles of the esophagus that propel chewed food from the mouth to the stomach. The risk of developing hiatus hernia, or protrusion of the stomach through the diaphragm separating the chest from the abdomen, increases with each year of age and affects fifty percent of all persons by their seventieth year. It may be associated with symptoms of **reflux esophagitis**. The incidence of **gallbladder disease** and **gastritis** also increases with age. The secretion of pepsin, a digestive enzyme of the stomach, which begins to decline in the thirties, levels off around the age of sixty. At that time, however, the production of hydrochloric acid in the stomach declines. Decline of another enzyme, lipase, makes digestion of fatty foods more difficult. Vitamins and minerals are often deficient because of inadequate nutrition or poor eating habits; numerous studies show that older people, particularly those who eat alone, tend to lose interest in the planning and serving of nutritionally balanced meals. In some cases, symptoms of disorders associated with aging are treated by the simple procedure of correcting nutritional deficiencies. Vitamins and minerals often may not be absorbed properly from the intestine, particularly B vitamins, vitamin K, iron, and calcium. Loss of muscle tone and control of the anal sphincter muscles can lead to constipation with fecal impaction or **fecal incontinence**, or both. Intestinal obstruction becomes an increasingly common cause of **abdominal pain**, and the most frequent cause of bowel obstruction in persons over the age of sixty is a hernia, resulting in entrapment of the bowel in the muscle layers of the abdomen. The risk of intestinal cancer also increases, sometimes presenting constipation and abdominal distention as the only symptoms of the obstructive growth in the bowel. The gastrointestinal changes frequently require careful diagnosis that includes the use of X-ray films made following a barium meal or a barium enema.

Genodermatoses   Skin abnormalities that are inherited. Examples include freckles, seborrheic keratoses, xanthomatosis, and some forms of eczema, psoriasis, and hair loss.

Genu valgum   A medical term for knock-knee, in which the legs curve inward. The condition can develop as an effect of **osteoarthritis** of the knee joint, resulting in cartilage loss on one side of the joint.

Genu varum A medical term for bowleg, in which the legs curve outward. The deformity can result in **osteoarthritis** if there is cartilage loss on one side of the knee joint with instability of the joint.

Geriatric dermatoses Skin changes that are associated with the aging process. General changes include development of wrinkles, increased pigmentation, and a widespread atrophy involving nearly all types of cells in all layers of the skin, resulting in dryness and itching. Although oil glands of the skin do not atrophy, their function diminishes in relation to the decline in androgen (male sex hormone) production by the gonads and adrenal glands. Specific forms of dermatitis that occur with increased frequency are **senile** and **seborrheic keratoses**, purpura, pedunculated fibromas, and senile hemangiomas. *See also* **Androgen, Dry skin.**

Geriatrics A branch of medicine that specializes in the diagnosis and treatment of diseases and disorders associated with aging.

Gerontology The study of the causes and effects of aging, including all medical, psychological, economic, and sociological aspects, on both the individual and society.

Gerontoxon *See* **Arcus senilis.**

Gerontic nurse A nurse who specializes in the care of geriatric patients.

Gerstmann syndrome A disorder marked by difficulty in distinguishing left from right and an inability to identify the fingers of one's own or another person's hands. The condition, which is believed to involve damage to the dominant side of a person's brain, also may result in an inability to read written material, or to read, write, or use numbers in calculations.

Giant cell arteritis *See* **Temporal arteritis.**

Gingivitis Inflammation of the gums (gingiva), usually due to accumulation of plaque and calculus along the gum line, poorly fitting complete or partial dentures, or nutritional disorders. Other factors may include mouth breathing, which tends to cause dryness and irritation of the gums; hormonal disorders; or the use of certain medications.

Glaucoma   A serious visual disorder caused by abnormally high fluid pressure within the eyeball. More than a dozen forms of glaucoma have been described but all are caused by the same defect, an obstruction that prevents normal drainage of fluid that circulates in the front chamber of the eye. As this fluid accumulates in the eye and pressure builds up, delicate structures within the eye, including the ending of the optic nerve, are damaged. The effects are insidious because in *chronic glaucoma* there are few warning symptoms until vision is partly destroyed. Like high blood pressure, glaucoma can develop without pain or discomfort and is often discovered during a routine medical examination. The earliest signs are the development of "tunnel vision," seeing "halos" around electric lights, and difficulty in dark adaptation (the adjustment the eyes make when one goes from a lighted room into an unlighted area). *Acute glaucoma,* however, may begin with sudden severe eye pain, accompanied by nausea and vomiting. The most common complication of both chronic and acute glaucoma is the loss of the peripheral, or outer, portions of the field of vision, which gradually diminishes until the disorder is diagnosed and brought under control with medications, such as eyedrops that relieve pressure within the eyeball, and/or surgery. If uncorrected, vision eventually deteriorates to total blindness. The damage is not reversible, although further deterioration can usually be slowed or stopped entirely by diagnosis and treatment. The risk of glaucoma increases with age, and it is recommended that all persons over the age of forty have their eyes checked periodically in order to detect early signs of the disease. Eye tests for glaucoma are also recommended for younger persons who experience vague visual discomfort and require new eyeglass prescriptions at frequent intervals.

Glioblastoma multiforme   The most common primary brain tumor of older adults, reaching a peak in frequency after the age of forty-five. The tumor may develop in nearly any part of the brain and tends to grow rapidly. Symptoms may vary somewhat with the area of the brain affected but generally include headaches, vomiting, and mental changes. The person may experience visual difficulties, urinary incontinence, or loss of the sense of smell. Personality and behavioral changes, such as drowsiness, lethargy, or other behavioral signs, often precede the physical complaints. There may be convulsive seizures. Women are more likely than men to develop this type of brain tumor. Treatment may include surgery, radiation, and chemotheraphy.

Glioma   A tumor of the glia cells, which form the structural tissues of the brain and spinal cord, as distinguished from cells involved in nervous system functions. *See also* **Glioblastoma multiforme.**

Glomerular filtration rate   A medical term for the rate at which substances in the blood, mainly waste chemicals and excess water, are filtered by tiny units (glomeruli) in the kidney, while most water and essential nutrients are reabsorbed. Kidney function begins to decline after the age of forty, and up to 40 percent of the glomeruli are gradually destroyed or impaired. Thus, the kidney of an older person may be only 60 to 70 percent as effective as the kidney of a younger person in adjusting to changes in the balance between electrolytes and fluids, as when salt or water intake is disrupted. A decrease of 30 to 40 percent in glomerular filtration rate can affect the heart, kidneys, brain, and other organ systems. *See also* **Fluid balance.**

Glossitis   A painful inflammation of the tongue that usually is marked by a reddish eruption at the tip or along the sides. In some cases, there may be ulcerations, whitish patches, or a pale smooth surface. Causes vary widely and can include diseases such as pellagra and anemia; excessive use of alcohol, tobacco, or spicy foods; mechanical irritants such as the rough surface of a natural tooth or of dentures; or an allergic reaction to a toothpaste, mouthwash, breath freshener, or food additive. Treatment usually requires avoiding any substance that irritates the tongue and the use of topical anesthetics, painkillers, ointments, and appropriate medications.

Glossodynia (burning tongue)   A form of glossitis in which the person has a painful sensation of burning in the tongue but no evidence of a disease or injury of the tongue. Middle-aged women who may be suffering from a systemic disorder, such as anemia, diabetes mellitus, or a nutritional deficiency, are affected most frequently.

Glucose tolerance test   *See* **Diabetes mellitus.**

Goiter   An enlargement of the thyroid gland. It can occur in association with **hyperthyroidism, hypothyroidism**, or in a normally functioning thyroid gland. There are about twenty different kinds of goiters. A *euthyroid,* or simple, *goiter* is a common form of the abnormality and results from a thyroid hormone deficiency that may be due to a lack of iodine in the diet. Ironically, it also may be caused by an intake of large doses of iodine, which has the effect of reducing the normal activity of the thyroid gland. Other causes may include the use of certain drugs or foods, particularly turnips, that may interfere with normal thyroid gland functions. A *toxic diffuse goiter* occurs with hyperthyroidism (Graves' disease) and is characterized by exophthalmos, or bulging eyeballs; an enlarged thyroid gland that may appear as a large lump in the neck; rapid heartbeat; a tremor in the hands and fingers; profuse sweating; and skin eruptions. The thyroid gland enlargement associated with hypothyroidism is sometimes identified as an *endemic goiter.* It has become relatively uncommon in North America since iodine has been added to table salt, thereby reducing the risk of a serious iodine deficiency in the typical American diet. Several types of goiters are caused by inherited metabolic disorders that interfere with the body's utilization of iodine.

Gout A form of acute **arthritis** caused by an accumulation of uric acid crystals in the joints and tendons. Men are more often afflicted than women; only 5 percent of gout patients are women, usually postmenopausal. The basic symptom is a warm, red, tender, acutely painful, swollen joint. A typical attack begins suddenly, often during the night, may be accompanied by chills, fever, and a rapid heartbeat, and can easily be mistaken for a serious infection. The first attack often involves a single joint, such as the big toe. Later attacks may involve any of several joints, from the toes and knees to the fingers and shoulders. Gout patients are more susceptible than the general public to deposits of uric acid crystals in the kidneys, which may lead to **kidney stones**. Diagnosis is based on X-rays of joints, finding of urate crystals in microscopic examination of a body tissue sample, and the response of the person to colchicine, a specific gout remedy. Treatment of gout is based on medications to control inflammation and prevent the formation of uric acid crystals, ample liquid intake, a change in diet to eliminate foods that contribute to high uric acid levels in the blood and, as in other forms of arthritis, a reduction in body weight, if necessary.

Granuloma A tumor or other growth containing granular elements, such as the nodules that occur with tuberculosis. Granulomas often develop in the skin as a reaction to a foreign substance, such as paraffin, talc, or chemicals in cosmetics. A type of granuloma not associated with a foreign substance is *granuloma annulare,* a common, benign type of skin eruption with a group of tiny nodules that form a circle. It often disappears without treatment. *Granuloma faciale* is a type of granuloma that tends to appear on the face in the form of small brownish pimples or plaques. Men who are middle-aged or older are most commonly affected. The cause is unknown, and the granuloma may disappear without treatment.

Graphanesthesia An inability to recognize letters, numbers, or similar patterns traced on the skin, as on the palm. In a person with no evidence of other illnesses, this condition is regarded as a symptom of a lesion of the part of the brain controlling size, shape, texture, and visual images.

Graves' disease   *See* **Hyperthyroidism.**

Gray hair   Hair that is gray or white because of the absence of pigment. Although it is commonly associated with aging, the loss of pigmentation may begin in early adulthood for some individuals who have inherited this trait. Graying of the hair also can be associated with certain disorders or diseases, such as anemia and vitiligo. The cause of graying hair is a decrease in the number of cells (melanocytes) in the hair roots that manufacture melanin, the substance that gives color to hair and skin. By the age of fifty, about half of all people show signs of graying.

Grimacing   An involuntary movement of the facial muscles. It may occur as a tic and may be either organic in nature or an expression of tension. When organic, a grimace can be a sign of **encephalopathy, chorea,** or a reaction to **dopamine** medication.

Guillain-Barré syndrome   A neurological disorder characterized initially by muscular weakness and a loss of sensation in the fingers and toes. It is believed to result from an immune reaction involving the peripheral nerves. Most cases occur following an infection, vaccination, or surgery. The disease varies in severity and can be fatal if it involves the brain or respiratory muscles. Guillain-Barré syndrome is difficult to diagnose because many of the symptoms resemble those of botulism, insecticide poisoning, or poliomyelitis. The symptoms include a dry mouth, fever, muscle tenderness and weakness, loss of some reflexes, hypotension, headache, nausea, and vomiting. The muscle weakness frequently moves upward through the body from the legs to the trunk, face, and arms. The acute condition is a medical emergency, requiring constant maintenance of breathing and other bodily functions. Recovery is a lengthy process, often taking months, and may be followed by surgery to correct musculoskeletal abnormalities resulting from the disorder or by retraining in activities of daily living, or both.

Gum changes with aging   Alterations in the gingival (gum) tissues that occur as a consequence of diminished blood circulation, making them more vulnerable to disease or injury. A loss of tissue elasticity and atrophy of the alveolar bone forming the tooth socket contribute to periodontal disease and loose teeth. Studies show that 90 percent of the population over the age of sixty-five have some degree of periodontal disease associated with changes in gum tissues. However, the condition does not begin with older adults; some early signs of changes in the gums may appear before middle age.

Gynecological changes with aging Changes in the female reproductive system that occur in the years following menopause. The changes are generally the result of diminished functioning of the ovaries, the primary source of the female hormones estrogen and progesterone. The changes include loss of pubic hair and subcutaneous fat around the vulva. There is some atrophy of Bartholin's glands near the vaginal opening, resulting in reduced natural lubrication. There may be drying of the skin outside the vagina and the appearance of grayish plaques, accompanied by pain and itching. The vagina becomes smaller in length and diameter and loses elasticity. Vaginal secretions are reduced, membranes lining the vagina are thinner, and inflammation of the membranes is more likely. The condition of *atrophic vaginitis* may require estrogen treatments. Vaginal changes also contribute to **dyspareunia**, or painful intercourse, which may be relieved by the use of supplementary lubrication. However, the vaginal environment no longer supports the colonies of microorganisms, such as *Candida,* that are a frequent cause of vaginitis in a younger woman. An estimated 25 percent of older adult women, particularly those who have experienced multiple pregnancies, are likely to suffer uterine prolapse, cystocele, rectocele, or a related form of herniation of the pelvic organs. In about 10 percent of such cases, the pelvic relaxation produces discomfort or other symptoms, including stress urinary incontinence. *See also* **Androgen, Androsterone, Sexual function changes with aging.**

H

Hair changes with aging   The rate of hair growth, density, color, and other factors that are related to the aging process. The graying of hair is due to a gradual loss of pigment-producing cells (melanocytes) in the hair roots. It is estimated that half of the total population will see some graying of their hair by the age of fifty. Premature graying of hair is influenced by heredity and is not directly related to aging. Hair that is on the head loses its coloring at a faster rate than other body hair, in part because it grows faster, so that gray hairs replace the pigmented hairs earlier. Hair follicles, the microscopic tunnels in the skin from which hair grows, atrophy or are destroyed by fibrous tissue growth as one grows older, so that there is a gradual loss of total hair. The decrease occurs in hair growth throughout the body and includes hair in the pubic and armpit (axillary) areas as well as scalp hair. By the age of sixty, an estimated 30 percent of women, and a smaller proportion of men, will have lost all of their axillary hair. Women may lose axillary and pubic hair at a faster rate than men of the same age because body hair growth is influenced by a female sex hormone (estrogen), which diminishes after the menopause. During the process of balding, the thick scalp hairs are gradually replaced by fine, downy (vellus) hairs, and sometimes even the vellus hairs vanish. Women also may experience balding, which does not appear to be related to sex hormone changes, and the loss of scalp hair is not as extensive or as complete as in male balding. An effect that is the opposite of balding occurs on the ears of men when vellus hairs are replaced by the thicker, scalplike hairs as they grow older.

Hallucinations   Vivid illusions seen or heard by a person in the absence of any actual object or agent that would produce the visual or

155

auditory stimulation. The hallucinations of older adults may also include illusions of touch, taste, and smell sensations and may be associated with sleep disturbances, occurring at about the time the person falls asleep. Hallucinations in younger people are usually associated with psychiatric disorders, including bizarre delusions of grandeur or the hostility experienced by schizophrenic or bipolar (manic-depressive) patients. In older adults, hallucinations may occur as a result of frequent use of medications or withdrawal from them, impaired vision, brain diseases or injuries, including strokes. They may also be related to personal fears and guilt feelings. The hallucinations are similar to vivid dreams, and in cases where it has been possible to record brain waves of persons experiencing hallucinations, the electroencephalograph (EEG) recordings showed brain-wave patterns similar to those produced by dreaming.

Hand changes with aging   The effects of normal tissue alterations and degenerative diseases, such as rheumatoid arthritis, on the hands as a part of the aging process. A common result is enlargement of the joints of the finger bones, with gradual loss of range of motion and increasing deformity. Deformities include enlarged areas of bone or cartilage at the joints. The enlargements, or nodes, may be painful. There may also be tenderness and swelling of the soft tissues of the fingers. The changes may affect the ability to use the hands in certain daily tasks. Normal tissue changes include diminished subcutaneous and epidermal tissues, resulting in a loosening of the skin and increased transparency, making the blood veins in the hands more prominent. Pigmented macules, sometimes called "age spots" or "liver spots," tend to increase in number, particularly on surfaces exposed to sunlight; they represent an increase in and irregular distribution of the number of pigment-producing melanocytes in the skin. Fingernail growth rate declines by 50 percent after the thirties, and nail surfaces develop lengthwise ridges. The nail of the older adult also may become more opaque and it gradually loses the half-moon shaped lunula at the base of the nail.

HDL   An abbreviation for high-density lipoprotein, a protein that occurs in the blood in association with **cholesterol** and **triglycerides**. HDL is assumed to have beneficial effects by helping remove cholesterol from the arteries and transporting it to the liver to be stored or excreted. *See also* **LDL**.

Headache   Any pain in the head. Headaches are usually a symptom of another disorder. They are sometimes divided into two basic categories: headaches that are *extracranial,* or a symptom of an abnormality outside the skull, and those that are *intracranial,* or caused by a condition within the skull. Extracranial headaches are most frequently the result of sustained contractions of muscles of the neck and shoulders. Intracranial headaches may be vascular, caused by distention or inflammation of blood vessels of the head, or a sign of a disorder involving tissues of the brain or other parts of the central nervous system, such as the cranial nerves that extend to the eyes, ears, and parts the head. Because a headache usually is not accompanied by any physical signs, such as bleeding or swelling, the diagnosis often depends on analysis of the symptoms and factors that can either provoke or relieve the symptoms. Such factors may include the position of the head and body, the effect of coughing or straining, emotional tension, allergic reaction, constipation, nausea, or dizziness that may accompany a headache.

Migraine is one of the most common forms of headache, affecting 10 percent of the general population. It is believed to be an inherited condition since more than two-thirds of migraine patients have first or second-degree relatives who also experience migraine headaches. Migraine is due to a blood vessel disorder that causes a temporary interruption of blood flow to a part of the central nervous system, resulting in pain and often preceded by prodromal symptoms, such as flashes of light. For some persons, migraine symptoms begin to subside after middle age; for others, migraine does not begin until they are in their fifties. Migraine is frequently averted or relieved by the use of medications, including aspirin or similar analgesics, caffeine or similar drugs that help contract distended blood vessels of the brain, and by maintaining an erect position.

A severe headache in an older adult, particularly one that begins suddenly, is often a sign of a serious condition such as a **stroke, temporal arteritis, glaucoma, brain tumor**, or **meningitis**. A stroke caused by the hemorrhage of an artery in the brain usually causes severe pain and loss of consciousness; it is most likely to occur to a person over the age of fifty. When glaucoma is a cause of a headache, blurred vision or other eye disorders usually develop before the onset of head pain. Headaches caused by high blood pressure or brain tumors tend to occur most often in the morning, whereas headaches associated with stress or eyestrain are most likely to develop in the evening.

Muscle tension headaches are usually felt at the back of the head, and they are often accompanied by tenderness in the neck and shoulders. The pain is frequently described as "like a vise" or a "tight band" that causes cramping, aching, and soreness. However, the headache is not accompanied by throbbing and is not aggravated by coughing, straining, or shaking the head. It is relieved by hot packs, massage, and aspirin. Occasionally, a person may experience a combination headache, such as a muscle tension headache that is secondary to a migraine, in which case both types must be treated in order to end the painful symptoms.

A *sinus headache* that involves a frontal sinus (in the forehead, over the eyes) may be relieved by keeping the head in an upright position. A headache caused by a problem in the maxillary sinus (in the cheekbones below the eyes) usually is improved by lying down. A pulsating headache may be due to **hypoglycemia, fever,** a lack of oxygen, an excess of carbon dioxide, caffeine withdrawal, or a hangover. *Cluster headaches,* like migraines, are caused by a blood vessel disorder. They are so named because they occur in clusters of attacks, each attack lasting from fifteen to forty-five minutes and repeating several times a day or a week, followed by long periods in which they do not reoccur. Cluster headaches usually affect only one side of the head, produce a severe, throbbing pain, and may be accompanied by flushing of the skin of the face, nasal congestion, and a flow of tears. A cluster headache is also known as a *histamine headache* because the symptoms can be produced by an injection of histamine into the carotid artery of the neck.

A headache that has persisted for months may be less serious than one that begins suddenly in a person who rarely has a headache, except if the cause of a persistent headache is an intracranial tumor or other disease. Treatment of cluster headaches is the same as for migraines. Caffeine, which is often used to relieve headaches, can also be the cause of head pain, because of a rebound effect that occurs when the caffeine wears off.

Hearing aid   An electronic device designed to compensate for a hearing loss, usually by amplifying sound. It consists of four parts: a *microphone* to gather sound vibrations; a *transducer* that converts the sound waves into electrical signals; an *amplifier* that raises the intensity of the electrical signals; and a *receiver,* placed in or close to the ear, that translates the electrical signals back into sound waves. In the traditional electronic hearing aid, the microphone, transducer, and amplifier are contained in a small unit that may be carried in a pocket, usually in the chest area. Some women conceal the microphone in a brassiere. The microphone is connected by a thin wire extending to the receiver, which is concealed in an earpiece. More sophisticated miniaturized hearing aids are available with all components built into eyeglass frames. Even smaller self-contained hearing aids have been developed with all components built into the earpiece. The smallest hearing aid, called a *cochlear implant,* consists of a tiny receiver that is implanted through the skin and bone behind the ear. Eight electrode wires extend from the receiver to the cochlea, the part of the inner ear that collects sound vibrations and sends the impulses to the part of the brain that interprets them. The microphone is a tiepin-size device that can be clipped to a shirt or blouse. However, it is not effective in restoring hearing to those whose hearing loss is due to a failure of the auditory nerves leading to the brain. The smaller self-contained units frequently help the hearing loss patient to overcome self-consciousness about appearing in public while wearing a hearing aid. The person who avoids the use of a hearing aid increases the risk of social isolation and loneliness in the later years of life.

Hearing aids are available for certain patients with both sensorineural and conductive hearing losses. They can be adjusted to receive certain sound frequencies rather than all frequencies, and they can be designed to receive sounds in "stereo" rather than from a single direction. This last feature is important because persons with normal hearing can tell the direction from which a sound is coming by the fraction of a second difference in the time it may take for each ear to detect the same sounds. But hearing aids should not be expected to restore normal hearing, and a choice should be based on specific need.

A hearing aid should be fitted by an audiologist, a health professional trained in the testing and measuring of hearing disorders. A hearing aid may be needed only to compensate for the loss of the ability to hear certain sound frequencies, such as high frequencies. If the hearing aid is needed for conversation, it should be designed for face-to-face dialogue within the range of sound frequencies and intensities generally used for human voice communication. There is usually a period of adjustment necessary after receiving a hearing aid, much as one must adjust to wearing bifocal or trifocal eyeglasses. The hearing loss patient should also practice lip reading to accompany use of the hearing aid. *See also* **Hearing loss.**

Hearing loss   A diminished sensitivity to sounds. The condition is usually subdivided into *conductive deafness,* caused by disease or injury affecting the part of the ear that transmits sound vibrations of the air to the surface of the inner ear, and *sensorineural,* or nerve, deafness that is due to injury or disease involving the structures of the inner ear or the nerves that carry signals from the ear to the part of the brain that translates the signals into sounds. Most people experience some degree of hearing loss as they grow older, beginning in early adulthood. Sounds in the higher frequencies are affected first, then the lower frequencies. The individual may lose the ability to hear a telephone or doorbell ring or to hear the higher-pitched voice of a woman. The person with a hearing loss may lose interest in social contacts because of the difficulty of hearing conversations. Because the hearing loss that occurs with aging (**presbycusis**) is so gradual, the person often is not aware of the change and may feel rejected or isolated without understanding the cause. This isolation can have serious psychological consequences, including resentment, suspiciousness, and depression. In some instances, symptoms of hearing loss, such as apparently ignoring questions or giving inappropriate responses because questions are not clearly understood, may be mistaken for signs of mental illness.

For many workers, hearing loss is caused by the intensity of noise in the workplace. Exposure to sustained noises at levels of 85 decibels and above (around the level of a vacuum cleaner) can cause permanent damage to the inner-ear structures. The noise level in many factories is greater than 100 decibels, which is the amount of noise produced by a subway train. The noise intensity of jet aircraft and some military guns can produce ear pain as well as hearing loss. Other causes of sensorineural hearing loss are viral infections, the use of aspirin or certain other drugs, and head injury. Hearing-loss problems due to conductive disorders, such as a ruptured eardrum or an abnormality of the tiny bones (ossicles) between the eardrum and the inner ear, can often be remedied with surgery. Many, but not all, hearing loss difficulties can usually be corrected with a **hearing aid.**

Heart attack   See **Myocardial infarction.**

Heart block   Any of several abnormal conditions of the heart in which the electrical impulse needed to cause contractions of the heart muscle is unable to travel over the usual route of conducting fibers, beginning with the natural pacemaker in the right upper heart chamber (atrium). The disruption can result in an irregular rhythm in which the atria and the lower heart chambers (ventricles) have different heartbeat rates, as in *incomplete heart block; a partial heart block,* in which some but not all of the impulses fail to reach the ventricles; or a blockage in some but not all of the fibers, causing a loss of coordination so that the two ventricles beat at different rhythms *(parasystole).* Causes include infections, reactions to drugs, **coronary artery disease**, or damage to the heart muscle. Heart block can result in episodes of weakness, dizziness, loss of consciousness, and convulsions. Heart block that causes loss of consciousness can be very serious, requiring emergency resuscitation efforts, as the event usually results in an interruption of the normal flow of oxygenated blood to the brain. The condition can often be corrected by installation of an electronic pacemaker in the patient's body to regulate the heartbeat or by a change in medication, if a prescribed drug is found to be a factor. *See also* **Arrhythmia, Bundle-branch block, Sinoatrial (SA) block.**

Heartburn   The painful burning sensation that rises upward from the stomach toward the neck. A frequent symptom of indigestion, it is commonly caused by a reflux of contents from the stomach, but it may also be a sign of a **myocardial infarction** (heart attack). *See also* **Esophagitis, Hiatus hernia.**

Heart changes with aging   Anatomical and physiological alterations in the heart that often occur with aging, resulting in a loss of ability to make the sudden adjustments necessary to maintain appropriate blood flow under normal conditions as well as under such stressful situations as surgery, accidents, and illness. Numerous studies have found that heart performance at rest is not significantly altered by age in a healthy person. But even apparently healthy persons are likely to show age-related deterioration in exercise stress tests. Although the heart of an older individual is often able to adjust to new and changing physical demands, it may require more time to make the adjustment without the risk of such symptoms as **angina pectoris** or dizziness or fainting due to an inadequate blood flow to the brain. Most older people undergo the same type of basic changes in the cardiovascular system, but not all older persons experience the same symptoms because of individual differences and such influences as genetic factors and lifestyles.

The amount of blood that can be pumped per minute by the heart decreases with age at an average rate of nearly 1 percent a year. The lining of the heart and the valves thicken, and rigid, waxy, fibrous substances accumulate in the heart. There is a loss of elastic muscle fiber but an increase in stiff fibrous tissue in the sinoatrial node that controls the rate and rhythm of heart contractions. A decline in the number and function of pacemaker cells in the sinoatrial node, along with alterations in the fibers that relay impulses from the node to heart muscle tissues, leads to disruption of the normal beat, so that **arrhythmia, fibrillation, flutter,** and **heart block** occur more frequently in older individuals.

The changes in heart valves contribute to **heart murmurs** and **endocarditis.** The symptoms produced by the various changes in heart structure and function may include palpitations, fatigue, sleep disorders, chest pain, dizzy spells, sudden loss of consciousness, and drops in blood pressure. In some cases, the lungs and kidneys may also be affected. Although heart disorders still are a leading cause of premature deaths in industrialized countries, countless lives have been saved or extended through the development of modern medications, including **beta-adrenergic blockers**, devices such as electronic **pacemakers** and artificial heart valves, and surgical techniques that permit replacement or repair of damaged heart tissues. The outlook for heart disease, particularly in the United States where the death rate has been declining in the past decade, has improved not only because of improved treatment but also, most experts believe, because of an increased public awareness of the influences of diet, exercise, smoking, and other lifestyle factors associated with heart disease.

Heart murmur   *See* **Cardiac murmur.**

Heat stroke   A life-threatening emergency caused by an inadequate response of the body's heat-regulating mechanism to high temperatures in the environment. Older adults are particularly vulnerable because of several changes in the body's ability to adapt to high temperatures as a result of the aging process. Normally, when the temperature of the environment exceeds that of the surface of the body, the body absorbs the external heat and responds to it by sweating. But sweating becomes more difficult as one grows older, because the sweat glands atrophy. If the humidity is high, any sweat secreted by the sweat glands in the skin will not evaporate. Because of cardiovascular changes, the heart is less able to respond to the stress of heat and **congestive heart failure** symptoms increase with heat and humidity.

The risk of death from heat stroke is increased for older persons with **diabetes, hypertension, cardiovascular disease, chronic obstructive pulmonary disease**, or respiratory illnesses. A wide range of medications interfere with the body's natural ability to sense heat and respond to it. These include diuretics, which cause excessive fluid loss; beta-adrenergic blockers, which block cardiovascular response to heat effects; and amphetamines, which alter the body's temperature-regulating mechanism. Studies have found that 80 percent of the victims of heat stroke are over the age of fifty.

Heat stroke is characterized by a body temperature that may rise to 106° Fahrenheit (41° Celsius), accompanied by a pulse rate of 160 to 180 per minute, headache, fatigue, and feelings of faintness or dizziness. The skin is hot, dry, and flushed, with no sweating. If emergency medical treatment is not given immediately, circulatory collapse and death may result. Emergency measures include cooling the body to a temperature of at least 101° Fahrenheit by any means possible while awaiting professional medical help.

Heat exhaustion differs from heat stroke and is usually associated with fluid depletion, often because of failure to drink enough water to offset the fluid loss through sweating. The important thing in treating heat exhaustion is to slowly and carefully restore enough fluid to assure a normal volume of blood and to keep the victim's head lower than the rest of the body so that as much blood as possible will reach the brain, thereby preventing permanent brain damage. The person with heat exhaustion will have symptoms of weakness, anxiety, profuse sweating, cold and clammy skin, a slow and weak pulse, and signs of a central nervous system disorder, such as disorientation and confusion, possibly followed by loss of consciousness.

Excessive heat exposure also may result in heat cramps, which are usually due to a loss of salt during profuse sweating. The condition is marked by muscle cramps, usually beginning in the arms and legs and eventually involving the abdominal muscles. The skin may be either hot and dry or cold and clammy, depending more upon the environment than the condition of the victim of heat cramps. Emergency treatment consists primarily of restoring body fluid and salt. Although heat cramps may follow strenuous activity in a hot environment, the condition also may affect those who are overdressed on a cold day or who may not be aware of the loss of fluid by sweating because they live in an environment that is so dry that sweat evaporates rapidly without leaving the usual moisture traces on the skin. Some diuretics, particularly those of the furosemide type, can contribute to the development of heat cramps by causing significant losses of sodium.

Heberden's nodes   Small, hard, bony swellings that sometimes form on the end joints of the fingers in **osteoarthritis** or other degenerative joint diseases. In the acute stage, the nodes may be tender or painful. They are most common in older women, and heredity is a factor in their development.

Hemangioblastoma   A tumor of the blood vessels of the brain, usually in the brain stem portion. It tends to occur mainly in middle aged persons and may produce signs and symptoms that vary with its precise location in the brain. The tumor is generally noncancerous, but it is in contact with the membranes covering the brain and may infiltrate adjacent tissues. The only treatment is surgical removal of the tumor, if it is accessible.

Hematoma   An accumulation of trapped blood in the skin or other body tissues. The pool of blood develops as a result of injury to a blood vessel or during surgery. A clot that may be tender or painful often results. In some cases, the pooled blood may cause pressure on neighboring tissues, as when a hematoma occurs in the brain, resulting in loss of consciousness or other signs of disability. When necessary and possible, the hematoma can be drained and the leaking blood vessel tied off. The symptoms are often treated with mild analgesics and hot applications. In most cases, the condition resolves itself spontaneously by reabsorption of the blood components, but occasionally a hematoma near the surface of the body may rupture and discharge the clot along with any blood that has not coagulated.

Hematomyelia   The presence of blood in spinal-cord fluid, usually indicating a hemorrhage with damage to central nervous system tissues following a spinal-cord injury. It is often accompanied by muscle weakness, diminished reflexes, and uncontrollable twitching of muscles innervated by the damaged nerves.

Hematuria   The presence of blood in the urine, which may indicate a disease in the kidneys, bladder, or urethra.

Hemianesthesia   A loss of feeling or sensitivity to touch on one side of the body. It is usually the result of a blood clot obstructing an artery in the brain stem and often affects the face or another structure in the head, such as the tongue or soft palate, on the opposite side of the body from the thrombus-blocked artery.

Hemiballismus   The involuntary "flinging" of an arm or leg on one side of the body as a symptom of chorea. The movements can be violent, sometimes causing injury to the affected limb and exhausting the patient. The symptom tends to occur in older adults afflicted by a blood-vessel disorder near the base of the brain. If the disorder is on the right side of the brain, the flinging involves the left arm or leg, and vice versa.

Hemicrania   A pain, such as in migraine, that affects only one side of the head.

Hemiparesis   Partial paralysis on one side of the body. *See also* **Hemiplegia.**

Hemiplegia   Paralysis on one side of the body. Hemiplegia can result from **stroke**, cerebral palsy, multiple sclerosis, or other disorders and can influence one side of the body in various ways, depending upon the part of the central nervous system affected. It may affect one side of the face, one leg, one arm, or any combination. In a case of *alternate hemiplegia,* an arm on one side and a leg on the other side of the body may be affected.

Hemorrhage   The loss of a significant amount of blood in a relatively short period of time. The blood loss may be external, flowing out of the body from a wound, or internal, as in a brain hemorrhage or a bleeding ulcer. A hemorrhage also may be marked by profuse bleeding from a body opening, such as the nose, mouth, anus, or vagina. The rate of blood loss is often more important than the site of the bleeding. The symptoms vary with the site of the hemorrhage but may include shock, a rapid pulse, thirst, pallor, dizziness, loss of consciousness, cold, clammy skin, and abnormal breathing. A brain hemorrhage may cause a sudden severe headache, stiff neck, and vomiting, followed by loss of consciousness or neurological changes, such as hemiplegia. If the hemorrhage is external, efforts are directed toward stopping the flow of blood by applying pressure to the nearest pressure point or to the wound itself, applying ice, and positioning the bleeding part of the body so there will be maximal blood flow to the brain.

In a gastrointestinal hemorrhage, a common complication of peptic ulcers, the person is likely to vomit blood and pass bloody or tarry stools. The person may complain of weakness and lose consciousness. The pulse increases to a rate greater than 80 or 90 per minute, and the systolic blood pressure may fall below 100. Because of fluid loss, the person may feel an extreme thirst that can be relieved with ice water, if a physician approves. The color of the vomited blood is sometimes an indication of the severity of the hemorrhage; bright red blood usually is a sign of fresh blood from rapid bleeding, while blood that has the appearance of "coffee grounds" is associated with bleeding slow enough to allow the action of digestive juices on it. Vomited blood frequently has a severe emotional impact on the patient, who usually believes he has lost considerably more blood than is actually represented by the reddish vomitus, and reassurance as well as treatment of physical symptoms is helpful. Severe bleeding from the gastrointestinal tract also may be the result of other abnormalities, such as the erosive effects of aspirin, alcohol, or other substances on the stomach lining; rupture of the esophagus; or cancer. Any hemorrhage is likely to be an emergency situation requiring immediate professional medical care.

Hemorrhoids (piles)   Varicose veins of the rectum or anus. The name of the condition is derived from that of the blood vessel involved, the hemorrhoidal vein that drains blood from tissues of the rectal area. Hemorrhoids are classified as internal or external, depending upon whether the affected part of the hemorrhoidal vein is located within the rectum or outside the sphincter muscle that controls the opening of the anus. Older adults frequently develop hemorrhoids as a complication of constipation and straining to defecate. Straining creates a great amount of pressure within the abdomen; the pressure is transmitted to the hemorrhoidal vein, causing it to become distended, or varicose.

External hemorrhoids may appear as a small reddish mass of skin outside the anal sphincter. External hemorrhoids may not cause any pain or bleeding unless a vein acquires a blood clot or ruptures. Small *internal hemorrhoids* may bleed during defecation. If they become enlarged, they may protrude from the anus and become constricted and painful. Pain with hemorrhoids is usually a sign of a prolapsed hemorrhoidal vein. In uncomplicated cases, the appearance of bright red blood that is not a part of a stool is an early sign of hemorrhoidal bleeding. There may be passage of mucus, itching, and skin irritation around the anus. While external hemorrhoids are easily visible to an examining physician, internal hemorrhoids that have not prolapsed may require proctoscopy as part of the diagnosis to determine the source of rectal bloodstains.

Treatment usually involves medications to lubricate and reduce the discomfort in the area while shrinking the hemorrhoid, the use of sitz baths, and moist hot or cold compresses. In severe cases, surgical methods are employed to tie off (ligate), remove, or destroy the varicosity with injected chemicals.

Hepatic encephalopathy *See* **Encephalopathy.**

Hepatitis An inflammation of the liver that destroys patches of liver tissue. It is caused by a bacterial or viral infection, parasites, alcohol abuse, certain drugs, or a transfusion of infected blood. The most common cause is an infection by one of the three major types of hepatitis virus: A, B, or non-A/non-B. The *type A* hepatitis virus usually enters the body through the mouth through the consumption of food or beverages contaminated by the feces of an infected person. Examples include shellfish contaminated by sewage in polluted waters or the handling of food or eating utensils by infected persons who have not washed their hands. Occasionally, the Type A virus is transmitted by direct contact, as through sexual relations, with a person who is infected.

The *type B* hepatitis virus is usually transmitted through the bloodstream, as with contaminated hypodermic needles used by drug abusers. Formerly, the Type B virus also could be acquired through the transfusion of contaminated blood, but this risk has been reduced considerably as a result of newer techniques for screening of blood donations. Like Type A, type B hepatitis also may be acquired from a sexual partner infected with the virus. The virus is found in the semen and saliva of infected males and is a relatively common sexually-transmitted disease among male homosexuals. Insects are a possible but rare source of a hepatitis virus infection. Studies indicate that hundreds of millions of people throughout the world have been exposed to hepatitis, and in some areas, particularly Asia, more than 10 percent of the local population may be carriers of the virus. In North America and much of Europe, the number of hepatitis carriers is estimated at less than one-half of 1 percent.

Non-A/non-B hepatitis is a less well known viral infection and may actually represent more than one disease agent. It is identified by the fact that it stimulates the production of antibodies that are neither "anti-A" nor "anti-B" substances. However, it appears to be transmitted through direct blood contact, as through transfusions, may be acquired from carriers who are asymptomatic, and produces signs and symptoms similar to those of type B hepatitis.

The symptoms of hepatitis may include loss of appetite, nausea and vomiting, an enlarged liver, abdominal discomfort, light-colored stools, dark urine, **jaundice**, and abnormal liver function. Older adults react differently to hepatitis than do younger people. They are more susceptible to Type B viral hepatitis and non-A/non-B viral hepatitis, and Type B is generally the more serious form of the disease. Viral hepatitis can be an insidious infection, producing symptoms that are easily mistaken at first for influenza. Jaundice, a clue to the liver disorder, is often one of the last symptoms to appear. The first symptoms may appear anywhere from two weeks to several months after contact with the virus. Recovery may require as little as two weeks in younger persons but as long as three months for older adults. Older persons have a much higher death rate from a viral hepatitis infection and often need to be hospitalized. Viral hepatitis cases must be distinguished from liver diseases due to drugs, alcohol, or other causes; identification of the specific viral antigen in a sample of the patient's blood may help to determine the specific cause. Also, the signs and symptoms of an acute viral infection tend to develop much more rapidly than those associated with the abuse of drugs or alcohol.

Treatment generally requires bed rest and a high-protein diet, with breakfast as the big meal of the day; the patient's appetite is better and there is less nausea in the morning. Type A infections generally resolve themselves within two months with conservative treatment. Persons in close contact with Type A patients should receive injections of gamma globulin as a preventive measure. Gamma globulin treatment is also advised as a preventive for those who plan to travel to areas of the world where the Type A infection is endemic. A vaccine is available for the prevention of Type B viral hepatitis. Type B infections may progress to a chronic asymptomatic state and, in some cases, may lead to **cirrhosis** and liver cancer.

Older adults are ten times as likely to suffer drug-induced hepatitis as those under the age of thirty-five. However, alcohol abuse is less likely to be a cause of hepatitis in older adults because alcoholism and average alcohol intake decline after the age of forty. In addition, fewer alcoholics survive into their forties, most having died from alcohol-related causes such as cirrhosis or accidents before reaching their forties.

Hereditary   Pertaining to a physical trait or condition that is transmitted by one or both parents to their offspring through their chromosomes. An inherited trait may be determined by a single gene on one of the chromosomes, a combination of genes, or genes that predispose a person to being susceptible to an influence in the environment. An inherited trait may also be conveyed by a chromosomal defect that occurs during maturation of an ovum or spermatozoon in the parent. A hereditary disorder is usually one that can be identified with specific genes and traced to one or more ancestors. *See also* **Familial.**

Hernia (rupture)   Any protrusion of an organ through the muscular wall that normally contains it. Causes can include weakness of a muscle wall, injury, pressure from a tumor, or degeneration of neighboring tissues. Among the most common sites of hernias are the inguinal (groin) area, the umbilicus (navel), and the abdomen beneath the breastbone (sternum), where the muscles are weak and may yield to the pressure of intestines or other internal organs. The danger is that the organ, or a portion of it, may become trapped between muscle layers, interrupting the blood supply and causing gangrene. Men are prone to inguinal hernias because the intestine can push through an opening in the abdominal muscle wall through which the spermatic cord passes. *See also* **Abdominal hernia, Herniated disk, Hiatus hernia.**

Herniated disk (slipped disk)   A condition in which the nucleus pulposus, the pulpy elastic center of the fibrous disk (intervertebral disk) separating two adjacent vertebrae, becomes abnormally compressed and is squeezed through the outer wall of the disk. Most frequently affected are men in their forties who have been doing work or exercise that requires bending and lifting, although some may trace the injury to a hard fall. The bulging nucleus pulposus then may press against a spinal nerve root and cause intense pain. The symptoms vary, depending upon which spinal nerve root is compressed as the result of the injury.

If it is the sciatic nerve, the pain (**sciatica**) may begin in the low back, or buttocks, and run down the legs. Any movement, including laughing or coughing, may aggravate the pain. The nerve pressure can also cause numbness in an affected body area. Muscle spasms in the low back (lumbar) region may prevent bending or rising. The pain may be relieved by lying on the side that is not affected and holding the painful leg in a flexed position. In some cases, the **knee-jerk reflex** may be lost. Treatment for mild cases includes bed rest, painkillers, application of heat to the affected area, and exercises to strengthen the spinal and abdominal muscles. When the injury is severe enough to result in loss of nerve or muscle function, surgery is usually recommended to relieve the condition. A herniated disk in the neck area can be complicated by the loss of muscle control below the point of injury, including loss of control of the bladder and bowel, resulting in **incontinence.** *See also* **Cervical disk syndrome.**

Herpes   Any of a group of inflammatory skin diseases, usually recurrent, having one or more blisterlike lesions, such as a cold sore, caused by the herpes simplex virus. The cause is a virus (herpesvirus), a member of a group of infectious agents that also includes infectious mononucleosis, cytomegalovirus, and genital herpes. The virus that causes cold sores, or fever blisters, is sometimes identified as herpes simplex virus *Type 1,* while genital herpes is generally an infection of a *Type 2* herpes simplex virus. Herpes infections are highly contagious and can be dangerous. Type 1 herpes simplex infections may spread to the cornea of the eye, causing *herpes simplex keratitis,* with inflammation and scarring of the cornea, leading to a loss of vision.

Genital herpes, usually spread by sexual contact, may result in redness, itching, and soreness of the skin and mucous membranes of the genitalia and around the anus. Some studies have suggested an association between genital herpes and cervical cancer in women. Herpes infections tend to become dormant, and relapses often occur, particularly when the resistance of the infected person is low. Exposure to sunlight may be a cause of a recurrence of Type 1 herpes simplex. A drug, idoxuridine, has been used in the treatment of herpes simplex keratitis, and acyclovir has been reported to be successful in relieving the symptoms of herpes infections. *See also* **Herpes zoster.**

Herpes zoster (shingles)   A viral infection that causes a painful skin eruption that follows the path of nerves lying beneath the skin. The virus that causes the infection is the same one that is responsible for chickenpox in children, and the disease seems to affect only those who have had chickenpox several decades earlier. The virus is believed to lie dormant in spinal nerve complexes, waiting to surface again when the person's resistance is low. The condition is most common after the age of fifty and is not contagious. It may also occur in an individual whose immune system has been depressed by cancer or by radiation or other treatments administered because of cancer. Herpes zoster affects mainly the nerves of the skin and surrounding tissues supplied by the infected nerve fibers, especially the chest, lower back, neck, and face, particularly along the route of a nerve supplying the eye. An attack of herpes zoster usually begins with a period of several days of chills and fever, sometimes accompanied by gastrointestinal discomfort. Then, chickenpoxlike eruptions appear along the nerve pathways, usually on only one side of the body. The inflamed areas can be highly sensitive and painful. In about five days, the skin lesions begin to dry and form scabs. Most patients then recover with no serious aftereffects, and they are immune from further attacks. In severe cases, particularly in debilitated persons, symptoms of **neuralgia** may continue after the disease has run its course. If the cranial nerves are involved, the patient may experience **headache, vertigo, Bell's palsy, meningitis**, hearing disorders, and damage to the corneas of the eyes. There is no specific treatment for herpes zoster, and therapy is generally directed toward the relief of symptoms, with mild analgesics, wet compresses, and prescription drugs.

Hiatus hernia (diaphragmatic hernia)   The protrusion of a part of the stomach through the diaphragm, the muscular wall that separates the abdomen from the chest. The condition is relatively common, affecting up to 50 percent of the population after the age of sixty-five. Hiatus hernia is symptomless in most persons, but others feel either a deep, steady pain or an occasional "burning" pain (**heartburn**) in the chest. There also may be some degree of irritation of the esophagus that results from regurgitation of stomach acid, which is actually the result of a weakening of the sphincter muscle at the junction of the esophagus and stomach. The symptoms can be brought on by any action that increases pressure on the abdominal contents, such as lifting a heavy load, coughing, sneezing, bending forward, straining to defecate, wearing tight clothing, swallowing air, or lying down after a meal. In severe cases, irritation of the esophagus can produce bleeding, which may not be apparent but may be detected in laboratory analysis of fecal samples. Dysphagia may result from the discomfort of swallowing solid foods through an inflamed esophagus.

Complications include the severely painful strangulation (entrapment) of the herniated portion of the stomach above the diaphragm; the development of fibrous growths (strictures) that block the opening through the esophagus and make swallowing difficult; inhalation of stomach contents that may be regurgitated during sleep; and ulcerations of the esophagus. The distress of hiatus hernia is often relieved by sitting or standing, and by raising the head of the bed by about ten inches so that gravity helps prevent the reflux of stomach contents into the esophagus. Hiatus hernia can be diagnosed with X-rays of the chest after the person has swallowed a barium mixture; often a hiatus hernia can be seen on X-ray films taken without the use of barium.

Treatment includes dietary changes, which also may help reduce body weight and abdominal pressure that forces the stomach into the chest; eating nothing within three hours of bedtime; eating a small evening meal; and taking an antacid an hour or two after a meal. Besides helping to neutralize the acidity of the stomach juices, the antacid has the effect of helping close the sphincter muscle at the bottom of the esophagus, so there is less chance of regurgitation of stomach contents. Because most antacids are effective for only two or three hours after taking them, many experts recommend other medications, such as cimetidine, that can control the production of stomach acid for a much longer period of time. The use of alcohol, coffee, chocolate, and fatty foods is often curtailed, as these tend to aggravate the symptoms of hiatus hernia. Alternative measures include drugs and surgery.

High blood pressure *See* **Hypertension.**

Hip fracture A break in the upper leg bone (femur) or, rarely, one of the bones forming the hip joint. Hip fracture is one of the most common types of injury experienced by older adults, usually as the result of a fall. Postmenopausal women are twice as likely as men to suffer a hip fracture, with their vulnerability to fracture increased by **osteoporosis**. The risk of hip fracture also is higher for persons with **rheumatoid arthritis, diabetes, chronic obstructive pulmonary disease, epilepsy**, and **adrenal gland** disorders because these diseases can lead to **osteoporosis** or **osteomalacia**. Other factors may include the use of certain medications and alcohol abuse. The chances of hip fracture increase rapidly with aging; after the age of sixty-five, the incidence grows at a rate of 20 percent per year.

The degree of injury and disability depends in part on the exact location of the fracture. A break below the neck of the femur is more easily repaired than one at the head, where it forms a joint with the hipbone. A break at the joint can also damage the blood vessels, resulting in the death of surrounding tissues, including bone tissue in the head of the femur. Hip fracture causes immediate pain that may be felt from the knee to the groin or thigh. The involved leg is shortened and turned outward. The skin over the hip may be discolored by bleeding beneath the skin. Early surgical repair of the damage is necessary. Total recovery depends on the degree of damage and on other factors, including rehabilitation and motivation of the patient to regain mobility. On the average, about twelve weeks are required for a hip fracture to heal, with up to eight weeks in traction. When the head of the femur is damaged, it is usually replaced with an artificial part made of plastic or metal.

Rehabilitation is an important step following repair of a hip fracture. Physical therapy and other techniques are employed to ensure recovery of a range of motion and muscle power in both the involved and uninvolved joints after several months of severely restricted weight-bearing and physical activity. Rehabilitation is also necessary in training the person to be as self-sufficient as possible in maintaining the activities of daily living. The rehabilitation period may include training in self-sufficiency while confined to a bed and wheelchair, then moving about with the help of crutches or a metal walker, without and then with weight-bearing activities. In the final phase of rehabilitation, the patient may use a cane as an aid in walking. In some cases, the involved leg may be shorter when healed, requiring a shoe lift or other prosthesis so that limping will not result. Active rehabilitation techniques have contributed significantly toward lowering the mortality rate among hip fracture patients. In the first half of the twentieth century, hip fractures frequently led to complications of pneumonia, embolism, and kidney disorders among persons immobilized for several months, and the death rate from the complications was around 35 percent.

Homeostasis   The automatic maintenance of equilibrium in the body's tissues, systems, and functions. Sensing and control mechanisms keep such functions as body temperature, blood pressure, heartbeat, breathing rate, acid-base balance, and glandular secretions within relatively normal limits despite wide variations in external stimuli or other environmental influences.

Honeymoon paralysis   A form of abnormal sensation (**acroparesthesia**) caused by entrapment of the median nerve at the elbow by forceful turning of the forearm, such as by holding an object in the crook of the elbow. Pressure on the median nerve produces a sensation of tingling or numbness. The popular name for the disorder is suggested by the position of the arm held as in a lover's embrace. Also called "pronator syndrome."

Hormone changes with aging Alterations in endocrine gland activity that are associated with the aging process. Some alterations that would be abnormal in younger persons, such as dry skin and thinning of the hair due to reduced thyroid gland activity, are regarded as normal for older adults with no history of a thyroid deficiency. However, it is in the production of sex hormones that the effects of increasing age are most obvious. Estrogen production greatly diminishes, causing gradual atrophy of the female ovaries, uterus, and vaginal tissues. In healthy males, the main sex hormone (testosterone) either remains stable or declines only slightly with aging. However, many older men who suffer from chronic illnesses have very low testosterone levels. The testes decrease in size and become firmer, but the quality of the sperm is only slightly affected. Most healthy men retain their reproductive capacity throughout life. Although libido and sexual activity may be maintained, the physiology of the sexual response changes with age. Older men tend to rely more on tactile stimuli (as opposed to younger men who rely on visual stimuli) to be aroused, and it takes them longer first to achieve an erection and then to achieve an orgasm (ejaculation). Also, the ability to have a second erection soon after an orgasm declines with age. Alcohol and medications commonly used by older adults may have a greater effect on sexual behavior than do the hormonal changes that occur normally in the aging process. *See also* **Estrogen, sexual function changes with aging.**

Hot flashes (hot flushes) A sudden, temporary sensation of warmth, usually in the face, neck, and chest, experienced by most women during or after the **menopause.** It is often followed by profuse sweating. The hot flashes are believed to be an effect of changes in hormone production on automatic mechanisms that control blood flow, but the exact cause is unknown. Hot flashes may be annoying and, for some women, disabling, and their intensity, duration, and frequency vary considerably. Some women do not experience hot flashes at all. For others, they may continue for up to five years after the menopause.

Huntington's chorea (Huntington's disease) A chronic, slowly progressive hereditary disease marked by nervous system degeneration. Although the disease may be diagnosed at almost any age, the onset of symptoms usually does not begin until after forty. Affecting both sexes, the disorder is marked by involuntary jerking movements **(chorea)**, a lurching gait, and accompanying mental deterioration that culminates in death. Symptoms that first appear after the age of fifty may resemble those of **Parkinson's disease**, except that the muscle rigidity of parkinsonism is usually absent. Death usually occurs within fifteen years.

Hydration The intake of an adequate amount of water to maintain a normal **fluid balance** in the body. Proper fluid intake is important in maintaining **acid-base balance**, avoiding the hazards of **acidosis** or **alkalosis**, and in maintaining the necessary fluid volume for blood and lymph circulation. The human body is approximately 60 percent water and requires an average intake of about 2.5 quarts per day, depending on the climate and the health of the person, in order to balance a similar amount of water lost through excretion, sweating, and breathing. A loss of 20 percent of the body's water without replacement can be fatal. Individuals taking certain medications require more than the average daily intake for proper hydration. Older people frequently become dehydrated without being aware of a significant fluid loss from **diarrhea, fever,** vomiting, **heat stroke,** or other causes. A low-grade fever (less than 100.5° F.) can account for an unperceived loss of a quart of fluid daily, while a high fever can result in a loss of two quarts of fluid each day. Some older people fail to maintain an adequate water intake by having an early dinner and drinking no fluids for the rest of the evening so as to reduce the urge to get out of bed during the night in order to urinate. They may not become thirsty and may not be aware that their bodies need more fluid.

Hydrocephalus A disorder marked by an accumulation of cerebrospinal fluid in one of the ventricles (open areas) of the brain. The type of hydrocephalus that affects older adults is called *normal pressure hydrocephalus,* to distinguish it from the condition that occurs in infants. When more than one ventricle is involved, the condition is identified as *communicating hydrocephalus.* The adult form of hydrocephalus is usually due to a hemorrhage, tumor, or brain infection that causes scarring or similar tissue damage, blocking the normal absorption of the fluid. The accumulation of fluid causes pressure on brain tissue, affecting such functions as walking and memory, and results in a shuffling gait and a declining ability to think clearly. The symptoms may develop gradually over a period of several months. As the condition progresses, there may be urinary incontinence. Because nerve control of the legs is affected, the person may spend much of his time in bed or sitting in a chair. Attempts at walking may appear clumsy and result in falls. Some patients can be treated by installation of a shunt that drains the excess cerebrospinal fluid from the brain.

Hypercalcemia A greater than normal amount of calcium in the blood, frequently associated with bone disorders such as **Paget's disease,** that cause a loss of calcium from the skeleton. The condition may also result from a hormone disease, particularly one involving an excess of thyroid or parathyroid hormone; excessive use of vitamins A and D; lack of physical activity due to immobilization; use of certain diuretic drugs; diseases such as tuberculosis; or an excessive intake of calcium and alkalis during treatment for a peptic ulcer. The major symptoms include fatigue, lethargy, weakness, thirst, and itching. There may also be nausea and vomiting, loss of appetite and weight loss, constipation, swallowing difficulty, and increased urinary frequency. Although hypercalcemia can occur at any age, it reaches a peak among men and women in their forties, and more than one-third of all patients are over the age of sixty. Because mild hypercalcemia, marked by symptoms of vomiting and increased urination, can lead to dangerous dehydration, increased intake of fluids is one of the primary steps in treatment of hypercalcemia. Therapy also involves control of the specific cause. An **electrolyte** imbalance often accompanies hypercalcemia, requiring replacement of such minerals as potassium and magnesium. Specific drugs are available to lower calcium levels in the blood and to halt the loss of calcium from bone tissue, depending upon the specific cause of hypercalcemia.

Hypercapnia   A condition of excessive carbon dioxide in the blood, as occurs in respiratory **acidosis**. *See also* **Hypocapnia.**

Hyperkalemia   An excess of potassium in the blood. A common cause of the disorder in older adults is dehydration associated with decreased kidney function. Symptoms are nausea, diarrhea, muscle weakness, and an irregular heartbeat. Uncorrected, hyperkalemia can lead to **cardiac arrest**, ventricular **fibrillation**, and death. Treatment depends on the severity and cause and may include medications and rehydration (replacement of body fluids).

Hypernatremia   An excess of sodium in the blood. The condition often develops in older adults who become dehydrated because of failure to drink enough liquids to maintain a normal fluid balance, particularly in situations of profuse sweating, vomiting, diarrhea, or frequent urination. The person may complain of thirst while showing drowsiness, lethargy, and confusion. If uncorrected, the condition may progress to stupor, seizures, and coma. Diagnosis is usually based on laboratory analysis of a blood sample, which determines the person's **electrolyte** balance, including sodium concentration. From the electrolyte balance, a mathematical formula can be used to indicate the amount of water needed to restore the person's normal state of **hydration**.

Hyperopia (farsightedness) A visual disorder in which the light rays reflected from an object fail to form a sharp image on the retina because of an abnormality in the lens or the shape of the eyeball. A defect in the lens due to aging *(acquired hyperopia)* or a disease, such as diabetes, bends the light rays entering the eye so that the rays strike the retina before they become sharply focused (the rays would theoretically be focused at a point beyond the retina). A similar effect results when the diameter of the eyeball, measured between the lens and the retina, is abnormally short *(axial hyperopia).* The hyperopic person receives a visual image that is indistinct. In some cases, the eye can automatically compensate for the error by the process of **accommodation,** in which the eye muscles can alter the focal length by changing the shape of the lens slightly. But accommodation also may be diminished as one grows older, and hyperopia must be corrected with eyeglasses or contact lenses that compensate for the individual errors in vision. Also called "hypermetropia" and "longsightedness." *See also* **Myopia.**

Hypersplenism An abnormal condition characterized by an enlarged spleen and a blood disorder that may include anemia, a deficiency of white blood cells, or a combination of blood cell disorders. Hypersplenism is usually associated with another disease, such as **amyloidosis, cirrhosis, sarcoidosis,** or **tuberculosis.** Symptoms include left-side abdominal pain, a feeling of fullness after eating a small amount of food, and bleeding beneath the skin and mucous membranes. The abdominal pain and premature stomach fullness are caused by pressure of the enlarged spleen against the stomach. Treatment is directed toward the underlying disease. *See also* **Felty's syndrome.**

Hypertension (high blood pressure) Blood pressure that is elevated above certain predetermined levels. It is usually measured as systolic and/or diastolic pressure, on three separate occasions to confirm that the elevation is persistent and not a temporary condition due to such factors as concern about undergoing a blood pressure checkup. Systolic blood pressure is the pressure produced in the arteries by the push of blood resulting from the contraction of the heart's left lower chamber (left ventricle). Diastolic pressure is the pressure of blood in the same arteries when the heart is relaxing between contractions. In younger adults, hypertension is sometimes defined as blood pressure that is persistently higher than 140/90, where 140 represents the systolic pressure and 90 the diastolic pressure. Some experts use a higher level of 160/95 as the benchmark for persons over the age of sixty-five. Hypertension cases are usually classified as *primary* (or *essential*), when the precise cause is unknown, or *secondary,* when the condition is the result of an underlying disorder, such as an **adrenal gland** tumor or a kidney disease.

More than 15 percent of the general population suffers from hypertension, and nearly 90 percent of those are afflicted with primary hypertension. Blacks are twice as likely as whites to develop hypertension, and the death rate from hypertension also is higher for blacks, although the reason for the difference is not yet known. Because it usually causes no symptoms, millions of people are not aware that they have the condition, which is usually discovered during routine medical examinations. Untreated, hypertension can lead to **coronary artery disease, congestive heart failure, stroke, aortic aneurysm**, and other cardiovascular diseases. The risk of such diseases increases with each year as one grows beyond middle age.

Secondary hypertension is treated by correcting the underlying cause. Treatment of primary hypertension depends mainly upon diet and drugs. Because older adults are more likely to experience adverse effects from drugs used to lower high blood pressure, doctors often try to encourage treatments such as weight loss and low-salt diets rather than drugs as a first step. Drugs used include **diuretics, beta-adrenergic** blockers, medications that suppress the body's neurotransmitter substances, which can raise blood pressure, and combinations of drugs. There is no "cure" for primary hypertension, and a drugs-and-diet regimen must be continued indefinitely to reduce the risk of stroke, heart attack, or other complications. Because the condition is generally symptomless, the hypertensive patient is also encouraged to learn to monitor his or her own blood pressure regularly with one of the commercially available devices sold for that purpose. The hypertensive person is also advised to report to a doctor periodically for more authoritative blood pressure testing. *See also* **Hypertensive crisis.**

Hypertensive crisis A condition of severe **hypertension** in which systolic blood pressure may be higher than 200 and diastolic pressure is greater than 120 (200/120). It is an emergency situation that requires immediate medical care to lower the blood pressure. The symptoms vary but may include severe headache, confusion, seizures, vomiting, partial paralysis, coma if the brain is affected, or intense pain in the chest and back if the extreme hypertension has caused an **aortic aneurysm**. A hypertensive crisis can also be triggered by consuming certain foods and beverages, such as aged cheese and Chianti wine, while taking **monoamine oxidase (MAO) inhibitor** drugs for the treatment of depression.

Hyperthyroidism A condition of excessive thyroid hormone secretion associated with a **goiter**, an inflamed thyroid gland, a benign thyroid tumor, or the use of iodine or thyroid hormone medications. Hyperthyroidism is sometimes accompanied by goiter, **exophthalmos,** or pretibial myxedema (a swelling of the legs); the condition is sometimes called **Graves' disease,** one of the most common of at least ten types of hyperthyroidism. The exact cause of hyperthyroidism is unknown, but the Graves' disease form is believed to result from genetic factors that affect the immune system. About one-third of all cases of hyperthyroidism occur in older adults, and women are afflicted with the disorder more often than men.

Hyperthyroidism may occur with a wide range of symptoms, some of which could be misinterpreted as those of a different disease. They may include a very rapid heartbeat **(tachycardia),** palpitations, atrial **fibrillation,** fatigue, weakness, mental confusion, and weight loss. Many symptoms associated with hyperthyroidism in younger patients are relatively infrequent in older adults, indicating that the type of hyperthyroidism that may afflict individuals over the age of forty differs in origin. The older adult often shows symptoms of depression and apathy as psychological effects. Treatment includes the use of antithyroid and **beta-adrenergic** drugs and radioactive iodine, which causes a gradual destruction of excess thyroid gland cells. Surgery may be recommended for patients with very large goiters or for those who cannot be treated with more conservative measures.

Hyperventilation   Abnormally deep and rapid breathing that leads to a depletion of carbon dioxide in the blood **(hypocapnia)** and respiratory **alkalosis.** Causes may include a **neurological disorder, hypoxia, hypoglycemia,** or exposure to toxic chemicals such as ethylene glycol or methyl alcohol. The condition also may be caused by an emotional disorder, such as anxiety, often with the person unaware of the abnormal breathing pattern. The rapid breathing causes faintness, tingling of the arms and legs, headache, blurred vision, and loss of consciousness. Hyperventilation caused by an emotional disorder can be relieved by having the person breathe into a paper bag, thereby inhaling the exhaled carbon dioxide and restoring the balance of blood gases.

Hypnotic   Any of a group of drugs used to induce sleep because they are able to produce partial or complete loss of consciousness. Hypnotics work by inhibiting the reception of sensory impulses by the higher brain centers, blunting the person's awareness of the environment, thus producing a hypnotic effect that helps induce sleep. Hypnotics are often combined with an analgesic to dull the feeling of any ache or pain that might interfere with sleep. Dangers of hypnotics include addiction and a cross-tolerance with each other and with alcohol: As a person becomes increasingly dependent upon any hypnotic, barbiturate, or nonbarbiturate, one of the drugs can be freely substituted for another to suppress withdrawal symptoms, and hypnotics can be used to suppress the withdrawal symptoms of alcoholism, or vice versa. Individuals who consume alcohol in more than moderate amounts may require a larger than usual dose of a hypnotic drug to induce drowsiness. Also, because alcohol and hypnotics can have a synergistic effect, they should not be used at the same time. Their combined effect can result in death.

Hypocapnia A deficiency of carbon dioxide in the blood, as may result from excessive rapid breathing (**hyperventilation**).

Hypoglycemia A deficiency of sugar (glucose) in the blood. The condition can result from several causes, including excess production of insulin by the pancreas or an overdose of insulin or oral hypoglycemic (antidiabetic) drugs in the treatment of **diabetes mellitus**. A common cause of hypoglycemia in older adults is the consumption of too much alcohol and not enough food. This results in a depletion of blood sugar due to an inadequate food intake and the alcohol's suppression of glucose synthesis by the liver. Some individuals may show symptoms of hypoglycemia after a few days of fasting or starvation. When a hypoglycemic person has the odor of alcohol on his or her breath, the condition is often mistaken for intoxication, and proper treatment is delayed. Hypoglycemia produces symptoms of fatigue, restlessness, irritability, weakness, delirium, and coma. There may be rapid and shallow breathing and a bounding pulse. Because the brain cells are heavily dependent upon a supply of sugar (glucose) for their functions, persistent hypoglycemia can cause permanent brain damage similar to that of oxygen starvation (anoxia) or death. Hypoglycemia can cause temporary periods of tremor, double vision, loss of muscle coordination, temporary partial paralysis, and difficulty in speaking or understanding speech. In some cases, hypoglycemia can mimic **epilepsy**. When a person shows the physical signs of hypoglycemia and responds to the intake of sugar or food, the diagnostic technique is also the treatment. When the hypoglycemic person is unable to swallow food, or even sugar in water or fruit juice, glucose may be administered intravenously.

Hypotension Abnormally low blood pressure. The term is often applied in identifying a condition in which the blood pressure falls rapidly when a person suddenly rises from a sitting or lying position *(orthostatic* or *postural hypotension)*. The shift of blood volume to lower parts of the body can quickly drain blood from the brain, causing a temporary feeling of faintness, a blurring of vision, falling, and, in some cases, a loss of consciousness. Factors that can aggravate the condition include a warm room, anemia, physical weakness, and a squatting position, which depletes the blood supply in the legs before rising. The cardiovascular system of a young person reacts quickly to compensate for the hypotension effect, but as one grows older this mechanism becomes impaired, so that a person who gets out of bed too quickly in the morning may fall on the floor. Getting out of a hot bath suddenly can have a similar effect. A number of medications, including antidepressants, blood vessel dilators, tranquilizers, and diuretics, as well as alcoholic beverages, can increase the risk of hypotension for some older adults. In some cases of hypotension, the drop in blood pressure does not occur until several minutes after the person first stands or until he begins walking. The person may then experience a **"drop attack,"** falling to the floor where he or she may remain, conscious or unconscious, until recovering from the effect. Mild cases of hypotension can usually be treated with drugs or by changing the dosages of medication that may contribute to the condition.

Hypothermia A condition in which the body temperature falls below 95° Fahrenheit (35° Celsius), usually as a result of exposure to cold weather or immersion in very cold water. Older adults are particularly susceptible to hypothermia in cold weather because of age-related impairments in the body's ability to compensate for temperature changes in the environment. Low body temperatures usually do not develop suddenly but are acquired through hours or days of exposure to cool temperatures, often in homes where the room temperature is between 60° to 65° Fahrenheit, perhaps in order to conserve fuel. The situation may be complicated by a diminished awareness of the temperature around one, poor nutrition, reduced physical activity, and an age-related loss of the shivering response to cold. Sedatives, certain other medications, and use of alcohol also contribute to a failed perception that the body temperature has fallen dangerously low.

There is further danger in that as the body temperature drifts lower, toward 90° Fahrenheit (32° Celsius), the individual becomes drowsy, apathetic, confused, and weak. Shivering is absent and the body is cold to the touch. Heart rate, blood pressure, and respirations are subnormal, and the person may fall into a stupor and then into a coma. Mild cases of hypothermia are often treated by placing the victim in a warm room and allowing the body temperature to rise gradually and normally. In severe cases, rapid rewarming may be achieved by placing the patient in a warm-water bath or by covering him or her with a heating blanket. Antibiotics and other medications may be given as needed;

antibiotics are often recommended as a preventive measure, under the assumption that the hypothermia patient may have acquired an infection before or during the period of abnormally low body temperature. Hypothermia is often misdiagnosed initially because a fever thermometer does not register readings below 94° Fahrenheit.

Hypothyroidism (myxedema)   A deficiency of thyroid hormone. The condition may develop as a result of loss of thyroid gland tissue, a tumor, or from impaired thyroid function, which may be due to disease or as a reaction to treatment for **hyperthyroidism**. Post-therapeutic hypothyroidism, following surgery or radioactive iodine (RAI) therapy for hyperthyroidism, is the second most common form of the disorder. The incidence of **iatrogenic** hypothyroidism (caused by hyperthyroid treatment) increases with the aging of the population, as does the risk of *primary* hypothyroidism, which is believed to be an **autoimmune** disorder. Although **goiter** is usually associated with hyperthyroidism, it may also be present in rare cases of hypothyroidism.

The symptoms of hypothyroidism (dry skin, constipation, loss of hearing, depression, intolerance to cold, and a general slowing of mental and physical activity) are subtle and often mistaken as "signs of aging." There may be weight loss, facial swelling with fluid accumulation (edema) under the skin, hair that becomes coarse and thick and tends to fall out, skin pigment changes, and brittle nails. In a few cases, particularly when primary hypothyroidism is involved, the person has a family history of thyroid disorders. Laboratory analysis of blood samples helps determine the type of hypothyroidism causing the symptoms.

Treatment of mild hypothyroidism is by slow replenishment of thyroid hormone over a period of several weeks; in almost all cases, thyroid hormone replacement must be continued for the rest of the life of the person. It may take several months to establish an optimum level of thyroid medications for a patient, and periodic blood measurements of thyroid hormone levels are recommended so that dosages can be adjusted. An excessive level of certain drugs may produce symptoms of heart disorders. A potential complication of hypothyroidism is myxedema coma, which is more likely to occur in cold climates. It can lead to severe **hypothermia** and death.

Hypovolemia   Abnormally diminished blood volume. The causes include **hemorrhage** and fluid loss from burns and from gastrointestinal disorders accompanied by vomiting and diarrhea. A reduction in blood volume of 15 to 25 percent usually causes rapid breathing and heartbeat, pale skin, and, in some cases, brain damage. A condition of hypovolemic shock, which could lead to death, will occur with a greater reduction. *See also* **Ketoacidosis.**

Hypoxemia   A condition of oxygen deficiency in the blood. It results in symptoms of confusion, weakness, rapid heartbeat, and feelings of faintness in mild cases, with loss of consciousness in severe cases. Causes may include **myocardial infarction**, pulmonary **embolism**, other pulmonary diseases, acute mountain sickness (breathing difficulty at high altitudes), or working in a confined space where the oxygen supply has been reduced. The term is sometimes applied to conditions caused by exposure to diseases and toxic chemicals that reduce the ability of the red blood cells to carry a normal proportion of oxygen molecules, or disorders involving substances, such as hydrogen cyanide, that prevent the tissue cells from utilizing the oxygen molecules carried to them by the blood. The condition may be complicated by respiratory disorders.

Hysterectomy   The surgical removal of the uterus. The operation may be performed to eliminate a uterine disorder (particularly near the end of a woman's fertile years or after the menopause) such as a prolapsed uterus, a cancer or a precancerous condition, severe endometriosis, hemorrhage, fibroids, or an intractable infection, such as pelvic inflammatory disease. The uterus may be removed through the vagina or through an incision in the abdomen. The uterus may be removed with the cervix, in a *total hysterectomy,* or with the ovaries, fallopian tubes, and associated tissues, in a *radical hysterectomy.* Total hysterectomy is more common in younger women who want to continue ovarian function and maintain natural estrogen levels, while a radical hysterectomy is done more often in women who are past their childbearing years or who do not want more children. In some cases, a hysterectomy may be the method of choice for sterilization when there is also a uterine disorder, or it may be combined with a cesarean section in which the fetus and uterus are removed together. Menstruation ceases with the removal of the uterus.

Hysteria (hysterical neurosis)   A psychological disorder usually marked by emotional disturbances and the expression of unconscious conflicts in terms of physical disabilities. The hysterical person may convert these conflicts into symptoms of paralysis, loss of vision, pain, lack of feeling in a part of the body, or other conditions. The physical disorders have no organic basis and are not substantiated by appropriate diagnostic tests. A person with hysterical blindness, for example, is found to have eyes that react normally to light, and the individual may show a remarkable ability to avoid harmful situations, such as bumping into objects. Hysteria is usually a chronic condition and occurs more frequently in women than in men. Treatment is individualized, but generally depends upon one or more forms of psychotherapy and may include psychoanalysis or hypnosis to explore possible causes in the subconscious. More conservative measures, such as family therapy or a change in the person's working or living environment, may also be employed.

I

Iatrogenic Any unintentional adverse health effect, physical or mental, that may result from treatment by a physician or surgeon. The term is sometimes broadly interpreted to include anxiety-related disorders that result from comments made by a health professional, as when a patient mistakenly believes he has heart trouble because of the questions asked by an examining physician. Examples of other iatrogenic disorders are a staphylococcus (bacteria) infection acquired during a hospital stay and hypothyroidism that results from a treatment for hyperthyroidism.

Ideational apraxia Loss of the ability to perform a sequence of related actions to their conclusion because of a failure to visualize the end result of these actions. The disorder is often due to a disease or injury affecting the dominant hemisphere of the brain, and the effect may be mistakenly dismissed as "absentmindedness." For example, the person may begin mixing ingredients for a meal but fail to follow through with the plan and do something entirely different.

Identity crisis The loss of the ability to perceive of oneself as a particular individual with a specific role in a society. The condition may develop in older adults during periods of confusion or disorientation. Recovery from surgery, particularly heart surgery, is frequently a period of disorientation and may even be accompanied by hallucinatory experiences. An identity crisis can be complicated by **dementia** or by reactions to certain medications that distort sensory perceptions. The term is also used to identify a form of anxiety experienced by late adolescents who find it difficult to make decisions regarding their role in society, career goals, sexual behavior, and religious and cultural loyalties.

Idiopathic Pertaining to a disease or other disorder that appears to have developed spontaneously or without a known cause. (Use of the term often persists after the cause of the disease has been identified.) Examples include idiopathic **hypotension**, idiopathic fibrosis of the lungs, and the idiopathic **dyskinesias**, or abnormal movements of the voluntary muscles that occur without an obvious cause.

Ileitis An inflammation of the ileum, the last segment of the small intestine before the beginning of the large intestine. It accounts for nearly one-third of the cases of regional enteritis. The condition affects both men and women and seems more likely to occur in certain families. The symptoms, which usually begin before the age of forty, include abdominal pain, fever, diarrhea, loss of appetite, and weight loss. **Crohn's disease** is a form of the disorder in which diseased segments of the ileum and other parts of the intestine, marked by ulcerlike lesions of the intestinal lining with underlying lymph nodules, are separated by normal areas of intestine. In complicated cases, there may be ulceration, abscesses, and adhesions. The disease is usually diagnosed with X-rays after barium has been introduced into the intestine. There is no known cure as yet for the chronic form of the disorder, but some relief of symptoms is offered by antibiotics, corticosteroids, and immunosuppressive drugs, special diets, and surgery. *See also* **Abdominal pain, Acute abdomen, Diverticulosis.**

Illusion A distorted sensory perception or a misinterpretation of a sensation or perception. An illusion may or may not be a normal sensation. The visual illusion of railroad tracks coming closer together in the distance is normal, as are illusions of time, in which events seem to pass faster or more slowly than is actually occurring. An older person may experience illusions as a symptom of a perceptual disorder, particularly when under stress or in an unfamiliar situation, or as the result of an organic brain disease. A moving curtain may be mistaken for a person entering the room, or an inanimate object may be seen as an animal or insect, while misidentification of individuals, with strangers mistaken for old friends or relatives, is relatively common. There also may be memory illusions, in which the older person may recall in detail past experiences of others as if they were his or her own, and a condition sometimes called "illusion of mastery" in which a person may feel in control of a situation as long as others are available to help in an emergency.

Immobility A loss of the normal ability to move the body or a limb of the body because of a disorder involving the muscles, bones, nerves, or cardiovascular system. Among the many conditions leading to immobility are **arthritis, osteoporosis, stroke, Parkinson's disease, angina pectoris, intermittent claudication**, visual impairment, pulmonary diseases, mental disorders, and the adverse effects of drugs. **Osteoarthritis**, and leg and foot problems, including **bunions, calluses**, and foot infections, are the most common causes of immobility among older adults. Psychological conditions, such as **depression** and fear of **falls**, may render many persons voluntarily immobile, leading them to spend much of their time in bed or in a chair. Sedatives, tranquilizers, and other drugs that cause drowsiness, lethargy, and loss of coordination can induce immobility in those who may be physically unimpaired. Immobility in itself can be a cause of deteriorating health in older adults, because lack of physical activity can lead to degenerative processes affecting many organ systems. With inactivity, muscle tissue atrophies, bones lose calcium, the skin is subject to pressure sores, the heart loses tone, emboli may form in the blood vessels, lung function deteriorates, appetite fails, and constipation develops, kidney stones form, and the risk of urinary infection increases. A number of metabolic disorders can result from immobility, including osteoporosis, **electrolyte** imbalance, and impaired glucose tolerance. In addition to deconditioning of the heart, immobility results in decreased blood volume; together the changes become a cause of **hypotension**, which can complicate efforts to make the person more physically active.

Immobilization paralysis A type of hysterical immobility in which a person is unable to move an arm or leg he or she believes to be paralyzed. The limb may have been injured and splinted previously but has now healed, although the patient fails to recognize that mobility has been restored. In a test for immobilization paralysis of a leg, the patient lies face up on a table and the examiner stands at the foot, holding the patient's heels, and asks him or her to lift the paralyzed leg. In a true case of paralysis, the heel of the healthy leg will press downward as part of the effort to lift the paralyzed leg. In hysterical paralysis, the unaffected leg does not press downward. If treated early, usually by psychotherapy, there is no significant wasting of muscle tissue as a result of **immobility** and no loss of deep reflexes, in contrast to paralysis due to organic causes.

Immune deficiency A lack of normal resistance to disease, due to failure of the body's immune system, particularly to infections, cancers, and a group of **autoimmune diseases** that includes **rheumatoid arthritis**.

The immune system is composed of a complex organization of antibodies that react with specific **antigens** (allergens) and cells that destroy invading organisms such as bacteria. It includes two types of white blood cells (lymphocytes) that provide the body's primary response to an infection. They are known as *B cells,* which acquire their ability to fight infections in bone marrow, and *T cells,* which derive their potential for resisting infections from the thymus gland. About 70 percent of the white cells circulating in the blood are T cells, and the remaining 30 percent are B cells. On contact with an antigen, a T cell undergoes a rapid cloning process, reproducing itself many times but in a variety of forms that attack antigens in different ways. Some forms secrete substances poisonous to bacteria; others destroy bacterial cell walls; and still others produce interferon, a substance that attacks viruses, or stimulate B cells to produce antibodies or immunoglobulins, proteins that are capable of neutralizing foreign substances in the blood.

The immune system normally identifies substances in the body as "self" or "nonself" (foreign), and attacks viruses, bacteria, or other foreign matter, including allergens. Some T cells serve as "memory cells," with an ability to recognize and react to a specific antigen that has appeared previously in the person's body. As one grows older, the immune system tends to lose some of its effectiveness, making older people more susceptible to infections that younger persons are usually able to resist. It is believed that immune deficiency also may account for the increased rate of cancers and some arthritic diseases in older persons, as defective or diminished immune factors become less able to distinguish between tissues that are "self" and "nonself" and to destroy abnormal or foreign tissue substances. The immune deficiency that occurs with aging has been measured in terms of both the quality and quantity of immune factors. The number of naturally occurring antibodies that resist bacteria is significantly lower. Because they acquire immunity factors from the thymus gland, the T cells decline as the thymus atrophies, beginning in early adulthood. By middle age, the thymus has shrunk to less than 20 percent of its original size, and by age sixty, its secretions, which are believed to stimulate immune activity of T cells, are no longer detectable. *See also* **Immunologic theory of aging.**

Immunologic theory of aging A concept that a breakdown of the body's immune system accounts for much of the aging process. Experts supporting the theory note that as one grows older, the body's resistance to infections declines. The B and T cell lymphocytes (white blood cells) of the immune system, which are primarily responsible for attacking and destroying bacteria, viruses, and other foreign substances that enter the body, diminish in number and activity as one grows older and no longer protect the tissues as in earlier years. In some cases, the immune system turns against the body's own normal tissues, misidentifies them as foreign substances, and attacks the tissues, producing **autoimmune diseases** in the form of some **cancers, rheumatoid arthritis**, and other degenerative diseases. *See also* **Immune deficiency.**

Impotence   The inability to achieve or to maintain a penile erection. True impotence has been further defined as an inability to maintain an erection strong enough to achieve vaginal penetration in at least three-fourths of attempts and for the condition to persist for two months or more, to distinguish the dysfunction from a temporary episode that may affect any adult male. The extent of sexual dysfunctions among older men is difficult to determine because of the reluctance of many men to seek medical help for the problem. However, various studies indicate that impotence is relatively rare before the age of forty-five but then becomes increasingly common, so that it may affect 50 percent of men over the age of seventy-five. This male sexual dysfunction may be due to any of a number of organic and psychological factors. In some cases, there is actually diminished frequency rather than actual impotence. Factors contributing to impotence include excessive use of alcohol, certain medications, monotony in the sexual relationship, a lack of privacy, anxiety about the ability to perform adequately, preoccupation with work or other problems, fatigue, and circulatory, neurological, or endocrine (hormone) disorders. Circulatory disorders, such as partial obstruction of blood flow to the ileofemoral (legs and lower pelvic) area, resulting in restriction of the flow of blood into the spongy tissue of the penis, are believed to account for a few cases of impotence in older men. **Neurological disorders**, caused by surgery, injury, alcoholism, or diseases such as **diabetes mellitus**, may be responsible for an additional 10 to 20 percent of cases of impotence. Nearly any medication that affects the **autonomic nervous system** may interfere with a man's ability to achieve an erection. These include barbiturates and other sedatives, tranquilizers, antihistamines, antidepressants, and many diuretics and other drugs prescribed for the treatment of **hypertension**. In some cases, a change in medication can solve the problem. Endocrine (hormone) causes include diseases of the thyroid, adrenal, parathyroid, and pituitary glands. Adequate production of testosterone (male sex hormone) by the testes is essential for maintenance of sexual potency. Reduced production of testosterone by the testes is a cause of impotence. In the diagnosis of the cause of impotence, one test is the ability of a man to have an erection while asleep. If he can achieve an erection during sleep, he is most likely suffering from impotence caused by psychological factors. One method of treating many cases of impotence caused by an organic disorder is the surgical implanting of a penile prosthesis, if the organic disorder fails to respond to other therapies.

Inanition   A condition of exhaustion caused by severe malnutrition, leading to structural and functional changes in the body's tissues and organ systems. Inanition may develop from fasting, **anorexia**, or dieting that does not provide for proper amounts of all necessary nutrients. The condition can also result from digestive or metabolic disorders that interfere with normal digestion and absorption of nutrients, or from diseases or injuries, particularly burns, that require increased amounts of certain nutrients daily. The major symptom of inanition is emaciation from severe weight loss. The skin becomes thin, dry, pale, and cold, and the hair is dry and loose. Because of weight loss, some bones may protrude through the skin. There is gonadal atrophy with loss of interest in sex, the heart becomes smaller and beats more slowly, and the breathing rate is reduced. The liver, intestines, and kidneys may be permanently damaged. Diarrhea is common and may be fatal. Treatment requires slow and careful restoration of body tissues and functions by small, bland, fat-free feedings until digestive function has been restored and diarrhea controlled.

Inappropriate antidiuretic hormone (ADH) secretion   An abnormal condition marked by a failure of the kidneys to excrete excess fluid from the body. As the name of the disorder suggests, the problem is caused by excessive secretion of the antidiuretic hormone, whose normal function is to help the body conserve water by causing the kidney to reabsorb fluid instead of excreting it. The malfunction can be caused by a number of factors, including a **tumor**, a lung disease such as **tuberculosis** or **pneumonia**, a central nervous system disorder such as **stroke**, or certain drugs, including sedatives, antidepressants, certain hypoglycemic agents used to treat diabetes, and nicotine. The condition results in a sodium deficiency in the blood (**hyponatremia**), with symptoms of nausea and vomiting, loss of appetite, drowsiness, irritability, muscle weakness, confusion, seizures, and coma. If uncorrected, the condition can be fatal. Inappropriate ADH secretion can occur at any age, but the risk increases as one grows older. Treatment is directed toward correction of the underlying cause, which may requiring discontinuing or changing a medication, reducing water intake, or the use of special drugs that increase water excretion without an accompanying loss of sodium.

Inborn error of metabolism   An abnormal health condition caused by an inherited lack of an enzyme needed for one or more steps of metabolism of a particular substance orginating in the diet. As a result, the person's body is unable to tolerate certain foods. Depending upon the particular enzyme that is missing, the disorders can range from mild to disabling to, in some cases, fatal. Poisonous by-products may accumulate in the body, producing symptoms of **diabetes,** mental retardation, a kidney disorder such as **Fanconi's syndrome,** muscle atrophy, lethargy, and skeletal abnormalities. Many inherited metabolic disorders have their onset in childhood, but others, such as **porphyria cutanea tarda** and hemochromatosis, both associated with iron metabolism, may not produce symptoms until middle age or later.

Incontinence   An inability to voluntarily retain urine or feces, usually because of a loss of control of the sphincter muscles that open and close the urethra or rectum. Incontinence may be due to a disease or injury involving the brain or spinal cord, or to many other conditions. *Urinary incontinence* is sometimes classified according to types and causes, such as stress, urge, overflow, functional, and total incontinence. *Stress incontinence* is marked by leakage of small amounts of urine that occurs during coughing, laughing, or sneezing and results from increased abdominal pressure in a person with sphincter weakness (urine is normally retained by maintaining a sphincter pressure that is greater than the fluid pressure of urine accumulated in the bladder). *Urge incontinence* identifies leakage of urine caused by an inability to delay urination after the urge to void develops, as when there is no easily available toilet. Urge incontinence tends to occur in persons with central nervous system damage, such as dementia or parkinsonism, or in those with a genitourinary tract disorder, including a bladder tumor, kidney stones, urethritis, or vaginitis. *Overflow incontinence* may occur in a person with an impaired ability to sense fullness of the bladder due to an anatomic obstruction, spinal cord injury, or the use of certain medications that affect the nervous system. Cases of *functional* and *total incontinence* are more likely to occur in institutionalized patients, particularly those with psychological disorders or impaired mobility who may be unwilling or unable to reach a toilet when the need arises. In some cases, involuntary urination occurs when a patient requires help from a hospital or nursing home attendant to reach a toilet but such help is late in arriving.

Urinary incontinence increases with age and is somewhat more common in women, who are more likely to suffer from sphincter or pelvic weakness. Urinary incontinence can range from occasional minor dribbling to a continuous flow. Effects of aging on the urinary bladder include a smaller capacity, a loss in the urethral sphincter function that normally helps retain urine in the bladder, and an increase in involuntary bladder contractions. In older women, the condition may involve a decreased level of estrogen, leading to **senile vaginitis** and painful or difficult urination, and a weakening of the pelvic tissues that often results from childbearing. In men, a complicating factor may be an enlarged prostate gland, which increases the urge to urinate, or weakness of the genitourinary structures following prostate surgery.

For some persons, the problem may be further complicated by **immobility** or infections of the urinary tract. Factors that are controllable include involuntary bladder contractions that can be treated with medications. Other drugs, particularly diuretics and sedatives, sometimes contribute to urinary incontinence by increasing the flow of urine into the bladder while diminishing the awareness of the need to urinate. Corrective measures may include the use of the newer launderable or disposable absorbent undergarments and bed pads, bladder-retraining programs (especially for persons affected by stroke or similar impairment), **Kegel exercises** for women, estrogens for women with urethritis and vaginitis, mechanical and electronic devices, and surgical repair of the bladder neck, which may be performed with a local anesthetic.

Some older persons with a serious problem of urinary incontinence also suffer from *fecal incontinence,* which is relatively uncommon otherwise. They are usually persons suffering from dementia or spinal cord or other nerve damage and who have a complete lack of control of the urethral or anal sphincters. In persons with organic brain disease, concomitant incontinence may begin occasionally at night and become generally constant as the mental condition of the person deteriorates. Fecal incontinence is also associated with **constipation**, abuse of laxatives, disease or damage involving the large intestine, and **neurological disorders**. Constipation can be a cause of fecal incontinence when impacted feces irritate the rectum, resulting in a release of fluid and mucus around the fecal impaction. Some of the same factors that contribute to urinary incontinence apply to fecal incontinence, because both conditions can be influenced by defects in coordination of nerve and muscle reflexes; diminished mental alertness due to drugs, dementia, or stroke; and physical difficulties in getting to a toilet.

Independent living   The ability to maintain self-sufficiency so that a person can perform all or most of the activities required for maintaining a home, occupation, or avocation, as well as mobility between the home and the outside world. *See also* **Activities of daily living (ADL).**

Indigestion   A popular term for any gastrointestinal discomfort that follows a meal. The symptoms, which are often vague, may include a sense of fullness, nausea, bloating, **gas,** or **heartburn**. There is often no organic cause for the discomfort, and stress or tension may be factors. Digestive system diseases that cause indigestion include **peptic ulcer, gallbladder disease,** or **hiatus hernia.**

Infarction An area of dead or dying tissue resulting from a circulatory disorder that blocks the flow of blood to the tissue, thereby depriving it of the oxygen required for its functioning. An infarction usually involves an interruption in blood flow through an artery, but it can also result from blockage in a vein that creates an area from which deoxygenated (used) blood cannot be carried away. A **myocardial infarction** (heart attack) causes an area of heart tissue to die. A brain (cerebral) infarction, usually the result of a **stroke,** can result in disruption of nerve tracts in the affected area. Infarction of the intestine can also occur, particularly in older adults, causing a cramping abdominal pain due to oxygen starvation of the cells of the bowel wall; as the cells die, gangrene develops and the intestine perforates, resulting in peritonitis. Treatment depends upon the degree of tissue damage, the age of the patient, and factors such as other illnesses.

Infection Any condition in which the body is invaded by bacteria, viruses, or other microorganisms, including rickettsiae, fungi, and parasites such as protozoa, that reproduce in the tissues with injurious effects. An infection may be localized or systemic (found throughout the body). It may be marked by pain, swelling, redness, heat, fever, and alterations in such normal functions as breathing or digestion. Environmental factors and underlying health conditions predispose older adults to certain types of infections. Older people are more likely to suffer from **immune deficiency,** resulting in lowered disease resistance and greater vulnerability to infections. Also, because they are likely to spend more time in hospitals or other health-care facilities than most younger persons, older adults are exposed to infections from bacteria that are **nosocomial,** or present in those health-care facilities.

Those with illnesses that require longer periods of confinement to bed or loss of mobility have the greatest risk of acquiring a nosocomial infection; the risk for those over the age of sixty-five is three times that of the general population. Nosocomial infections may follow surgery, as in some cases of **endocarditis** or bacteremia (blood poisoning), or from the use of invasive medical equipment such as catheters. Adding to the risk are alterations in physiological functions involving the lungs, skin, urinary bladder, and metabolism that are associated with aging. Underlying diseases such as **diabetes mellitus** increase the risk of infections of the bones, soft tissues, and urinary tract. Older men with enlarged prostate glands also are at greater risk of acquiring a urinary tract infection. Immunosuppressive therapy for a tumor or other cancers further increases the person's immune deficiency and risk of an infection. Viral infections that are most common among older adults include **herpes simplex, herpes zoster**, and **warts**. Other common skin infections include **erysipelas, candida**, impetigo, folliculitis, ringworm, and infected bed sores. For reasons not fully understood, the frequency with which certain strains of bacteria cause infections in older people is different from the prevalence of infection by the same bacteria in younger persons, particularly in cases of **pneumonia, urinary tract diseases, meningitis**, and **septic arthritis**. As in younger patients, antibiotics are the primary method of treating infections, but the older person may experience different, and frequently more serious, side effects.

Inflammation A natural reaction of body tissue to disease or injury, producing symptoms generally similar to those of an **infection**, including heat, redness, pain, and swelling. There also may be other generalized symptoms similar to those of an infection, such as headache, loss of appetite, and a feeling of discomfort. However, an inflammation is usually localized, whereas an infection is likely to be systemic (spread throughout the body). The heat, swelling, and redness are due to dilation of the blood vessels in the affected area, in response to the injury or infection. The source of the pain or other discomfort is usually due to the release of histamines or similar substances from tissue cells damaged by the inflammation.

Influenza A highly contagious viral **infection** that usually involves the respiratory tract. It tends to occur in epidemics that spread around the world, affecting millions of people, and often resulting in many deaths. Particularly vulnerable are older persons with **immune deficiency** or who have been weakened by other diseases or poor nutrition. The infection may begin slowly with symptoms of chills and discomfort, or suddenly with headache, muscle pain, and fever. The patient also may experience sore throat, weakness, cough, and chest pain. The illness usually lasts about one week, but recovery may take longer for older adults, particularly if they are afflicted with heart or respiratory disorders. **Pneumonia**, caused by the influenza virus or a secondary bacterial infection, is often a complication in older persons. Vaccines are available to provide immunity to current strains of the virus; because new strains emerge at frequent intervals, the vaccine is modified each year. Medical experts recommend that all persons over the age of sixty receive an injection of the newly modified vaccine early each autumn. Most deaths due to influenza each year occur in persons over the age of forty, who fall victim to secondary infections such as pneumonia. Treatment for influenza is directed toward relief of the symptoms. Antibiotics are not recommended, except to treat secondary bacterial infections, because they have no effects on viruses.

Initial insomnia A type of insomnia in which sleeping difficulty is greatest at the beginning of the night. The inability to fall asleep easily is usually due to tension or anxiety, and in some cases it can be caused by worries about falling asleep. *See also* **Insomnia.**

Innervation The distribution of nerve fibers in muscles, glands, or other body tissues.

Inpatient A person who is an overnight or fulltime patient in a hospital or similar institution, receiving more or less continuous supervision with diagnostic and treatment services, as distinguished from an outpatient, who does not require overnight care.

Insomnia An inability to fall asleep or remain asleep through the night. Insomnia may be physical or psychological in origin. Sleep patterns change as one grows older, and both periods of deep sleep and total sleeping time tend to be shorter than during one's younger years. This is a normal phenomenon and does not represent a change in one's health or well-being. Also, many persons misjudge the amount of time required for them to fall asleep (**initial insomnia**), as well their total sleeping time, with the result that they generally spend more time in actual sleep than they have estimated. Insomnia is often a symptom of an underlying problem, such as anxiety, physical pain or discomfort, drug reactions, the need to urinate at night, or **congestive heart failure** with a condition (orthopnea) that requires a person to sit or stand in order to breathe comfortably. Insomnia is a common symptom of **depression** in older adults, associated with early morning awakening. Individual needs for restorative rest vary considerably, and there is no specific "normal" requirement for sleep. Although there are many types of drugs offered to help induce sleep, including **sedatives** and **hypnotics**, both addictive and nonaddictive, authorities caution about dependence on such drugs. Such medications, in addition to their potential for physical dependence, may not help one obtain truly restorative sleep. Most drugs decrease one's periods of dreaming sleep, which is believed to be essential for normal mental health.

Instability Difficulty in standing or walking due to disorders in the sense of balance, a diminished sense of the position of the body in space, visual impairment, muscle weakness, or degenerative joint diseases.

Circulatory disorders, including **hypotension**, diseases such as **parkinsonism**, and **strokes** also may contribute to instability. *See also* Falls.

Intention tremor   An involuntary contraction of muscles that accompanies movements of the body associated with delicate or precise activities. The **tremor** usually increases as the movement nears completion of its purpose. It is seen in alcohol intoxication, tumors, and blood vessel disorders involving the brain stem nerve fibers. *See also* **Chorea, Finger-to-nose test.**

Intermediate care facility (ICF)   A hospital unit or nursing home that provides care for persons who are moderately ill, who require routine medical and nursing care, and who are not capable of **independent living**. An ICF may also offer physical and occupational therapy, social programs, and social services. Federal regulations may establish certain standards for the physical setting and medical and nursing requirements of an ICF in order for it to qualify for reimbursement of costs with government funds.

Intermittent claudication   A painful and sometimes disabling circulatory disorder that affects the legs and sometimes the arms, particularly in older men, during periods of exercise or exertion. It is caused by **arteriosclerosis**, which restricts the blood flow in the arteries of the legs or arms. The cause and effect are similar to the condition that causes **angina pectoris,** the chest pain associated with restricted blood flow in the coronary arteries of the heart. Insufficient blood flow to the muscle tissue of the legs results in oxygen starvation (**ischemia**) of the tissues, marked by painful cramps that often restrict walking. After a few minutes of rest, the symptoms disappear and walking can be resumed until the pain or weakness returns. Relief also may be obtained by the use of drugs that help relax the arteries. *See also* **Claudication.**

Intertrigo   A form of skin inflammation (dermatitis) that occurs in skin folds or where two opposing skin surfaces contact each other. The affected skin is red from heat and friction and may be macerated or eroded as a result of trapped moisture, particularly during warm, humid weather. Such skin surfaces may be infected by bacteria or fungi. The most common sites are in the armpits, under the breasts, in the anogenital region, and between the toes. Careful drying after bathing, followed by the application of prescribed lotions or powders, is the recommended treatment. The condition is most likely to affect persons who are overweight or who have **diabetes mellitus.**

Intervention   An action to protect a person from harm or to improve his mental or physical well-being, such as relieving pain, monitoring the breathing of a patient, or giving medications. *Crisis intervention* is a form of psychotherapy in which an individual or family receives professional help in coping with a crisis situation, such as the loss of several family members in a traffic accident or fire. *Behavior therapy* may be used as an intervention technique in the control of obesity or alcoholism.

Intervertebral disk   A cushionlike disk of cartilage and fibers that separates two adjacent vertebrae in the spinal column. The center of the disk contains a capsule of gelatinous fluid, the **nucleus pulposus**. As one grows older, degenerative changes often occur in the vertebral bones and the disks, causing compression of the disk or dehydration and sometimes collapse of the nucleus pulposus, which may bulge (herniate) through the outer shell of the disk. The bulging disk and bone spurs that develop press against the nerve roots of the spinal cord, causing pain or loss of feeling, and may lead to muscle wasting of the body area, with possible permanent injury. *See also* **Herniated disk, Sciatica.**

Intestinal obstruction   A painful blockage of the intestinal tract caused by a tumor, a loop of bowel trapped in a hernia, adhesions from previous surgery, or a large gallstone. The most common cause of intestinal obstruction in older adults is a trapped (strangulated) **hernia**. It is also frequently fatal. Pain, constipation, and abdominal distention are signs of an abdominal obstruction caused by a tumor. Although a gallstone one inch or more in diameter would not ordinarily pass into the small intestine through the bile duct, such large gallstones have entered the intestine through fistulas, causing obstruction. Treatment usually includes sedatives and/or analgesics to relieve symptoms, and surgery, which may be immediate in the case of a life-threatening emergency such as a strangulated intestine or a bowel **infarction**.

Intolerance   An inability to endure the effects of a drug, a food item, or a sensory input such as pain or intense noise.

Intoxication   A state of poisoning with accompanying abnormal behavior caused by the effects of a drug or chemical on the central nervous system or other organ systems. Although intoxication is commonly associated with the abuse of alcohol, similar effects can be produced by sedatives (especially in the elderly), drugs used in psychotherapy, and numerous substances used in industry, such as mercury, thallium, and lead. The behavior of some persons who have been exposed to such substances in large amounts or for a period of many years is similar to that observed in patients treated for **senile dementia**.

Intracranial Pertaining to the region within the skull.

Intracranial pressure A pressure buildup within the skull because of hemorrhage, tumor, or fluid accumulation. Because the skull is rigid and cannot expand to accommodate additional fluid or tissue, the pressure tends to crush the brain cells within it, resulting in neurological damage and sometimes death if it is not relieved. The condition can usually be reversed with surgery or drugs that reduce pressure within the skull, though damage to the brain is not always correctable.

Invalidism A preoccupation with one's health to the point of accepting the role of a chronic invalid, whether or not one is seriously ill or disabled. The person usually enjoys the attention and concern of others about his or her condition and welcomes being excused from responsibilities associated with being healthy and active.

Involutional Pertaining to a turning inward or decline associated with the aging process. It is sometimes applied to the depressive phase of **bipolar disorders** (involutional melancholia) that may occur during the menopausal period, marked by feelings of depression, guilt, and persecution.

Ipsilateral Pertaining to the same side of the body, such as a disability on the left side of the body associated with an injury or disease affecting the left side of the brain. When a lesion on one side of the brain results in a physical problem on the opposite side of the body, the condition is called "contralateral."

Iridocyclitis An acute inflammation of the iris and the front chamber of the eye. The symptoms include pain, tearing, blurred vision, and eye congestion with a discharge that may contain pus. The cause often is a viral or bacterial infection that has spread from another part of the body. Treatment is with medicated eye drops and other drugs.

Iron deficiency A condition caused by a lack of iron in the diet or an inability to absorb an adequate amount of iron from foods in the diet. Iron deficiency is relatively common in older adults, usually because of a choice of foods that are poor sources of iron and factors, such as tea-drinking, that inhibit the absorption of iron from foods in the digestive tract, and a deficiency in stomach acid secretion. A common effect of iron deficiency is anemia, which may be accompanied by feelings of fatigue and weakness. Iron is needed for the hemoglobin of red blood cells and makes it possible for the blood cells to transport sixty times as much oxygen as they could without iron. Because of menstrual blood losses, premenopausal women are particularly prone to an iron deficiency and may require almost twice as much iron in their daily diet as men or postmenopausal women. It is possible to have an iron deficiency condition while eating iron-rich foods because the body absorbs only a portion of the iron in foods eaten, depending upon the form in which the iron occurs in a food. Animal food sources, for example, are a better source of dietary iron than foods from plants because the iron in meats is in a form (heme) that is more easily absorbed than the iron (nonheme) in vegetables. However, when ascorbic acid (vitamin C) is included in a meal, absorption of nonheme iron is increased. Tea interferes with iron absorption because the tannic acid in tea binds the iron into an insoluble compound that is excreted. Calcium, phosphorus, and a substance in cereals (phytic acid) also can reduce the absorption of iron. Thus an older person who subsists largely on tea and bread or other cereal foods may be at high risk of developing iron-deficiency anemia.

Ischemia   A decreased blood supply to an organ or body part, causing oxygen starvation and often resulting in severe pain in the tissue. Examples include **angina pectoris, myocardial infarction,** or **intermittent claudication. Transient** (or temporary) **ischemic attacks (TIAs)** may occur in brain tissue without producing pain, but they usually cause such symptoms as vertigo, double vision, facial numbness, or feelings of weakness in the arms or legs. Ischemia also may account for the pain of a strangulated hernia, or it can occur in an arm or leg encased in a plaster cast, if the cast restricts the blood flow.

Itching   An annoying irritation of the skin surface that results in an irresistible urge to scratch the affected area. Causes usually include allergic reactions, various forms of skin inflammation (dermatitis), and insect bites. Also called "pruritus."

J

Jacksonian march A form of **epilepsy** in which a seizure begins in one part of the brain and gradually spreads to neighboring tissues, affecting parts of the body controlled by the brain areas involved. In a typical case, a seizure may produce symptoms of a numbness or tingling sensation that begins in the fingers and gradually spreads up the arm, or begins in a toe, gradually spreading up the leg. *See also* **Acroparesthesia.**

Jackson's law A rule of psychiatry that in **dementia** or deterioration of the mind due to organic brain disease, the higher and most recently acquired mental functions are the first to be lost.

Jactitation A medical term for the muscle twitchings, spasms, and restless body movements that may accompany a severe, feverish illness.

Jakob-Creutzfeldt disease A slow-virus infection of the central nervous system that causes a form of **dementia**, with symptoms that begin in middle age, many years after original exposure to the virus. Because of the amount of time that may elapse between contact with the virus and the appearance of the disease, the exact means of transmission of the virus is not known. It has been reported, however, that the disease can be acquired by contact with an infected person. Symptoms may include insomnia, drowsiness, fatigue, self-neglect, apathy, irritability, and disorientation. The person may lose speaking, reading, and writing abilities and be unable to perform simple tasks because of the loss of muscle coordination. There is progressive deterioration of most central nervous system faculties, with loss of vision, spasticity, tremors, and alternating involuntary contractions and relaxations of muscles. There is no specific treatment, and death usually occurs within a year after the onset of symptoms. Also called "Creutzfeldt-Jakob disease."

Janeway lesions   Small reddish patches or nodules in the skin of the palms, finger pads, or soles of the feet that are a symptom of bacterial **endocarditis** or an **aneurysm** caused by bacteria. The lesions frequently contain the disease organism that is the cause of the underlying problem. The patches or nodules may also involve bleeding beneath the skin. They are neither tender nor painful, although ulceration may occur.

Jar tenderness   A term used to identify the site of abdominal discomfort that may involve the lining of the abdomen (peritoneum). The term is derived from a test in which the person stands on his toes, with the knees straight, and then drops the heels suddenly to the floor. If jarring the body in this manner produces a rebound pain in the area of peritoneal inflammation, the location of the problem can be more easily determined.

Jaundice   A yellowish coloration of the skin, whites of the eyes, mucous membranes, and body fluids. Jaundice is usually caused by an accumulation of bilirubin (a bile pigment) in the blood. It is usually a sign of a disease of the liver, gallbladder, or pancreas. Bilirubin is produced by the liver in the course of breaking down red blood cells, and jaundice occurs when the bile ducts are obstructed or there is an excessive breakdown of these cells. Jaundice may be a sign of viral **hepatitis**. It also can indicate a tumor of the liver or pancreas, an obstruction of a bile duct, bacterial infections, or a reaction to a variety of drugs, including certain antibiotics and sulfa drugs, phenylbutazone, steroid hormones, and tranquilizers.

Jejunal ulcer   A **peptic ulcer** that forms in the jejunum, the portion of the small intestine between the duodenum and the ileum. *See also* **Duodenal ulcer.**

Joint alignment   The natural symmetry of the various parts of the human body in a standing or sitting posture. Many of the moveable parts of the body form geometric patterns. Injury or disease can result in a faulty alignment.

Joint disorders Degenerative and other diseases affecting the tissues of knees, hips, hands, feet, spine, and other body areas in which adjacent bone surfaces, normally cushioned with cartilage, are linked to permit movement. Arthritis or other joint diseases are the most common health complaint of persons over the age of fifty in North America and Europe. The most common of joint disorders is **osteoarthritis**, which eventually affects nearly all physically active individuals in varying degrees; those less likely to be affected are persons handicapped by **immobility**. Osteoarthritis, or noninflammatory degenerative joint disease, is caused by "wear and tear" on the cartilage surfaces of joints. After the age of fifty, more than 80 percent of all men and women show signs of joint degeneration on X-ray films. As aging continues, the number of persons with evidence of osteoarthritis increases to nearly 100 percent. Not all persons with X-ray evidence of osteoarthritis, however, experience pain or other symptoms of the disorder. Factors that aggravate symptoms of osteoarthritis are obesity, injury, poor posture, and repetitive work patterns (miners are likely to develop osteoarthritis of the knees and elbows, while construction workers tend to develop osteoarthritis of the elbow and shoulder joints).

Aging causes the cartilage to become thinner and less able to resist physical stress, and there is also a decline in the activity of cells that produce new cartilage. As the cartilage degenerates, bone surfaces rub against each other or bone spurs form from new growth of tissue, or both. The bone ends also undergo changes when injuries or excessive pressure cause minifractures; the damaged bone is replaced by harder bone material that is less resilient. **Heberden's nodes**, a form of osteoarthritis marked by bony spurs at the finger joints, tend to appear on the hands of some women in middle age. **Rheumatoid arthritis**, unlike osteoarthritis, is a systemic disease associated with an immune condition rather than a localized joint disorder. However, rheumatoid arthritis causes severe pain and stiffness in the joints. The onset of symptoms is usually in the thirties and forties, but rheumatoid arthritis reaches a peak in the fifties for women and a decade later for men. The frequency of new cases of rheumatoid arthritis and its more serious symptoms among women is associated with the **menopause**. Rheumatoid arthritis affects women more often than men by a ratio of greater than 4 to 1. Unlike osteoarthritis, which increases in incidence with age, rheumatoid arthritis in later life is often a continuation of the same disease that began producing symptoms when the patient was younger. When rheumatoid arthritis begins in an older adult, the onset of symptoms may be sudden or gradual. A sudden onset often results in involvement of joints of the upper part of the body, mainly the neck and shoulders. Gradual development of the disease in an older person generally results in stiffness or limited movement in the hands and feet at first and later spreads to the larger joints. When rheumatoid arthritis affects an older adult for the first time, the effects are usually less disabling than in a younger patient. However, symptoms of rheumatoid arthritis that first appear in an aged person may signal an underlying malignancy (cancer), requiring a medical evaluation. *See also* **Gout.**

K

Kegel exercises A system of exercises designed to strengthen the muscles of the pelvic floor. They are recommended as a method of preventing or treating urinary **incontinence** in older women who are capable of performing the exercises. Kegel exercises consist of repeated contractions and relaxations of the pubococcygeus muscle that controls the flow of urine. They may be performed while seated on a toilet. Contractions of the muscle interrupt the flow of urine and relaxations allow the flow of urine to resume.

Kellgren's syndrome A form of **osteoarthritis** that affects certain joints of the hands, feet, knees, and spine.

Keloid An overgrowth of scar tissue at the site of severe acne, a surgical incision, or a burn or other injury. Keloids tend to develop on the neck, back, and chest of susceptible persons. Unlike many ordinary scars, keloids are permanent, and various treatments have had limited success.

Keratectomy A surgical procedure performed to remove a scar or other small lesion from the cornea of the eye when the affected area is not large enough to warrant a corneal graft. It may be performed with only a local anesthetic.

Keratitis An inflammation of the cornea characterized by a loss of luster, blurred vision, and watery eyes. There may be a loosening of corneal surface cells, leaving small ulcers. It may be caused by irritation or infection, particularly a herpes infection.

Keratocanthoma   A solitary dome-shaped sore that may appear on the face, hand, or forearm of an older adult. It grows rapidly in size, reaching more than an inch in diameter, and develops a central crater. Untreated, it usually diminishes in size and disappears after a few months, leaving a small scar. Because it resembles a skin cancer, the growth is usually removed for biopsy.

Keratoconjunctivitis   An inflammation of both the cornea and the conjunctiva of the eye.

Keratoconjunctivitis sicca (dry eye disease)   An inflammation of the cornea and conjunctiva caused by loss of the ability to produce tears needed to prevent drying of the eye tissues. Symptoms of the tear (**lacrimal**) deficiency include a burning sensation and a feeling of a foreign body in the eye. There may be erosion of the surface tissue cells of the cornea and conjunctiva. The disease tends to affect women during and after the **menopause** and sometimes accompanies diseases such as **rheumatoid arthritis** and **systemic lupus erythematosus**. Treatments include the use of "artificial tears" to keep the cornea moist, soft contact lenses that can be moistened frequently, and, in certain cases, where the tear ducts are involved, surgery.

Keratoderma climactericum   Areas of skin overgrowth that appear on the palms and soles of some women around the time of **menopause**. The lesions resemble those of **psoriasis** and are sometimes diagnosed as that disorder. **Estrogen** has been used to treat the condition.

Keratosis   A change in the condition of the skin associated with the aging process that is marked by a flat, discolored overgrowth and thickening of a small area of the skin's surface. An **actinic keratosis**, or senile wart, is a precancerous skin growth that usually develops on an area of skin that has been exposed repeatedly to sunlight. Light-skinned people with blond or red hair who have worked outside for many years are at highest risk of developing senile warts. Another common form of the skin disorder is a **seborrheic keratosis**, which may appear as a waxy, brownish crust and may develop on covered as well as uncovered areas of the skin. A cancerous or precancerous keratosis generally appears to be firmly imbedded in the skin, while a noncancerous lesion often has the appearance of being loosely attached to the skin surface. However, any skin lesion that changes in size, shape, or color should be considered as potentially dangerous unless diagnosed as benign (noncancerous) by a physician.

Kernig's sign A test for **meningitis** in which the person lies face up with the hip and knee flexed at a ninety-degree angle. When the upper leg is held immobile, any attempt to extend the knee against pressure on the lower leg produces pain in the muscles at the back of the upper leg, which is a clinical sign of meningitis. The sign may be absent in some elderly patients.

Ketoacidosis A potentially dangerous form of **acidosis** caused by an accumulation of ketones, by-products of faulty carbohydrate metabolism in the body. Ketoacidosis usually occurs as a complication of **diabetes mellitus**. Symptoms include confusion, breathing difficulty, the fruity odor of acetone (a ketone) on the breath, dehydration, nausea, vomiting, and weight loss. If untreated, the condition most often leads to coma and death. Among older adults, ketoacidosis may also occur as a complication of other disorders such as **stroke**, heart attack **(myocardial infarction), intestinal obstruction**, or an infectious disease, so that early symptoms are often misinterpreted. Fatalities are more likely when ketoacidosis accompanies an **infection**. In older adults, 40 percent of the cases of ketoacidosis are associated with infections. Other causes of death associated with ketoacidosis include **thrombosis, hypovolemia**, and hypovolemic shock, which is caused by dehydration resulting from significantly diminished blood volume. Treatment of ketoacidosis consists of restoring **fluid** and **electrolyte balance**, giving insulin as necessary, and correcting the underlying disease.

Kidney changes with aging A decline in the structure and function of the kidney after early adulthood. As one grows older, the kidney gradually decreases in size by about 33 percent, the filtration function gradually slows by about 50 percent, and blood flow to the kidney declines at a rate of approximately 1 percent per year. The tissues that remain undergo a process of thickening and hardening that reduces their effectiveness. These changes are found in healthy older adults and apparently have little effect on the ability to maintain normal daily activities. The changes may be important, however, in the event of a stressful situation such as an infection or injury. The diminished filtration capacity may result in fluid accumulation or depletion and altered levels of sodium and other electrolytes, as in **hypernatremia, hyponatremia**, and altered **acid-base balance**. Prescriptions for medications may have to be altered to compensate for the reduced filtration rate. The kidney of the older adult may also be more vulnerable to the effects of an **embolus** or **thrombus**.

Kidney stone (renal calculus) A hard accumulation of calcium and other substances that forms in the urinary tract, causing severe pain, restriction or obstruction of urine flow, and increasing the risk of urinary tract infections. The stones (calculi) may range in size from fine gravel to more than an inch in diameter. Their exact composition may be influenced by such factors as the age, sex, hereditary, geographic location, diet, and any disease of the patient. Kidney stones in North American men are composed mainly of calcium and/or uric acid, while those composed of struvite (a compound of magnesium and phosphorus) are formed mainly in women. Men with **gout** are prone to develop uric-acid kidney stones. Struvite kidney stones are associated with urinary tract infections.

Kidney stones often produce no symptoms until or unless they cause irritation or obstruction at some point in the urinary tract, from the kidney to the bladder. An early sign may be blood in the urine. Pain may be felt in the back or the abdomen, or both, with fever, nausea and vomiting, and other gastrointestinal symptoms. Men are three times as likely to develop kidney stones as women, and they occur most commonly in the middle aged. The prevalence of kidney stones is greater than the actual number of persons treated as the stones are frequently found in autopsies, and very small stones are often excreted in the urine. Stones that are not excreted tend to grow larger, causing pain and obstruction. The largest and most dangerous stones, called "staghorns," develop from struvite calculi within the kidney and may completely fill the funnel-shaped renal calyx, which drains urine from a kidney into a ureter leading to the bladder.

Various techniques are used to remove stones, including surgery, introducing fluids to help flush out a stone, and a method (lithotripsy) in which sound waves are used to shatter the stones into fragments small enough to be excreted in the urine.

Kimmelstiel-Wilson disease A disorder caused by the degeneration of the glomeruli (the urine filtration units) of the kidney. The disorder may be a complication of **diabetes** with **arteriosclerosis** of the kidney (renal) artery. Symptoms include edema, high blood pressure, and the presence of a protein (albumin) in the urine.

Klüver-Bucy syndrome A disorder resulting from changes in the brain due to **atrophy** of certain brain tissues. It may develop during an intermediate stage, after the first two to four years, of **Alzheimer's disease**. Among the distinguishing symptoms are a loss of fear, an inability to recognize objects without touching them or placing them in the mouth, an inability to concentrate, and a voracious appetite.

Knee buckling   Sudden loss of control of the muscles that extend the leg and keep it straight, usually due to paralysis of the femoral nerve that innervates the muscles. A common cause of the disorder is **diabetes**. Buckling of the knee contributes to **falls** among older adults. Many persons afflicted with this condition learn to walk on level surfaces by utilizing alternative muscles, but they also may find it necessary to press a hand against the thigh of the affected leg. Climbing stairs is usually more difficult.

Knee-jerk reflex   A reflex action of the leg muscle (quadriceps) that contracts and extends the leg at the knee when a tendon just below the kneecap is tapped sharply. An overactive reflex or one in which the lower leg responds limply may be a sign of a **neurological disorder**. The knee-jerk reflex is tested in several different ways. The patient may sit on a chair or table, or lie face up. The legs may dangle freely, or the examiner may hold the foot or leg so as to feel the muscle contraction. Also called "patellar reflex."

Korsakoff's syndrome   A **neurological disorder** marked by symptoms of organic brain disease, including **amnesia** for recent events, confusion, and nerve inflammation. The causes can range from head injury, brain tumor, herpes infections, or **pellagra** to **alcoholism** and heavy metal poisoning. The person is disoriented in time and exhibits memory defects, which lead to **confabulation** in an effort to fill in the gaps of lost memory. The person is able to perform complex activities learned before the onset of the disorder but cannot learn simple new skills. The outlook depends in part on the cause of the disorder; cases due to head injury or a brain hemorrhage often recover, but if there is irreversible brain damage because of a brain infection or chronic alcoholism, the prognosis is poor.

Kraurosis vulvae   An extreme degree of **atrophy** of the female genitalia that may develop after the **menopause**. The vulva becomes thin, shiny, and yellowish white in color, and there is dryness and itching of the skin. The vaginal opening becomes constricted, and there is shrinkage of the vaginal canal. Kraurosis vulvae is often accompanied by a whitish inflammation of the skin in the genital area (**leukoplakia**), resulting in **fissures** and ulcerations, that often progress to cancer. Because the vaginal wall becomes very fragile, kraurosis vulvae can cause **dyspareunia** and can make an older woman vulnerable to serious injury if sexual intercourse is forced.

Kuhnt-Junius disease   *See* **Macular degeneration.**

Kussmaul's respiration (air hunger)   Breathing difficulty in which respirations occur in deep, regular, sighing paroxysms characteristic of diabetic **acidosis, uremia,** and coma. The rate may be slow, normal, or fast.

Kussmaul's sign   An increase in pressure and distension of the jugular vein in the neck when a person inhales. This is the opposite of the normal situation, in which there is a decrease in distension and pressure during inhalation. It is usually a symptom of a heart disorder, such as when blood flows abnormally into the membrane surrounding the heart (**tamponade**), or a disease of the lungs.

Kyphoscoliosis   A complication of **kyphosis** in which there is a sidewise curvature of the spine (scoliosis) in addition to the convex curvature that produces a humpback effect. The degree of distortion varies, but in serious cases the lateral curvature may form an "S" shape, and some of the vertebrae may be rotated out of normal alignment.

Kyphosis   A convex curvature of the upper spine, giving the person a humpback appearance. The term *kyphosis* is derived from the Greek word for humpback. Causes include **osteoporosis, rheumatoid arthritis, osteoarthritis, cancer**, rickets, birth defects, and certain infectious diseases, such as **tuberculosis**. Kyphosis can result from the collapse of a single vertebra of the spinal column. Treatment may consist of wearing a brace or undergoing surgery for **spinal fusion**, as well as attending to the underlying condition.

L

Laboratory test results, changes with aging Variations from "normal" values that often occur in results of laboratory tests of blood, urine, or certain organ systems of older adults. In **glucose tolerance tests,** performed to detect possible evidence of non-insulin-dependent **diabetes mellitus** that often begins after the age of forty, blood sugar levels of an older individual are generally higher both before and after the start of the test, as compared to test results of younger persons. For an older individual, the higher blood sugar levels are not necessarily evidence of the onset of diabetes but may simply reflect a typical decline in function of the pancreas, the organ that is the source of insulin. Also, as with other aging body organs, pancreatic function may appear normal in a "resting" state, but the organ might fail a "stress test" by being unable to handle a diet containing excessive amounts of carbohydrate. It is estimated that half of all older persons would show abnormally high blood sugar levels if their laboratory test results were compared to what is considered "normal" for a younger person.

The presence in urine of abnormal amounts of albumin, a protein molecule, can be a sign of changes in blood pressure or kidney structure, or both, resulting in the leakage of protein through the kidney membranes. Serum albumin levels are usually lower in older persons than in young patients, but a very low reading is likely to be a sign of a chronic disease. However, the presence of another protein, globulin, in laboratory test results tends to increase as one grows older.

Maximum breathing capacity declines with age, and several changes that occur in breathing-ability tests, as well as in electrocardiograms of heart function, may actually be normal for an older person rather than signs of disease. Because older adults are more likely to suffer from a lack of body fluid (**dehydration**), a number of items in a laboratory test report, particularly those relating to **electrolytes**, may show deviations from what is regarded as normal for the general population. Certain medications also can alter results of laboratory tests. Some **diuretics**, for example, can cause levels of uric acid or blood sugar to appear abnormally high, while heart tonics and medications for **parkinsonism** can distort results of thyroid-function tests. Some changes also may be affected by variations in hormones between men and women. Blood levels of calcium and phosphate are increased in women after the menopause, while the same substances show a steady decline in men of the same age groups.

Labyrinth In medical terminology, the inner ear, a series of bony cavities in either side of the skull containing, in addition to the hearing apparatus, organs that regulate the body's sense of balance. Disease or injury involving labyrinthine structures can result in **vertigo, Ménière's disease**, and sensorineural **hearing loss**.

Lacrimal Pertaining to tears or the tear drainage system of the eye. Tears are produced in the lacrimal gland above the eye, flow across the eyeball, and drain through openings in the inner margins of the eyelids, and then flow into the nose through a nasolacrimal duct. *See also* **Keratoconjunctivitis sicca.**

Lactose intolerance In adults, a digestive disorder that may include bloating, gas, nausea, diarrhea, and cramps, which is experienced by persons who lack the enzyme that breaks down milk sugar (lactose) molecules into carbohydrate units that can be absorbed in the intestine. The condition affects most adults over the age of forty-five to some degree, with the exception of persons of northern European ancestry who still retain the needed enzyme. In Orientals, blacks, American Indians, and many persons of southern European descent, production of the enzyme begins to decline during their teenage years. Many older adults with lactose intolerance are able to tolerate small amounts of milk daily as well as hard cheese, yogurt, and other dairy products in which the lactose has been chemically altered.

Lacunar infarction An abnormal condition in which the small arteries of the brain form small cysts (lacunae) that block the blood flow to an area of brain tissue. These obstructions may not always produce typical stroke symptoms, but in some cases they are the source of small **strokes** that affect only one or a few nerve functions. Depending on the site of the infarction, or obstruction, symptoms may vary from paralysis of the eye muscles to a general clumsiness or to a loss of the ability to speak clearly. A lacunar infarction often escapes detection during diagnosis because it is too small or too deep in the brain to be detected by usual examination techniques. The condition may be associated with **hypertension**.

Lagophthalmos An inability to close the eyelids completely. Causes include facial nerve paralysis, thyroid disease, or the effects of an injury or surgery affecting the eyelids. If uncorrected, the defect can lead to exposure **keratitis** of the cornea.

Lamellar cataract A type of **cataract** in which the lens of the eye has alternating layers of opaqueness and clarity. The vision may not be seriously affected.

Lamellar keratoplasty A surgical procedure for replacing the outer layers of the cornea of the eye with corneal tissue from a donor.

Laminectomy A surgical procedure in which the bony arches of one or more vertebrae are removed to relieve pressure on the spinal cord. The operation is done in cases of injury or to correct the problem caused by a herniated or "slipped" cartilage disk between two vertebrae. If it is necessary to remove bone from several vertebrae, surgeons may fuse some of the remaining vertebrae in order to preserve stability of the spinal column. The operation is performed under a general anesthetic, and the patient is required to lie flat for the first few days of recovery to hold the spine in correct alignment. *See also* **Herniated disk.**

Laryngeal cancer A cancer that develops from tissues that form the lining of the larynx. The cancer usually appears after the age of fifty and is almost twenty times as likely to occur in men than in women. It tends to develop in persons who use alcohol and tobacco. A common symptom is persistent hoarseness accompanied by a sore throat and difficulty in swallowing and breathing. Small tumors of the larynx are sometimes controlled by radiation; more serious cases require surgical removal of the affected tissues.

Laryngectomy The surgical removal of the larynx, usually performed to prevent the spread of a cancer of the larynx. Depending upon the extent of the cancer growth, the surgeon may remove just the vocal cords or the entire larynx along with the surrounding throat cartilage and the epiglottis at the back of the throat. After the larynx is removed, the rest of the trachea (windpipe) is sewn to the skin of the throat to allow normal breathing to continue. The patient learns to use "esophageal speech," in which gulps of air from the esophagus are forced through the mouth to form speech sounds.

Lasègue's test A test for **sciatica** or a **herniated disk** that stretches the sciatic nerve by having the person raise a leg while the hip is flexed and the leg is straight. A healthy person can usually move the leg through a ninety-degree range without pain, but those with sciatica encounter pain when the leg is moved through a range of just thirty or forty degrees.

Latent deficiency syndrome A borderline malnutrition condition, which is common in older adults. The person may consume just enough of the essential nutrients to avoid any signs or symptoms of a vitamin or other deficiency disease but fail to maintain a sufficient nutritional reserve to avoid overt malnutrition condition in the event of injury, serious infection, or surgery.

Lateropulsion A type of walking disturbance that occurs in some **parkinsonism** patients, in which they use their feet to move sideways instead of forward.

Laxatives Substances employed to ease the passage of fecal material from the rectum in order to correct or prevent a condition of **constipation**. Laxatives are usually foods or drugs that either increase the bulk of the bowel contents, lubricate the inner walls of the bowel, increase the fluid content of the intestine, or irritate the lining of the bowel so as to increase its muscular activity. Laxatives are misused by some individuals who mistakenly believe that "regularity" in bowel movements is essential for good health. Actually, the transit time for the passage of fecal material through the bowel varies widely between individuals and among members of different populations. Excessive use of laxatives can result in a "lazy bowel" condition, in which the digestive tract becomes dependent upon laxatives in order to produce a bowel movement, and constipation occurs in the absence of laxatives. Also, some laxatives are harsh and potentially damaging to the digestive tract. Alternative measures include diets that ensure an adequate intake of water and **fiber** and the use, when recommended by a doctor, of stool softeners.

LDL An abbreviation for *low-density lipoprotein,* one of a group of food substances composed of combinations of fat and protein molecules.

Low-density lipoproteins are associated with the development of **athero-sclerosis** and **cardiovascular** disease because they transport **cholesterol** and other fats, particularly **triglycerides,** through the bloodstream, thereby accounting for the link between LDLs and heart disease. Another type of lipoprotein, *high-density lipoprotein* (**HDL**), has essentially the opposite effect in that it helps remove cholesterol from artery walls and carries it to the liver where it can be stored or excreted. Generally, the proportion of LDL in the body increases with excess body weight and lack of exercise. Women are believed to be protected from diseases of the heart and blood vessels by a higher proportion of HDL to LDL before the menopause. After the menopause, blood levels of LDL in women rise to about the same level as in men.

Left-heart failure A heart disease involving a defect in the left side of the heart that causes pulmonary congestion, retention of sodium and water, and fluid accumulation in the body extremities (**edema**). The right side of the heart may continue to function normally for a while, although failure of one side of the heart eventually affects both sides since they are part of the same blood-pumping circuit.

Legionnaire's disease A form of bacterial **pneumonia** that occurs in sporadic outbreaks, with symptoms of high fever, a dry cough, chest pain, chills, and diarrhea. The cause is a bacterium that grows in watery areas, including hot water tanks, shower heads, and air conditioners, as well as lakes and creeks. There is no evidence that the disease is transmitted from one person to another. It is acquired by inhaling air contaminated by the bacteria. Legionnaire's disease was named after an epidemic that occurred in Philadelphia in 1976 during a veterans' convention. Other outbreaks have since been reported at sites such as hotels and hospitals where a number of people have gathered. Older adults appear particularly susceptible, and the death rate for persons fifty-five and over is double that of younger adults. Treatment is with antibiotics.

Leiomyoma uteri A fibrous tumor of the muscle wall of the uterus. It occurs most frequently in women near the end of their childbearing years. A noncancerous tumor, it usually appears as multiple nodules on the inner surface of the uterus. The tumor often develops without symptoms and is discovered during a routine pelvic examination. In other cases, it may be a cause of excessive bleeding during menstruation, leading to anemia. A leiomyoma may grow rapidly as a result of the use of estrogens. The tumor is usually removed by dilatation and curettage (D & C).

Lentigo   A flat tan or brown spot on a skin surface, usually resulting from exposure to the sun, that appears in middle age or later. A lentigo may resemble a freckle but usually is derived from pigment cells deeper in the skin than those that produce freckles. Any lentigo should be examined by a doctor because a third of such pigmented areas eventually evolve into skin cancers *(lentigo-malignant melanomas)*.

Leriche syndrome   A circulatory disorder caused by an **embolism** or other obstruction at a point in the abdominal aorta (the main artery of the body) where it branches into left and right segments leading to the legs. The blockage results in **intermittent claudication**; pain in the buttocks and thighs that may continue even at rest; numbness and coldness of an affected leg; loss of normal skin color in the leg; and **impotence** in the male. Temporary relief may be provided by cooling the leg, and by sleeping with the affected limb uncovered or hanging out of the bed. Treatment usually requires surgical removal of the offending blood clot, which may be done under a local anesthetic. Untreated, the condition may progress to gangrene of the foot.

LES   An abbreviation for lower esophageal sphincter, the ring of muscles at the lower end of the esophagus where it empties into the stomach. The LES normally closes the end of the esophagus so that reflux, or regurgitation, of stomach contents will not occur. When the LES fails to function properly, particularly as a complication of **hiatus hernia**, gastric acid can back up into the esophagus and throat.

Lesion   Any tissue abnormality, which may appear as a sore, injury, boil, ulceration, rash, wound, or scar. A lesion may be *malignant* (cancerous) or *benign* (noncancerous) and can occur on the skin or in an internal organ or tissue. The incidence of skin lesions increases with age, particularly when the person has been exposed to the sun for many years as a result of outdoor work or recreation. Lesions that may start as benign, such as certain moles, must be monitored for changes in color, size, and shape, which can signal that they have become malignant. A lesion that appears firmly implanted in the skin is usually more dangerous than one that seems to be only on the surface. Examples of internal lesions include brain tumors, **peptic ulcers**, and **myocardial infarctions**.

Lethargy   A condition of drowsiness, stupor, apathy, or sluggishness.

Leukemia   A form of cancer marked by excessive production of white blood cells that are abnormal in appearance and function.

These white blood cells (leukocytes) proliferate throughout the body, but because of defective development they are less effective than normal leukocytes in destroying bacteria. Red blood cell formation may also be affected. Several forms of leukemia affect older adults more frequently than younger persons. *Chronic lymphocytic leukemia,* for example, begins to appear in the fourth decade of life and reaches a peak among persons in their sixties. More than two-thirds of patients with *acute myelogenous leukemia* are over the age of fifty. Symptoms of leukemias depend in part on the type but may include fatigue, fever, generalized discomfort (malaise), frequent nosebleeds, bleeding under the skin, pain in the upper left part of the chest, and tenderness under the breastbone.

The specific treatment depends upon the type of leukemia and the needs and responses of the patient to particular therapies. Diagnosis is made on the basis of detailed blood cell examinations and studies of bone marrow. Chronic myelogenous leukemia, for example, is usually marked by the alteration of two chromosomes in the nuclei of bone marrow or blood cell nuclei. Chronic lymphocytic leukemia is often diagnosed on the basis of the proportions of various types of cells in the blood and bone marrow. Because most anticancer drugs are extremely potent, their use may be postponed until the leukemia shows definite signs of progression; overtreatment may be more dangerous than lack of treatment when chronic leukemia has been diagnosed. In addition to anticancer drugs, therapy may include radiation, the use of corticosteroid drugs, and blood transfusions. Although leukemia is a progressive disease, treatment of patients with chronic forms may reduce symptoms and prolong life for many years. The eventual cause of death is usually an infection.

Leukonychia   White spots that develop in the nails. The causes vary from air bubbles to immature skin or nail cells. No treatment is necessary for the condition.

Leukoplakia   A disorder of the mucous membranes, marked by white patches on the lips, tongue, and linings of the mouth, the throat, and similar surfaces. Although *oral* (mouth) *leukoplakia* affects mainly men over the age of forty, the condition also may affect the female genitalia *(vulvar leukoplakia),* particularly in older women. Leukoplakia lesions are often painful and in some cases may progress to cancer. Treatment includes elimination of substances that may cause irritation of the plaques, such as tobacco, drugs, or hot, spicy foods, and surgical removal of any lesion that could become cancerous.

Leukorrhea   A white discharge from the vagina. It may be copious, irritating, and foul-smelling. Diagnosis usually requires a pelvic examination and microscopic examination of a sample of the discharge. Treatment often consists of antiseptics and antibiotics to control bacterial or fungal infections. When leukorrhea occurs with **senile vaginitis,** the cause may be that tissues of the vagina are much less resistant to infections. In addition to antibiotics, treatment in such cases may include the use of creams or ointments containing the female sex hormone **estrogen.**

Libido   Sexual desire, a term derived from the Latin word *libidines,* meaning "lust." Sexual desire should not be confused with sexual performance, which may vary widely among different individuals because of many psychological and physiological factors. *See also* **Impotence, Sexual function changes with aging.**

Lichenification   A thickening and hardening of the skin due to irritation. It is usually marked by rough, slightly raised patches. A foot callus is an example of lichenification.

Lichen planus   A chronic skin disease characterized by small, flat, purplish patches that are often crossed by grayish lines. The condition is accompanied by intense itching. The eruptions can occur anywhere on the skin but are most frequently found on the wrists and legs. There may be alternating periods of eruptions and remissions. Lichen planus is not contagious, but the eruptions can become the sites of secondary infections, usually as a result of scratching. Treatments consist of antihistamines to reduce the itching sensations and medicated lotions. Although lichen planus outbreaks can persist for months at a time, they have no direct effect on the general health of the person.

Lifespan   The length of life of an individual or the average length of life of a population or species. The maximum human lifespan of around 100 years has changed very little over the ages, though a much larger percentage of the population now survives to that age, and the *average* length of life has increased because of the control of infectious diseases and improved public health. However, the oldest individuals in ancient Greece and Rome, according to historical records, occasionally reached the tenth decade of life if they survived the diseases of childhood and youth.

Ligament   A white, shiny band of connective tissue that is attached to bones or cartilage to help hold a joint together. Ligaments are flexible and slightly elastic. Ligaments lose their elasticity and resiliency with aging.

Limb girdle-trunk paresis   A form of partial paralysis resulting from lack of oxygen reaching the brain, as may happen during interruption in heart function, in which the affected brain tissues are those where nerve cells control muscles of the trunk and the pelvic and shoulder areas. Those parts of the body are weakened as a result of the oxygen deficit, but brain centers controlling the hands, feet, and face are spared. *See also* **Pelvic disorder, Shoulder girdle.**

Limp   An abnormal hobbling gait that favors one side, usually in an effort to avoid pain, such as from **sciatica** or **intermittent claudication**. It may also be caused by muscle weakness or foot problems.

Lipidosis   Any skin disease associated with a fat metabolism disorder. *See also* **Xanthelasma, Xanthoma.**

Lipoma   A noncancerous tumor composed mainly of fatty tissue. It may appear as a skin cyst. It is usually harmless, but if prominent it may be removed for cosmetic reasons.

Liver cancer   A carcinoma of the liver, which may be *primary,* if it originates there, or *secondary,* if cancer cells from another site, such as the skin, ovary, breast, kidney, lung, pancreas, stomach, or intestine, have migrated (metastasized) there. Primary liver cancer is much less frequent in North America and Europe than metastatic carcinoma. Primary cancers tend to appear during or after middle age, affect men almost ten times as often as women, and are often associated with exposure to cancer-causing industrial chemicals such as arsenic or vinyl chloride. Other factors may include nutritional deficiencies, eating foods contaminated by mold, and a previous condition of **cirrhosis**. Some primary liver cancers also have been linked to copper deposits in the liver in cases of Wilson's disease. Symptoms include weakness, loss of appetite, mild jaundice, pain in the upper abdominal area, and abdominal bloating. Diagnosis is sometimes made indirectly, as through radioactive scanning techniques, but many doctors prefer direct examination of liver tissue through **biopsy** or exploratory surgery. Treatment is by surgery to remove cancerous tissue and by chemotherapy. The outlook for recovery is poor and often depends on how far the cancer has spread.

Liver changes with age　The effects of aging on the size and functions of the liver, the organ responsible for most of the body's chemical activities, including metabolism of proteins, fats, and carbohydrates; regulation of blood sugar; processing of blood components; manufacture of bile, and the converting of poisonous substances into less harmful materials that can be excreted. A person's liver size, which is a fairly constant 2.5% of the total body weight throughout earlier years, begins to decrease after the age of fifty. Around the age of seventy, it begins to decrease more rapidly. Because of the reduction in heart output that accompanies aging, blood flow to the liver diminishes. The conversion and excretion of certain drugs are slowed, and in some instances there appears to be a relationship between drug metabolism and the use of tobacco as the decreased rate is found in smokers but not in nonsmokers. Persons over forty appear to be more susceptible to some liver diseases. There is a smaller risk of acquiring Type A viral **hepatitis** but a greater chance of contracting either Type B or non-A/non-B viral hepatitis. Drug-induced hepatitis is more common among individuals over forty, at a rate that is four to seven times that of persons under the age of thirty-five, depending upon the specific medication. Alcoholic hepatitis is less common, partly because the average intake of alcohol diminishes after the age of forty and there is less alcohol abuse among older persons, with only about 5 percent of older men and women identified as "heavy drinkers."

Liver spot　A popular term for any area of abnormally dark skin pigmentation that may appear on the hands, arms, or face, including an area of brownish pigmentation (chloasma) that may occur on the face of some women using hormone pills. Also called freckle, lentigo, keratosis.

Locomotion　The act of motion or of moving from one location to another. It is usually assumed that the movement is made possible by one's own physical resources or power. Locomotion can be by wheelchair as well as by walking.

Longevity　The number of years an average person of a particular age can expect to continue living, as determined by statistical tables based on mortality rates of various population groups. Factors that influence longevity may include sex, heredity, nutrition, lifestyles, and medical care. *See also* **Lifespan.**

Long-term care Continuous medical and personal care that is provided for those who lack some capacity to take care of themselves because of chronic illness, debility, lack of mobility, mental illness, or confinement to a bed or wheelchair. Persons requiring long-term care may be patients in a nursing home or those who have been returned to their own homes after a period of hospitalization but who require home health care during an extended period of rehabilitation or convalescence.

Lordosis A deformity of the spinal column that results in its being bent backward so that the back of the person appears hollow or concave. It is the opposite of **kyphosis**. Lordosis may develop as an effort by the body to counterbalance a protruding abdomen or as a result of rickets or other disorders affecting the spine.

Low back pain *See* **Herniated disk, Lumbago, Osteoporosis, Sciatica.**

Lumbago A popular term for any mid or low back pain.

Lumbar puncture The introduction of a hollow needle into the spinal cord in the lower back (lumbar) region for diagnosis or treatment of disorders of the central nervous system. The needle may be used to withdraw samples of cerebrospinal fluid; to reduce fluid pressure within the brain and spinal cord; or to inject drugs, a spinal anesthetic, or a dye that will produce shadows outlining brain or spinal tissues for diagnostic purposes. Also called "spinal tap."

Lung cancer Any cancer of that portion of the respiratory system between the windpipe (trachea) and the air sacs (alveoli) of the lungs. Symptoms usually are a persistent cough, **chest pain**, sputum that is streaked with pus or blood, breathing difficulty, and frequent bouts of respiratory diseases such as **pneumonia** or **bronchitis**. There also may be weight loss, fever, and weakness, particularly in advanced cases. About three-fourths of lung cancers are associated with cigarette smoking. It accounts for 27 percent of all cancer deaths in the United States. Lung cancer associated with cigarette smoking is the most common form of cancer among both men and women in the United States. Other possible causes are exposure to asbestos, radiation, nickel, petroleum products, arsenic, beryllium, chromium, and other industrial chemicals. Studies show that the risk of lung cancer from exposure to industrial chemicals is increased considerably if the worker is also a cigarette smoker. Lung cancer occurs in more than a half-dozen different forms, depending upon the type of tissue cells involved, the particular site (bronchi or alveoli), and whether the cancer is primary (originating in the lungs) or secondary (carried to the lungs from a cancer in another part of the body via the blood or lymph vessels). Early diagnosis is difficult because early tumor stages may not be visible on X-ray films, and the typical symptoms are not manifested until the disease is well established and may have already spread by metastasis to other parts of the body. (Primary lung cancers are often found by doctors tracing the source of a secondary cancer in another body area.) Treatment may include surgery, radiation, and chemotherapy. Untreated, a patient with primary lung cancer may live only nine months; treated, there is a 13 percent chance that an average patient may survive an additional five years. However, the five-year survival rate is as high as 40 per cent for patients with slow-growing tumors that can be removed in the earliest stages of the disease.

Lung changes with age   Alterations in lung capacity and function that are associated with the aging process. Many of the changes in lung capacity and airflow rates are due to the loss of elasticity of the lung tissue and to alterations in the tiny air sacs (alveoli) that give the lung its spongy characteristics. The changes in the alveoli reduce by about 25 percent the surface area available for the absorption of oxygen and the discharge of carbon dioxide with each breath. The stiffening of lung tissue also diminishes the ability to exhale carbon dioxide, requiring intensified breathing to accomplish this. Oxygen intake, meanwhile, decreases at a rate of approximately 1 percent per year and more in persons who are not physically active. Chest muscle tissue also atrophies. **Osteoporosis** leading to spinal compression, **kyphosis**, and lumbar **lordosis** may also affect the breathing capacity of the older person. The changes in lung function make the older adult much more vulnerable to respiratory infections and the effects of environmental pollutants. There is a much higher incidence of respiratory diseases among individuals over the age of forty.

Lupus   *See* **Systemic lupus erythematosus.**

Lymph   A relatively clear fluid that is similar to blood plasma with most of the red blood cells and many of the protein molecules removed. Lymph is formed in tissue spaces throughout the body as a result of chemical activity within the body's trillions of cells, following delivery of oxygen and nutrients to the cells by the capillaries. Lymph contains mainly white blood cells, fat globules, and waste products of cell metabolism, which are collected by a network of lymph vessels (the lymphatic system) and drained back into the blood circulation after passing through a filtering system of lymph nodes, or glands. The lymph nodes also serve as storage sites for lymphocytes, specialized white blood cells of the body's immune system that attack and destroy bacteria and other foreign substances.

Lymphadenopathy An enlarged or diseased lymph node. A swollen or inflamed lymph node may be tender, hard, smooth, irregular, or feel warm. This abnormal condition of a lymph node is a sign of vigorous activity by lymphocytes defending the body against an **antigen** or foreign protein substance. The location of the involved node is usually a clue to the site of a disease or infection that causes the condition, as when swollen lymph nodes in the neck accompany a sore throat.

Lymphangioma A noncancerous skin tumor that may appear as a group of small blisterlike eruptions, which is composed of a mass of dilated lymph vessels. Though harmless, it is usually removed for cosmetic reasons.

Lymphocytic choriomeningitis (LCM) An influenzalike viral infection that is transmitted through exposure to dust or food that has been contaminated by the gray house mouse. The disease affects mainly adults during the winter months with symptoms of fever, weakness, muscle pains in the lower back area, headache, nausea, loss of appetite, and a feeling of faintness. Complications include potentially serious brain inflammation, **arthritis**, skin rashes, inflammation of the testes, swollen salivary glands, and the symptoms may last from several weeks to several months. There is no specific treatment. Older adults are particularly susceptible to central nervous system inflammation, which can be fatal.

Lymphoma A general term for a tumor of the lymph tissue that is usually, but not always, cancerous. A typical lymphoma appears as a painless enlarged lymph node, often in the neck or chest area, accompanied by weakness, weight loss, fever, and anemia. Untreated, the disease may spread to the liver and spleen, which become enlarged, the skeletal system, and the digestive tract. Lymphomas are usually treated with radiation and chemotherapy, with a cure rate that ranges upward to 95 percent for Hodgkin's disease lymphomas given early therapy. Of the various types of lymphomas, persons over the age of forty are affected most often by Hodgkin's disease and **mycosis fungoides**.

M

Macula   A medical term for any small spot, usually distinguished by a color that differs from its background. The term is most commonly used to identify the *macula lutea,* or "yellow spot" on the retina of the eye, the central vision area near the connection between the retina and the optic nerve leading to the visual centers of the brain. It is the point of greatest visual acuity.

Macular degeneration   A form of vision loss that occurs after the age of fifty because of deterioration of the surface of the **macula**. Central vision becomes blurred, while peripheral vision remains normal. It is a major cause of blindness in older people. The condition is usually caused by a fluid leak under the retina in the area of the macula, which is followed by bleeding and scar formation in the retina. Some cases of macular degeneration occur without a fluid leak because of changes in the cells of the retina. Women are affected by macular degeneration more often than men. Total blindness does not usually occur, even after central vision is completely lost, because peripheral vision continues to permit those daily activities that do not require the ability to see details. A self-test for macular degeneration can be done by simply looking at objects known to have straight lines, such as the lines between bathroom tiles or along door frames. The test should be done by covering first one eye, then the other. If the straight lines appear to curve or if there is a blank spot, the condition should be reported without delay to an ophthalmologist.

Macule   A flat, well-defined area of skin that is of a different color than the surrounding skin. It is usually at the same level, neither depressed nor raised, as the rest of the skin and less than half an inch in diameter. A freckle or a **lentigo** may be a macule.

Magnetic apraxia   A condition in which a person moves across a floor by sliding the feet rather than lifting them and taking steps. He or she may need to stand in one place for a while before beginning **locomotion**. The magnetic apraxia patient also may require some support for crossing uneven surfaces, such as thresholds, curbs, or even the edge of a rug, to prevent falls. The condition may be associated with a **brain tumor, hydrocephalus, senile dementia**, or a cerebrovascular disease. *See also* **Apraxia.**

Major tranquilizer (antipsychotic drug)   A drug that is intended primarily to reduce the emotional reactions of persons being treated for a psychosis, such as **schizophrenia** or the **manic state** of a **bipolar disorder**, with a minimum effect on the person's consciousness, as distinguished from the traditional calming effects of sedative-type medications. Major tranquilizers do not "cure" a patient, but they can help restore his or her ability to function adequately in the **activities of daily living**. There are three main categories of major tranquilizers: *phenothiazines,* the original antipsychotic, or neuroleptic, drugs introduced in the 1950s; *butypherones,* which are sometimes used to treat patients who do not respond to the effects of phenothiazines; and *thioxanthenes,* which have been used in patients who fail to respond adequately to the use of either phenothiazines or butypherones. Each type may also be a drug of choice for a specific form of psychosis, one being preferred over the others for treating a paranoid or nonparanoid schizophrenic patient. Each type of major tranquilizer may also have advantages over the other types in avoiding adverse side effects that may result from the use of such drugs. For example, one patient may be unable to tolerate a particular major tranquilizer because of a heart condition, while a second patient with a similar diagnosis may require a different major tranquilizer that will not aggravate a liver impairment. A physician may prescribe several types of antipsychotic drugs before determining which drug most effectively controls the patient's symptoms with the fewest adverse side effects.

Older adults are generally more sensitive to the effects of major tranquilizers and usually receive smaller initial doses than younger persons with the same condition. Also, because apparent psychological abnormalities in older adults, such as insomnia and confusion, may actually be due to a medical problem, an effort is usually made at first to treat any underlying physical disorder. A major tranquilizer may often be the cause of confusion, tremor, restlessness, **tardive dyskinesia,** or other effects in an older person. Antipsychotic drugs in each of the major categories are capable of triggering symptoms of **parkinsonism** or of worsening the condition of a person with true **Parkinson's disease**. Butypherones and thiothixene, a form of thioxanthene, have been known to cause permanently disabling side effects and are usually not prescribed for older persons when there are alternative medications that are less hazardous. *See also* **Minor tranquilizers.**

Malabsorption   The defective absorption of nutrients in the small intestine. Examples include a failure of the intestine to absorb the folic acid and vitamin B_{12} needed for the maturation of red blood cells, resulting in anemia, weakness, and fatigue; and **celiac disease**, which is marked by an inability to tolerate foods containing wheat gluten. Causes of malabsorption also can include diseases involving the pancreas, liver, or bile ducts; intestinal infections; the use of various medications, including antibiotics; the use of alcohol or mineral oil; and certain foods containing chemicals, such as oxalates, that bind with nutrients so they are excreted rather than absorbed.

Maladaptation   Failure of an individual to make necessary adjustments to changes and pressures of the external world. Examples may include a person with few if any outside interests who is forcibly retired after many years of service to a company, the sudden death of a spouse, or the loss of income requiring a move to a less desirable neighborhood. Illness may be a cause of maladaptive behavior, which can in turn increase the severity of the illness. The victim may retreat from reality, displaying behavior that may be self-defeating.

Malaise   A general feeling of discomfort, uneasiness, tiredness, or of being sick.

Malalignment   Any improper alignment of the skeleton or other body tissues. A malalignment of the weight-bearing bones of the body can result in disorders of gait, such as limping, lurching, or the knock-knee or bowleg effects caused by uneven loss of cartilage in the knee joints due to **osteoarthritis. Osteoporosis** can lead to compression fractures of the spinal column and abnormal curvature of the spine.

Male climacteric (male menopause)   A type of midlife crisis that some men undergo, often linked to a psychological complex of aspirations unrealized, a sense of time passing, and youth past. There may be some symptoms of depression. However, many authorities doubt the reality of the condition and regard it as an artificial analogy to the true physiological process of the female menopause. Unlike the female climacteric, male sex hormones continue to be produced during the male midlife crisis, although there may be some gradual decline with aging, and many men retain some degree of fertility throughout their adult lives. The term has also been used to identify a period of reduced sexual desire and activity, accompanied by a drying of the skin, reduced **metabolism**, and other functional changes in the older male.

Malignant   Pertaining to something that is particularly harmful or dangerous, as a tumor that is cancerous.

Malignant hypertension   An acute, severe form of high blood pressure caused by a blood circulation disorder in the kidneys. The lining of the arterioles (small arteries) in the kidneys becomes thick and fibrous, eventually obstructing the blood flow and destroying the blood vessels. Diastolic blood pressure (the low number in a blood pressure reading) may rise above 120, or 30 points above the "normal" maximum. Symptoms include headaches, blurred vision with bleeding and fluid leakage from the retinas of the eyes, plus various other disorders resulting from circulatory damage to tissues in the brain, heart, kidneys, or other organs. Causes or contributing factors include heredity, obesity, stress, excessive use of table salt, and use of oral contraceptives. The disorder tends to affect men over the age of forty, but women may experience the symptoms before they are forty. Untreated, malignant hypertension is usually fatal within one year. Treatment involves a special diet and drugs. *See also* **Hypertension.**

Malnutrition   Any abnormal health condition due to a deficient, excessive, or unbalanced intake of food elements or to a failure of the body to absorb or utilize certain food elements. The risk of malnutrition increases for older persons who for reasons of low income, solitude, fear of leaving home, frailty, poorly fitting dentures or missing teeth that make chewing difficult, an inability to cook, or a lack of basic knowledge of nutrition fail to receive an adequate intake of the nutrients needed to maintain good health. It is not uncommon for a diagnosis of **senile dementia** to be made in an older person whose condition is actually due to malnutrition. The term is often used to identify persons suffering from deficiency diseases, such as scurvy, rickets, or iron-deficiency anemia, but it may also be applied to cases of **obesity** or **malabsorption**. Malnutrition may also be an effect of alcohol abuse.

Malum coxae senilis A medical term for **osteoarthritis** of the hip.

Malum gleni senilis A medical term for **osteoarthritis** of the shoulder.

Manic-depressive illness (bipolar disorder) A neuropsychiatric disorder marked by a dominant mood of euphoria or depression but sometimes alternating between the two extremes. It is sometimes identified as an affective disorder because it is marked by displays of unusual affects (moods), from morbid depression that will not respond to normal reassurances to manic states of unrealistic optimism, overconfidence, and delusions of grandeur. Although bipolar affective disorders may begin as early as the teenage years, they can be diagnosed at any age, and depressive forms of the condition tend to increase with aging. Accurate diagnosis of a bipolar disorder is often more difficult in an older adult because the condition is likely to be complicated by a physical illness, side effects of medications, decline in vision and hearing, or social isolation. Some experts also believe that an older adult is more likely than a young person to mask an affective disorder with complaints of pain or discomfort. Factors that may contribute to manic-depressive illness include heredity, tumors, stressful life events, adverse effects of drugs, infections, hormone disorders, and malnutrition. *See also* **Depression, Manic State.**

Manic state A psychological condition marked by elation, excessive activity or restlessness, talkativeness, racing thoughts, and a tendency to irresponsible acts, such as buying sprees and reckless driving. The person in a manic state also may show aggressive irritability and hostility, experience **hallucinations**, and may act in an impulsive and dangerous manner without being aware that his or her behavior could be hazardous. The manic state can be especially dangerous when the patient is paranoid, with delusions that include ideas of being persecuted by an individual or group. *See also* **Manic-depressive illness.**

Manipulation Any treatment, such as massage, that is performed with the hands. Manipulation is often used in rehabilitation techniques to increase the range of motion of an arm or leg that has been partially or completely immobilized or to correct a faulty position of a part of the body, such as an abnormal spinal curvature.

Marche à petits pas A shuffling gait with short mincing steps, as observed in persons with **parkinsonism** or the effects of brain damage due to small **strokes**.

Marin Amat syndrome **A neurological disorder** in which involuntary contractions of the facial muscles cause the eyes to close when the person opens the mouth or chews food.

Massage The therapeutic manipulation of soft tissues of the body. There are nearly two dozen types of massage techniques used for various specific disorders, including friction, vibration, stroking (effleurage), kneading (petrissage), and tapping (tapotement).

Mastectomy The surgical removal of one or both breasts, usually performed to remove a cancer. In a *simple mastectomy*, only breast tissue is removed. In a *radical mastectomy*, chest muscles underlying the breast and lymph nodes in the adjacent armpit (axilla) area of the affected side are removed along with the breast. In a *modified radical mastectomy*, the entire breast and nearly all of the axillary lymph nodes are removed, leaving the chest muscles intact. The precise procedure depends in part on the extent of cancer spread in the area and the agreement of the woman involved, usually resulting in a collaborative decision between the patient and the surgeon. The trend toward collaborative surgical decisions has been accompanied by a reduced frequency of radical mastectomy procedures. Studies indicate that the outlook for recovery is about the same when the more conservative modified mastectomy procedure is chosen. The surgery may be supplemented by hormonal therapy, chemotherapy, and/or radiation therapy. The missing breast can be replaced with a flexible plastic implant after an interval of about six months following surgery. An alternative procedure for some cases is a *lumpectomy*, in which only the part of the breast actually invaded by cancer cells is removed. Some authorities oppose lumpectomies on the grounds that breast cancer is seldom confined to only one part of a breast.

Melanoma, malignant A cancer that develops from the pigment cells (melanocytes) of the skin. Melanomas are more common in persons with fair skins and light-colored eyes. They usually develop from a pigmented mole. However, they can develop from melanocytes in otherwise normal skin as well. Exposure to sunlight is believed to play an important role in the development of melanomas, but the lesions may also occur on skin areas rarely if ever exposed to sunlight. The cells that develop into malignant (cancerous) melanomas may be present in the skin from birth but do not make an appearance until later adulthood. Any mole or spot on the skin that appears suddenly or that spreads, turns darker, forms a crust or ulcer, or bleeds should be examined promptly by a dermatologist. With early detection, diagnosis, and treatment by surgical excision, a cure rate of nearly 100 percent is possible for this potentially fatal form of skin cancer. *See also* **Lentigo.**

Melena (black stool)　Feces that are abnormally dark because they contain digested blood. The condition is usually a sign of bleeding in the stomach or small intestine. (Bleeding in the lower bowel may result in red-colored feces, which should be differentiated from black.) The source may be swallowed blood from the nose or throat or bleeding from a point in the digestive tract, as well as cancer, peptic ulcers, or other life-threatening conditions that require immediate attention by a physician. It is not unusual for gastrointestinal bleeding to be caused by aspirin or other drugs that may irritate the lining of the stomach. Iron supplements, when taken by mouth, can also result in darkened feces, but this condition should not be confused with the effects of internal bleeding.

Memory loss　Diminished ability or failure of the ability to recall past events or experiences because of any of a wide range of possible factors, including diseases affecting the brain tissues, psychological disorders, malnutrition, and side effects of drugs. Memory loss may be total or partial. It may affect only recent events or only past events. Types of organic brain damage that may contribute to memory loss include **arteriosclerosis** of the brain, **stroke**, injury, or **Alzheimer's disease.** Memory loss in a case of **Korsakoff's syndrome**, a brain disorder associated with alcoholism, is attributed to a deficiency of a B vitamin. Psychological disorders include **amnesia**, sometimes identified as a type of "isolated memory loss" because only a certain part of the past cannot be recalled, and **confabulation**, characterized by the creation of false information about past events when the person cannot actually recall details of the past. Types of memory loss that are temporary or reversible include those associated with epileptic seizures, head injury, **malnutrition, hypoglycemia,** use of alcohol or medications, or diseases such as **uremia** or **hypothyroidism.** Memory loss is usually permanent when it involves destruction of functional brain tissue, as can result from multiple strokes, brain tumor, or Alzheimer's disease.

Ménière's disease　A disorder of the inner ear, affecting the sense of balance and also producing some degree of hearing loss. Symptoms include attacks of **vertigo** accompanied by nausea and vomiting, a fluctuating hearing loss that gradually worsens, and a constant or intermittent ringing or buzzing in the ears (**tinnitus**). Patients also complain of a feeling of "fullness" in the affected ear, and some report profuse sweating during the attacks, which may last from several minutes to several hours. The exact cause is unknown. Persons afflicted with the disease prefer to move cautiously, since any sudden movement can trigger or aggravate the sensation of vertigo. Treatment usually includes drugs, a low-sodium diet, and surgery, if necessary. When possible, neurosurgery is performed to sever nerves associated with the vertigo symptoms without affecting the sense of hearing. In cases where hearing has already been lost and the vertigo is disabling, the inner ear structures may be removed.

Meningitis An inflammation of the layers of thin membranes (meninges) that cover the brain and spinal cord, usually caused by a bacterial, viral, or fungal infection. Meningitis also may be caused by a tumor or chemical irritation. The term **encephalitis** is commonly used to identify a viral inflammation of the brain, while *cerebritis* specifies a bacterial inflammation of brain tissues. Viral forms of meningitis also may be called *aseptic meningitis.* Typical symptoms include a severe headache, pain and stiffness in the neck, fever, and vomiting. Older adults are likely to show signs of altered mental functions. Other diseases, such as **diabetes mellitus, tuberculosis**, syphilis, and infections of the lungs or urinary tract, may increase the risk of meningitis in older adults. Older adults are also increasingly susceptible to meningitis caused by bacteria that cause pneumonia. Diagnosis of the exact cause is based on the age and medical history of the patient, examination of a blood sample and a sample of cerebrospinal fluid obtained from a lumbar spinal tap, and physical examination of the person. The physical examination may indicate how an infecting organism may have entered the brain or spinal cord, as through a head injury or an ear infection. Treatment is with antibiotics for bacterial infections, the choice depending on the specific organism involved. Therapy in cases of viral meningitis is more difficult, but an antiviral drug, cytosine arabinoside, is available for infections due to the **herpes simplex** virus. There is no specific drug for other viral infections of the meninges, and treatment is limited to relief of the symptoms.

Menopause A term that is used both to identify the final menstrual period in a woman's life and to delineate the entire transitional phase preceding, during, and immediately after the end of a woman's fertile years. The final menstrual period for the average woman is in her fifty-first year. For a reported 10 percent of women, menopause occurs a decade earlier in life. The age of onset of the menopause does not appear to be affected by race, body size, nutrition, health, or socioeconomic factors. One study found that the average age at menopause has not changed since medieval times, although the average age for a girl's first menstrual period has been diminishing at a rate of more than three months every ten years for the past century. As the menopause approaches, the ovaries gradually stop secreting the female sex hormone estrogen. Estrogen levels decline, and the time between menstrual periods grows longer until they cease altogether. Levels of both female and male sex hormones in the woman decline as a result of the menopause, although hormone production does not cease completely. The ovaries and uterus shrink; the breasts decrease in size and weight. The gradual decline in estrogen levels, which is erratic rather than constant, causes gradual atrophy of the external genitalia. There is a loss of pubic hair, and some masculine-type facial or body hair may appear because it is no longer suppressed by high blood levels of estrogen. The risk of cancer of the reproductive organs, with the exception of the cervix, increases, and many women experience **hot flashes**. Because estrogen provides some protection against bone loss, **myocardial infarction, stroke,** and **arteriosclerosis,** postmenopausal women are more susceptible to these conditions and to **osteoporosis** than are younger women. Despite anatomical and physiological changes, menopause does not necessarily alter female sexual function or **libido.** Nor should it mark the end of a productive and active life. With an average lifespan of nearly seventy-eight years for women, they can expect nearly thirty additional years of life after the menopause.

Metabolism   The physical and chemical changes that take place in the body, including the conversion of food substances into energy, that allow essential life processes to go on. The term is commonly applied to those processes that occur when the human body converts proteins, fats, carbohydrates, and minerals into chemical forms that the body uses to build and repair tissues. The term *basal metabolism* refers to the minimum number of calories of energy (about 1,500 calories per day) needed to maintain these processes in a resting human being. Metabolic requirements diminish as one grows older. A person at age forty-five needs 10 to 15 percent fewer calories than were needed at twenty-five; and at age sixty-five, 20 to 30 percent fewer calories than at twenty-five.

Metastasis   The process whereby cancer cells spread from their original site to other parts of the body, usually through the blood or lymph vessels. Cancers that develop as a result of metastasis are identified as secondary cancers to distinguish them from the original, or primary, cancers.

Microaneurysm   A tiny dilation in a capillary that may appear as a red dot in the skin, on the retina of the eye, or other body tissues. It frequently occurs in clusters. Microaneurysms of the retina are a clinical sign of **diabetes mellitus**. On the skin, microaneurysms may be tiny thrombi (blood clots) and a sign of a serious systemic disease.

Middle age   A nonspecific term for a period of life with both psychological and physiological interpretations. For some individuals, it is a recognition that youth is over. For others, it is largely ignored. In some cultures of the world, middle age is identified as the period of life that begins around the age of forty; in some cultures middle age does not begin until after the age of sixty. It is also regarded as a period of lower energy levels and the first signs of certain health deficits. It may also be a time when many individuals reshape their perspectives regarding work, marriage, and the future. Middle age also borders on the periods some describe as young-old, as distinguished from old-old and late maturity, which is marked by a feeling of release from earlier responsibilities of establishing oneself in a secure occupational and social position in the community.

Migraine   *See* **Headache.**

Milk-alkali syndrome   A condition of **hypercalcemia**, or abnormally high levels of calcium in the blood. It can develop in persons who continually consume excessive amounts of absorbable antacids, particularly in the form of calcium carbonate and sodium bicarbonate. They have symptoms of nausea, headache, vomiting, constipation, abdominal pain, swallowing difficulty, and urinary tract disorders. Untreated, the condition may lead to kidney damage. Symptoms diminish when the intake of antacids and calcium ceases.

Minor tranquilizer (antianxiety agents)   A family of drugs with a mild sedating or anxiety-reducing effect used to treat persons suffering from anxiety or tension. They are not useful in treating cases of psychosis. They are also helpful in relieving the anxiety that often accompanies a physical illness, such as gastrointestinal or heart disorders. They may be used in some cases of epilepsy. An example are the *benzodiazepines,* the most widely used of the minor tranquilizers, which are prescribed in the treatment of alcoholism, as anticonvulsants, and as muscle relaxants. *See also* **Major tranquilizer.**

Miotic   Pertaining to small eye pupils. A miotic drug reduces the size of the pupils.

Mitral valve   The heart valve that separates the left upper heart chamber (atrium) from the left lower chamber (ventricle) and prevents blood from flowing backward during heart contractions. Changes in the mitral valve that may occur with aging include hardening (**sclerosis**) of the valve, valve **prolapse**, and other defects. Such defects can result in blood pressure changes, backflow of blood, increased workload for the heart, and pain in the chest or left armpit. Other problems may be sensations of heart palpitations, fatigue, breathing difficulty, and faintness. Depending upon the specific type and degree of damage, treatment may be with medications, with open heart surgery to repair the defect, or by replacement of the mitral valve with an artificial valve. Persons with artificial mitral valves must usually take anticoagulant drugs and other medications, such as antibiotics, as needed, before undergoing dental work.

Mobility   The ability of a person to move the body or a body part without assistance. Patients with musculoskeletal, mental, or neurological disorders are sometimes graded for mobility on a scale ranging from complete independence to complete dependence, as in a person who is in traction or bedfast because of a serious condition. In between are stages of being able to move about in bed, to move from the bed to a chair, to move about in a wheelchair, and to be able to stand without assistance.

Mole   A usually pigmented area of skin, flat or elevated, sometimes occurring as a cluster of nodules. Some moles lack pigment and are flesh-colored. A mole may look like a wart and may or may not contain hairs. Moles can appear anywhere on the body but tend to occur most frequently on the head and neck. They are present on almost every adult, though they can seem more prominent on some persons than others. Some moles are harmless, but others may suddenly grow in size, change color, or undergo other changes that may be signs of cancer. Any mole that undergoes a sudden change should be examined by a physician. Also called "nevus." *See also* **Melanoma.**

Monilial infection   An infection of the skin or mucous membranes by a yeastlike fungus. A genital infection by the *Candida albicans* fungus results in **vaginitis**. Older adults are increasingly susceptible to monilial infections of the mouth because of a thinning of the tissues and decreased salivary gland activity, plus effects of **dehydration**. They are also more likely to suffer from vitamin A deficiency and to be using antibiotics that destroy microorganisms that would ordinarily compete with and suppress fungi on body tissues. The condition may be complicated by **diabetes mellitus**. Treatment is with antifungal medications, which may be taken by mouth or applied as creams or lotions, depending upon the site of the infection.

Monocular diplopia   Double vision that occurs with only one eye, usually in association with a **cataract** or a defect in the cornea.

Monoamine oxidase (MAO) inhibitors   A group of drugs, sometimes called "psychic energizers," used to treat **depression**. They inhibit an enzyme, monoamine oxidase, that occurs naturally in the body, but which can become overly active and destroy nerve impulse transmitter substances, such as dopamine, that are needed for normal mental activity. Authorities believe that destruction of the nerve transmitter substances results in a reduced level of mental activity, leading to a form of depression (endogenous) that is produced from within the body rather than by an external event (exogenous), such as a crushing disappointment. The MAO inhibitors have been used primarily to counteract this situation by, in effect, inhibiting the inhibitor. However, because of the complex chemical relationships between MAO inhibitors and substances in many foods and medications, serious adverse reactions can occur when MAO inhibitors are taken with certain foods and beverages, particularly aged cheeses and Chianti wine, that contain a chemical called tyramine. People who do not use MAO inhibitors may not be affected by such foods, but those using the medication may experience sudden, dangerously high blood pressure (**hypertensive crisis**). A similar reaction can occur from taking certain medications, ranging from nasal decongestants to barbiturates, or certain drugs of abuse, such as cocaine, at the same time as MAO inhibitors. MAO inhibitors remain in the body tissues for a long period of time, and a reaction can occur up to two weeks after the use of the antidepressant drug has been discontinued.

Moon type   A printing method that produces large-type letters that are raised so they can be read by touch by blind or visually impaired persons. The lines of type run alternately from left to right, then right to left, and so on, so that finger contact with the embossed letters is nearly continuous. The system, developed in England, is learned more easily than the braille method by persons who lose their sight later in life.

Morbidity   Pertaining to disease and usually applied to statistics showing the number of persons afflicted with a particular health disorder for a specific population, such as the number of cases per 1,000 or 10,000 people. *See also* **Mortality.**

Morphea A form of **scleroderma,** or hardening and thickening of the skin. It is usually localized rather than widespread and may be treated with physical therapy or hormone injections to prevent it from developing into a disabling permanent tissue contraction.

Mortality Pertaining to death and usually applied to the death rate for a particular health condition, such as the number of pneumonia deaths per 1,000 or 10,000 people. *See also* **Morbidity.**

Motility Pertaining to the ability of something to move spontaneously or involuntarily. The term is commonly applied to describe the movement of food through the digestive tract, as in *gastric motility* or *intestinal motility.*

Movement disorder Any disabling condition, such as muscle weakness or paralysis, that results in **immobility** of a person. *See also* **Mobility.**

Mucormycosis A fungal infection of the nose, sinuses, or eyeball socket. It develops rapidly, particularly in persons with diabetic **acidosis** or disorders of the immune system, and is frequently fatal.

Multi-infarct dementia A form of mental deterioration that can occur in older adults as a result of repeated small circulatory accidents in the brain, such as small brain hemorrhages or obstructions in the blood vessels supplying certain areas of brain tissue. The infarcts can result in alterations in behavior, **memory loss,** loss of ability to make proper judgments, or inability to think in abstract terms. Multi-infarct dementia also can account for gait abnormalities, partial paralysis, and loss of the ability to detect sensations of touch or other stimuli in various body areas.

Multiple myeloma A cancer involving the blood-cell forming areas of the bone marrow that produces an excess of protein substances such as immunoglobulins. There may be **anemia, hypercalcemia,** kidney damage, and loss of resistance to infections. The disease is progressive, tends to affect primarily men in their fifties, and is usually fatal. The cancer invades the "flat" bones of the body, such as the ribs, skull, pelvis, and the vertebrae, producing effects that resemble the damage of **osteoporosis.** Symptoms include bone pain, kidney problems, pallor, weakness, fatigue, and susceptibility to bacterial infections. Bones often break spontaneously. Treatment consists of chemotherapy, radiation, pain-killers, and antibiotics, which may prolong survival for two to three years.

Murmur   An abnormal heart sound detected with a stethoscope. The sound, which may range in tone from a blowing to a rasping noise, is caused by the movement of blood through the heart and its adjacent large blood vessels. A murmur may be a sign of a heart valve defect or an abnormal constriction or dilatation of a blood vessel, but it may not be associated with any cardiovascular defect.

Muscle changes with age   Alterations in muscle tissue associated with the aging process. There is a general loss of muscle mass as a person grows older; much of the muscle tissue is replaced by fat deposits, so that the gradual change is more easily detected in strength tests than in physical appearance. The decrease occurs both in terms of the number of muscle fibers and in a smaller average diameter of individual muscle fibers. Microscopic studies of the muscle tissues of older adults also may show a loss of contact between muscle fibers and the nerve fibers that normally transmit the impulses required to produce muscle contractions. The loss of muscle bulk and strength with age is usually not great enough to interfere with the ability of most older adults to carry on their usual **activities of daily living**.

Musculoskeletal disorder   Any disease or injury affecting the structure or function of the muscles, bones, joints, tendons, and ligaments of the body. The disorder may result in a loss of locomotion or the ability to perform labor or daily living activities. Examples include **bursitis, Dupuytrens's contracture, osteoarthritis, rheumatoid arthritis, gout,** and **osteoporosis**.

Mutation theory of aging   A theory that tissue cells gradually deteriorate through errors that develop in structure and functions of the cells, including changes in the chromosomes of the cell nuclei that are reproduced when the cells divide. The errors may occur through exposure to radiation, such as cosmic rays or ultraviolet light from beyond the atmosphere, chemicals in the environment, or drugs, or be the result of spontaneous mistakes that may occur in any of the hundreds of chemical reactions that take place during normal cellular metabolism. Daughter cells may inherit defective enzymes or other cellular components and fail to function properly. Cells that normally do not reproduce, such as brain cells, simply die or cease working when they acquire such defects. Other theories of aging suggest the presence of a genetic clock that limits the number of times a body cell can reproduce or replace itself; a built-in lifespan limit, particular to each species, which may be related to the number of calories burned in a lifetime; and the occurrence of "free radicals," molecules with an extra electrical charge that interact with vital body chemicals and render them useless; and the gradual breakdown of the **immune system**, leading to increased susceptibility to infections and increased risk of cancer and other diseases that would have been suppressed by the immune function in earlier years.

Myasthenia gravis   A disease characterized by severe muscular weakness caused by a failure of nerve impulses to produce muscle contractions. It affects women more often than men, particularly those over the age of forty. It is associated with either a lack of a nerve transmitter chemical (acetylcholine) or the presence of an enzyme that destroys the nerve transmitter substance. There is evidence of an **immune system** failure that contributes to the faulty nerve transmission. The disorder begins with weakness and fatigability of the face and neck muscles, causing difficulty in chewing, swallowing, and talking; and with visual problems, such as seeing double. As the disease progresses, the loss of facial muscle function results in drooping eyelids and absence of facial expressions. Symptoms generally increase toward the end of the day. The disorder may spread to other parts of the body and interfere with other functions, particularly breathing. In acute cases, death may result from respiratory failure. Diagnosis is based on **electromyography** (a method of testing muscle contractions with electricity) and injection of a drug (edrophonium) that causes a brief improvement in the condition. The condition responds to drugs that inhibit cholinesterase, an enzyme that destroys acetylcholine. Treatment also includes bed rest or restricted activity, a diet that minimizes the need for chewing, and other medications.

Mycosis fungoides   A form of **lymphoma** that begins as an itching skin disease and eventually spreads to other parts of the body, including internal organs. It is generally fatal. The disease usually affects persons over the age of fifty. In the initial stage a red, scaly rash appears that resembles **eczema** or **psoriasis**. Some of the patches of eruption become raised and appear to heal but are followed by nodules and ulcerated plaques that may produce secondary infections. The survival period for most persons is over seven years. Treatment is with radiation and chemotherapy, which are most effective in the early stages.

Mydriatic Pertaining to drugs (mydriatics) or other agents that cause dilation of the pupil of the eye. Pupils normally increase in size when light intensity is reduced. Mydriatics usually cause an increase in the pressure within the eyeball and are sometimes used in tests for **glaucoma**.

Myeloma A type of bone tumor that invades the bone marrow. *See* **Multiple myeloma.**

Myocardial Pertaining to the muscle tissue (myocardium) of the heart.

Myocardial infarction (MI) (heart attack) Damage to an area of heart muscle from an interruption of blood flow through a coronary artery supplying the heart. Interruption of the normal blood flow, caused by an obstruction in the artery, causes immediate oxygen starvation that leads to death of the affected heart tissue. The symptoms are a crushing, viselike pain that may radiate to the left arm, neck, and jaw. The pain is steady and is not relieved by rest or the medications normally used to treat **angina pectoris,** which presents some of the same symptoms. The pain may continue for hours if untreated. The skin is usually cold and moist, and there is sweating and pallor. The patient frequently experiences nausea and vomiting. Breathing difficulty, shock, and heart failure can occur within minutes of the onset of symptoms, so emergency professional medical treatment is essential. Any person with symptoms that suggest a possible myocardial infarction should seek immediate help. Half of all myocardial infarction patients die within two and a half hours of the first symptoms. Most MI patients have a preexisting condition of **atherosclerosis** of the coronary arteries. **Thrombosis** is a common complicating factor; nearly one-fourth of all sudden fatal heart attacks are due to a coronary artery thrombosis. Emergency treatment includes injections of morphine to relieve pain, reduce the workload of the heart, and dilate the coronary arteries. Medications may also be administered to compensate for shock and a sudden drop in blood pressure. Anticoagulants may be given to reduce the risk of additional blood clots in the coronary arteries, and other drugs administered to stabilize the heartbeat. Additional measures include bed rest, low-calorie, low-sodium diet, and gradual physical reconditioning.

Myoclonus Any rapid, irregular, involuntary jerking movement of the muscles, as the shocklike involuntary contractions experienced when one is drifting into sleep.

Myoglobinuria   The presence of an iron-containing pigment (myoglobin) in the urine. Myoglobin tends to color the urine red and may be mistaken for blood in the urine. It is a substance similar to the hemoglobin in red blood cells and occurs naturally in muscle tissue. The myoglobin may be forced out of muscle tissue and excreted in urine as a result of strenuous physical exercise, crushing injuries, and other conditions.

Myokimia   Slow, quivering contractions of a few muscle fibers. It occurs frequently in the facial area, as in the twitching of an eyelid during periods of stress or fatigue. Temporary myokimia is generally harmless, but if it persists, the condition may be a sign of a central nervous system condition and should be investigated.

Myopia   Nearsightedness. It is usually due to an elongation of the eyeball or to a defect in the refractive ability of the lens, so that images are focused at a point in front of the retina rather than on the surface of the retina. Lens errors in older adults are usually the result of an increase in the size of the lens, caused by old lens fibers accumulating in the nucleus of the lens. As the nucleus becomes more compact, its refractive power changes. The condition is corrected by prescription lenses (eyeglasses or contact lenses) that compensate for the refractive error of the natural lens.

Myotonia   A muscle spasm that follows a voluntary contraction of the muscle, as when the fingers fail to relax immediately after shaking hands with another person. Myotonia often occurs in cases of swallowing difficulty, as when a person feels that food is stuck in the throat because the muscles of the esophagus fail to relax after swallowing. When the condition threatens to become disabling, treatment may require surgery, medications, or physical therapy, or a combination of procedures.

Myringitis   Inflammation of an eardrum.

Myxedema   *See* **Hypothyroidism.**

N

Nail changes with aging   Alterations that occur in the fingernails and toenails as one grows older. The rate of nail growth begins to decline after the age of thirty, and the rate of decline is faster in men than in women until their fifties, when nail growth rate is approximately the same for both sexes. The nails also become dull, opaque, and sometimes discolored as one ages. Ridges develop along the length of the nail, and layers of nail may break off occasionally. The half-moon shaped, lightly colored area near the base of the nail (lunula) gradually disappears. Some changes in tissues beneath the fingernail are due to exposure to sunlight; because nails are transparent, the sun's radiation can damage sensitive skin tissues beneath the nail. Changes in toenails and adjacent tissues are usually caused by impaired blood circulation to the toes. Age changes in the nails also include an increased susceptibility of the tissues to fungal infections.

Narcolepsy   A **neurological disorder** that results in chronic excessive daytime sleepiness or an irresistible desire to sleep at inappropriate times or places. The affected person also usually goes into immediate, deep sleep. Symptoms may begin in adolescence or early adulthood, but the condition occurs most frequently among hypertensive middle-aged men who are overweight and who also may be bothered with sleep **apnea**, a condition of breathing difficulty while sleeping. The person may also experience symptoms of sudden muscle weakness after normal emotional excitement such as laughter or anger. Persons affected by narcolepsy are most likely to fall asleep under conditions that normally cause drowsiness, as after a meal or during a period of boredom. However, a narcoleptic episode also may occur when alertness is important, as when driving a car or operating machinery. Narcolepsy also affects women, whose symptoms may begin to appear before middle-age. Diagnosis is based in part on results of **electroencephalographic** studies of electrical activity in the brain. Treatment is with drugs that stimulate the central nervous system.

Natriuresis The excretion of large amounts of sodium in the urine. Increased sodium excretion may be induced with drugs as part of the therapy for some conditions such as kidney and metabolic diseases, or it may occur as a result of use of **diuretic** drugs, certain hormone disturbances, **cirrhosis**, or diabetic **acidosis**. Serious loss of sodium is less common in the older adult than excessive sodium levels. The condition may result in **hyponatremia**, marked by headache, confusion, weakness, and fatigue.

Nausea An unpleasant sensation marked by the urge to vomit. It may or may not lead to actual vomiting. Nausea occurs with motion sickness, vertigo, emotional upsets, gallbladder disorders, certain diseases of the central nervous system, early pregnancy, intense pain, food poisoning, radiation exposure, some drugs and anesthetics, and viral infections. Nausea also may be caused by unpleasant sights, tastes, or odors. Nausea due to food poisoning is usually self-limited and requires no particular treatment after the offending food or other substance is ejected or removed. Nausea with vomiting that is persistent can lead to dehydration with loss of **electrolytes** and may require emergency medical care. Treatment is with tranquilizers, sedatives, antihistamines, or other medications, depending upon the cause of the condition and individual sensitivities to the drugs.

Nearsightedness *See* **Myopia.**

Neck pain Discomfort or pain in the region of the neck that can be a symptom of numerous disorders. Diagnosis is often aided by determining whether the pain is aggravated by chewing or swallowing or by moving the head or shoulder. Pain affected by chewing or swallowing may involve the salivary glands, the thyroid gland, the lower jaw, one of the carotid arteries of the neck, or conditions such as tonsillitis, cancer of the larynx, or **esophagitis**. Neck pain that is increased by head movements may be caused by **wryneck** (torticollis), spinal **arthritis**, viral inflammation of the neck muscles, **meningitis**, or a herniated spinal disk. A herniated disk may also cause pain when there is no movement of the head or shoulders. **Herpes zoster**, poliomyelitis, a spinal cord tumor, or **erysipelas** are also sources of neck pain that is not affected by movement of the head or shoulders. In some cases, neck pain may be **referred** from **headaches, angina pectoris,** or other causes.

Neoplasm A medical term for any new tissue growth, such as a tumor or cancer. Cancers are usually identified as malignant neoplasms to distinguish them from noncancerous (benign) growths.

Nephritis Any inflammation of the kidneys. The term is sometimes modified to denote a specific type of kidney disorder, as *glomerulonephritis* refers to an inflammation of the urine-filtering units (glomeruli) of the kidneys. A common cause of nephritis is a bacterial infection, often acquired through catheters or other instruments inserted into the urethra during a medical or surgical procedure. The bacteria may travel back through the bladder and ureters to infect the kidney. One form of such an infection, *acute bacterial pyelonephritis,* is marked by chills, fever, nausea, vomiting, and flank pain. There may also be bladder irritation, causing increased urgency and frequency of urination. Diagnosis is by symptoms and laboratory examination of the urine. Antibiotics are used to treat the infection, the specific type depending upon the species of bacteria involved. Glomerulonephritis may follow a streptococcal bacterial infection and may be more difficult to detect in an older adult because the symptoms are less specific than in a younger person. The symptoms may include nausea, malaise, joint pains, and lung congestion, and the condition is often mistaken for another illness, such as a complication of congestive heart failure. Nephritis leading to severe kidney damage may require treatment by **dialysis.**

Nephroangiosclerosis A disease caused by hardening of the small arteries of the kidney and associated with **hypertension**. The disease usually occurs around the age of forty in some persons with high blood pressure (hypertension), particularly those whose **diastolic** blood pressure is greater than 120. Symptoms include headaches and blurred vision. The heart is usually enlarged, and red blood cells appear in the urine. Treatment involves drugs to lower the blood pressure and dialysis, if necessary because of kidney damage.

Nephrosclerosis A hardening and thickening of the kidney tissues, leading to interruption of blood and oxygen flow to the kidney. This condition results in the degeneration of the urine-filtering units (glomeruli) and their replacement with fibrous tissue growth. It is usually a complication of **hypertension**. Treatment requires drugs to lower the blood pressure.

Nephrotic syndrome An abnormal condition of the kidneys characterized by the presence of excessive amounts of proteins and fats in the urine (proteinuria) and accumulation of fluid (**edema**) in the body tissues. In older adults, nephrotic syndrome may accompany diseases such as **diabetes mellitus, polyarteritis, amyloidosis,** or **cancer.** The condition involves changes in the kidney's filtration process, so that large molecules, such as proteins, which normally are retained and returned to the blood circulation, are allowed instead to slip through the pores of the filters and into the urine. There are over fifty known causes of nephrotic syndrome, all resulting in the abnormal excretion of protein in the urine. Diagnosis of a specific form of the disease is based on evaluation of symptoms and laboratory tests. Treatment is directed toward relief of symptoms and correction of the underlying cause, such as elimination of an infection, removal of a toxic substance in the environment, or desensitization of a person whose nephrotic syndrome may be associated with poison ivy, insects, pollens, or other **allergens.** Therapies include moderate restriction of salt intake, increasing the protein content of the diet, exercise routines, increasing the excretion of sodium and water, and the use of corticosteroids or other drugs.

Nervous system changes with aging Alterations in the central nervous system and peripheral systems associated with the normal aging process. Studies of the brains of older adults who have died in accidents or from other causes not involving the nervous system show a gradual loss of nerve cells, particularly in areas affecting voluntary and involuntary muscles. There are also degenerative changes in the nerve fibers, some of which lose their contact with muscles they normally control. There is a loss of synapses that help transfer nerve impulses between nerve cells, depletion of neurotransmitter substances such as acetylcholine, and loss of receptors that would normally be stimulated by the neurotransmitters. These losses and changes account for many of the disorders of behavior, mobility, and other neurological functions observed in older individuals. Because mature nerve cells are unable to reproduce themselves, any damage or loss is irreversible. However, nervous system changes with aging need not affect mental function significantly if there is no other disease process involved. Some diseases and disorders affecting the nervous system that are often associated with aging, such as **parkinsonism, stroke, multi-infarct dementia, herpes zoster,** and **temporal arteritis,** are usually secondary to other disorders and are not the result of normal aging effects on nervous system tissue.

Neuralgia   Severe stabbing pain in a nerve or along a nerve pathway caused by any of a variety of disorders affecting the nerve tissue. With aging, changes in the nerves makes them more susceptible to inflammation or irritation that can result in neuralgia. *See also* **Neuritis, Sciatica, Trigeminal neuralgia.**

Neurasthenia   A nonspecific lay term sometimes used to describe a condition of fatigue, insomnia, aches, pains, and general debility due to an emotional rather than a physical disability or disorder.

Neuritis   Inflammation of a nerve. The condition produces different effects depending on the location of the nerve. Some of the signs and symptoms are **neuralgia**, tingling, numbness, paralysis, muscular atrophy, and defective reflexes. There are a variety of causes for neuritis, including **anemia, vitamin deficiencies**, nerve compression, injury, infections, and **peripheral vascular disease. Bell's palsy** and **herpes zoster** are forms of neuritis.

Neuroleptic   A medical term for a tranquilizer or other drug used to treat a psychosis or other mental disorder.

Neurological disorder   Any disease or injury affecting the structure or function of a part of the nervous system, including the brain and central nervous system, peripheral nervous system, and the autonomic nervous system. Examples may include disorders of speech, behavior, and memory, **parkinsonism, Alzheimer's disease**, loss of sensitivity to pain or temperature, abnormal gait or reflexes, and impairment of senses, such as vision or hearing.

Neuroma   A general term for a tumor that develops in nerve tissue.

Neuromuscular disorder   Any disease or injury that affects normal functioning of nervous system control of muscular contractions, such as **myasthenia gravis, myotonia**, and **polymyositis**.

Neuropathy   Any abnormal condition of a nerve or nerves of the body. Neuropathy is a frequent complication of **diabetes mellitus**, particularly in older persons, and may be marked by either pain or loss of sensation in the feet, loss of reflexes, **orthostatic hypotension**, and difficulty in emptying the bladder when autonomic nerves are affected. Older persons are also prone to nutritional neuropathy, in which both the brain and peripheral nerves may function abnormally because of a deficiency of certain vital food elements, particularly B complex vitamins, in the diet. Some older persons with metabolic or nutritional neuropathies have been mistakenly diagnosed as having **Alzheimer's disease**. Other forms of neuropathy include **impotence** due to autonomic nerve dysfunction, and nerve inflammation caused by lead poisoning.

Neurosis   A psychological or behavioral disorder marked by anxiety and other severe emotional symptoms, such as obsessions, compulsions, or morbid fears (phobias), or by health problems that are exaggerated or occur in the absence of any evidence of actual disease or injury, such as hysterical paralysis. Neurosis is generally distinguished from psychosis by the absence of such characteristics as gross personality disorganization, total lack of insight into one's symptoms, loss of contact with reality, incoherent thought and speech, and inability to make accurate evaluations of perceptions. Also called "neurotic disorder."

Nevus   *See* **Mole.**

Nosebleed   *See* **Epistaxis.**

Nocturia   An increased or excessive urge to urinate during the night. For many adults, the need to interrupt sleep to urinate once during the night is normal. An increased urge beyond the normal frequency may be a sign of a urinary system disorder. It also may be the result of consuming excessive fluids or alcoholic beverages before bedtime.

Nocturnal myoclonus   Sudden, sometimes violent, movements of the arms or legs during sleep. The person may be awakened briefly by this body movement, or be unaware of the kicking or striking out but experience a soreness of the arm or leg in the morning. The condition tends to occur in older adults and may be related to other conditions, including epileptic seizures, **Alzheimer's disease**, drug reactions, circulatory lesions of the brain, viral infections, and metabolic disorders such as **uremia.**

Nodular vasculitis   A skin disorder that tends to affect some middle-aged women, resulting in chronic painful **nodules** on the calves of the legs. The cause may be an inflammation of tiny blood vessels (capillaries) in the skin and associated with **arthritis** or a related disorder. Treatment includes rest, painkillers, heat, and correction of any underlying disorder such as a drug or food reaction.

Nodule A small lump or solid mass that occurs most commonly beneath the surface of the skin. It is usually smaller than a half-inch in diameter. Nodules are often a sign of a disease or disorder such as **arthritis**. An enlarged lymph node (gland) may appear as a nodule. Nodules also may occur on internal tissues, as those that develop on the vocal cords of individuals who use the voice excessively. A lump that is larger than a nodule is usually called a tumor.

Nosocomial infections Infections that are acquired as a result of being a hospital patient. The infection may be acquired from viruses or bacteria present on diagnostic or therapeutic equipment, disseminated through a ventilation system, or carried by hospital personnel who have had previous contact with an infected patient. Endotracheal tubes and catheters are a common source of nosocomial infections. **Hepatitis** may be acquired from transfusions or other blood products such as fibrinogen or from the reuse of hypodermic needles. In addition to viruses that cause hepatitis and **herpes zoster**, staphylococcus bacteria are a frequent source of nosocomial infections. Because hospitalized patients usually have low resistance to infection due to disease or injury, they are particularly vulnerable. Many of the typical hospital procedures, including use of preventive antibiotics; wearing of masks, gowns, and rubber gloves; and isolation of certain patients, are intended to reduce the risk of nosocomial infections.

Nuclear sclerosis An early stage of **cataract** formation due to aging, characterized by hardening or density at the center of the lens of the eye. It also contributes to **myopia** by changing the refractive power of the lens.

Nucleus pulposus The pulpy elastic center of the pad of fibrous tissue between vertebrae (intervertebral disk). The nucleus loses resiliency with aging, and when compressed by injury or severe exertion, it may squeeze through the outer wall of the disk. The result is a herniated, or "slipped," disk. *See also* **Herniated disk.**

Nummular eczema A skin disorder characterized by coin-sized patches of pimples or blisterlike eruptions. The eruptions tend to appear on the arms and legs and cause severe itching. Scratching the eruptions generally leads to infections. The condition is aggravated by low indoor humidity during winter. Treatment may include a change in diet, medications, and avoiding excessive use of soap and water on the skin, particularly during the winter months. Also called "nummular dermatitis."

Nutrition   The process of providing the body with the food elements necessary for growth, repair, and maintenance of body structures and functions. It includes the consumption, digestion, absorption, and metabolism of proteins, fats, carbohydrates, minerals, vitamins, and water. A deficiency or excess of one or more of the essential food elements can result in **malnutrition**. Nutrient requirements do not decrease with aging. While older people may need fewer calories because of metabolic changes and decreased physical activity, the nutritional quality of their diets should be higher in proportion to the number of calories consumed.

Nutritional amblyopia   A type of gradual vision loss that occurs in adults as a result of deficiencies of B vitamins, particularly thiamine, and excessive use of alcohol and tobacco. It is an irreversible organic disorder for which there is no effective therapy except for correcting the underlying cause at the earliest signs of the defect.

Nystagmus   An involuntary, rhythmic oscillation of the eyeballs. The movements may be lateral, vertical, rotary, or mixed. It may be one of the symptoms of **vertigo**, multiple sclerosis, or of a brain lesion, and it frequently accompanies an inner ear (labyrinthine) disturbance that causes a loss of balance.

O

Obesity An accumulation of fat that is excessive for a person's age, sex, height, and body build, or an abnormal proportion of fat cells in the subcutaneous tissues of the body. The guidelines for defining obesity vary somewhat according to different experts, who regard a gain of either 20 or 25 percent above the "ideal" or average weight for a particular height, body build, and sex as obese. Because the person with an "ideal" body weight already has a body that is 25 percent fat, adding an additional 25 percent justifies the classification of obese. Most of the height-weight tables used to gauge ideal body weight are compiled by insurance companies; others have been developed by government agencies, using data from such sources as measurements of military personnel. The tables can be misleading since they may be based on information about younger people who buy life insurance, soldiers, or other special groups, rather than the general population. Obesity can also be calculated from tape measure readings or the use of calipers to measure skinfold thickness on the back of the upper arm or over the lower ribs of the chest.

The underlying cause in most cases of obesity is an intake of calories (in the form of food) greater than are utilized in work, exercise, and basal metabolic needs. A person gains approximately one pound of body weight for each 3,500 calories consumed beyond the body's needs. An excess of just 100 calories per day can result in an accumulation of more than ten pounds of body weight each year. Causes of obesity are complex and may include family eating patterns, which may or may not be complicated by genetic factors; the period of life in which fat accumulation begins; psychologic influences that may lead to overeating

247

as a response to emotional stress; a sedentary life style; and social factors. Despite the importance of body weight on health and longevity, there is a lack of scientific research data that might provide good answers about the various causes. Most animal species experience some weight gain with aging, but authorities do not agree as to the amount of human weight gain that can occur without increasing the risk of disease, disability, or death. Also, the effect of obesity on longevity is hard to measure because the data are clouded by other factors. For example, cigarette smokers tend to weigh less than nonsmokers of the same sex, age, and height, but smokers do not increase their lifespans by losing weight. In general, premature death occurs most frequently among the persons at either end of the height-weight scales, the fattest and the leanest. Excess fat is a complicating factor in numerous diseases, particularly among women in **gallbladder disease, uterine cancer,** and **osteoarthritis**. Obesity also is associated with a number of serious disorders, including **hypertension, diabetes mellitus**, and **coronary artery disease**.

Obsessive-compulsive neurosis   A personality disorder marked by anxiety and depression. The person has persistent thoughts or impulses that may be recognized as senseless and repugnant but are not produced voluntarily and seem to invade the consciousness. The person may attempt to ignore or suppress the thoughts, but there is a mounting tension that is relieved only by yielding to the compulsion, which may have certain fixed rules. The person may manifest the condition through excessive orderliness, demands for perfection, cleaning up after others, and, in some extreme cases, sorting, counting, checking, and similar repetitive tasks that may help relieve tension. The behavior is not an end in itself but appears intended to produce or prevent some future unrelated situation. Also called "obsessive-compulsive disorder."

Obtundation   A state of impaired consciousness somewhere between drowsiness and stupor. Although the person may respond to questions and react to painful stimuli, he or she appears to be lethargic and the mental processes are slowed. The condition may result from taking tranquilizers or sedatives or be caused by a head injury or an abnormal condition such as a stroke.

Occlusion   Any closure or closing of a passageway of the body, such as the blockage of a coronary artery by a blood clot. The term is also used to describe the position of the teeth when the upper and lower jaws meet. *Visual occlusion* may refer to a **cataract** or other defect that obstructs the normal passage of light rays through the lens of the eye.

Occupational neuroses Involuntary muscle contractions associated with certain jobs in which workers may be required to perform skilled movements under stress. The involuntary muscle movements may occur as tics, cramps, tremors, aches, or sudden weakness. Those commonly affected include typists, watchmakers, ballet dancers, pianists, violinists, and seamstresses.

Ocular Pertaining to the eye or vision.

Ocular pemphigus A chronic degenerative disease of the eye surfaces that tends to affect older adults with blistering and scarring of the mucous membranes of the eyes. There is severe drying of the eye surfaces. Adhesions then form between the eye surfaces and the lining of the eyelids. The cornea becomes opaque and vision is lost. There is no cure for the disorder.

Oculogyric crisis A condition in which the eyeballs become fixed in the same position for several minutes to hours, usually as a symptom of **parkinsonism** or **encephalitis**. The effect also can be produced by certain medications, such as tranquilizers, that cause an upward fixed stare, or by certain types of brain damage that result in a downward fixed stare.

Odynophagia A medical term for painful swallowing. It is usually characterized by a severe burning sensation and is often associated with inflammation of the esophagus. It also may produce the sensation of food being stuck in the throat. *See also* **Dysphagia.**

Olfactory sense impairment Diminishment or loss of the sense of smell. Some degree of olfactory acuity is lost during the aging process because of a diminished number of nerve fibers or receptor cells in the nasal cavity. The condition may also be due to a brain tumor, nasal obstruction, or psychological factors.

Oligospermia An abnormally low density of sperm in the ejaculate. It is associated with decreased sperm production and can result in a loss of fertility in older men. It may be caused by a varicocele (varicose vein in the scrotum) or occur without known causes.

Onychorrhexis A medical term for the lengthwise ridges that develop on fingernails and toenails as one grows older.

Oophorectomy The surgical removal of one or both ovaries. The operation may be performed to remove a cyst, abscess, or tumor of the ovary, or to supplement treatment of **breast cancer** or severe endometriosis when estrogen produced by the ovaries appears to aggravate the condition. The ovaries are often, but not always, removed as a part of a **hysterectomy**. If both ovaries are removed before the menopause, estrogen may be given to ease any adverse effects of suddenly induced menopause.

Oophorosalpingectomy An **oophorectomy** in which the fallopian tube is removed along with the ovary.

Open angle glaucoma The most common type of **glaucoma**, caused by gradually increasing fluid pressure within the eyeball due to a defect that interferes with normal drainage of excess fluid. *See also* **Glaucoma.**

Ophthalmia Any inflammation of the eye, affecting either the outer membranes (conjunctiva) or the deeper structures, or both.

Ophthalmoplegia The paralysis of a part or all of the eye muscles. The term may apply to paralysis of extra-ocular muscles that move the eyeball or to loss of function of the internal eye muscles, such as those that control the size of the pupil. Ophthalmoplegia may occur with **diabetes, myasthenia gravis**, and **botulism**.

Oral cancer A cancer of the mouth, including the lips, gums, palate, and tongue. Oral cancers increase in frequency after the age of forty and are often associated with the use of alcohol and tobacco or with poorly fitting dentures. Lip cancers may also be caused by exposure to the sun and wind. Early symptoms may include a change in color of the mucous membrane, which acquires an area of whitish or red overgrowth of tissue (**leukoplakia**). The discolored spot may appear as a painless ulcer that does not heal. Pain is often a later symptom of an oral cancer. Treatment may include surgery, radiation, and chemotherapy, depending upon the stage of cancer growth and whether the malignancy has spread to the nearby lymph nodes.

Orange peel breast A term sometimes used to describe the appearance of the skin of a breast with prominent hair follicles and pores.

There is usually fluid accumulation beneath the skin. The condition may be a sign of **cancer.** Also called "pigskin breast."

Orchiectomy The surgical removal of one or both testes in the male. The operation may be performed in the treatment of cancer of the testes, or in cases of injury involving the testes, and in the treatment of prostatic cancer. Orchiectomy in the treatment of cancer usually involves the removal of the inguinal (groin) lymph nodes and adjoining tissues as well as the testes. The condition results in sterility.

Organic brain disorder Any mental or behavioral disorder, temporary or permanent, that involves changes in the structure and function of brain tissues, as distinguished from psychological or behavioral disturbances that may be due to neuroses or emotional problems. Causes include **stroke, arteriosclerosis** of the brain, lead poisoning, injury, or brain tumor; but the exact cause may not be known. Among the symptoms are memory failure, disorientation, emotional disorders, **dementia,** and **delirium.**

Orthokinetics A technique for treating a **neuromuscular disorder** by stimulating the sensory nerves with an outside influence such as heat, cold, or gentle pressure.

Orthopnea Breathing difficulty that occurs when lying down. The rate of breathing may be either slow or rapid, and the person may appear at times to force respirations. Relief is obtained by sitting or standing. The disorder may be missed by an examining physician who sees the patient only in a sitting or standing posture. The condition can be a symptom of **angina pectoris, pneumonia, emphysema,** or other heart or lung problems.

Orthosis Any device applied to a person with a **musculoskeletal disorder** for supportive or corrective purposes, such as braces, splints, collars, or corsets, as distinguished from a *prosthesis,* which replaces a missing body part.

Orthostatic hypotension *See* **Hypotension.**

Osteitis deformans *See* **Paget's disease.**

Osteoarthritis (degenerative joint disease) The most common form of **arthritis,** in which one or more of the cartilage surfaces between two bones forming a joint undergoes degeneration. Weight-bearing joints, including the spinal column, are most commonly affected, along with the hip and knee. For reasons not clearly understood, osteoarthritis rarely affects the ankle joints. Virtually everyone who lives beyond early adulthood eventually experiences the effects of osteoarthritis; exceptions are some individuals who are bedfast or are otherwise restricted in physical activity. Signs of joint deterioration usually appear on X-ray films long before the person experiences pain, the most common symptom. X-ray evidence of the disease has been found in nearly 85 percent of Americans over the age of fifty-five. Pain is often a late symptom, being preceded by stiffness after rest or brief morning stiffness and limitation of mobility. Hands often develop bony enlargements (**Heberden's nodes**) in the finger joints. Other characteristics of the disorder are changes in posture, mobility, and gait, when the person favors the affected joint and walks with a limp or lurch, tilting the body over a weakened hip or dragging an affected leg rather than allowing the body weight to rest on it. Loss of cartilage can account for a scraping or crackling noise produced by movement of an affected joint. Uneven loss of cartilage can alter the stance, giving the appearance of bowleg or knock-knee. Muscles, tendons, and ligaments are eventually affected, leading to muscle atrophy and contractures. These soft tissue changes, in turn, may aggravate the original problem of osteoarthritis. Osteoarthritis is occasionally complicated by the presence of other arthritic diseases, particularly **rheumatoid arthritis** and **gout**. Osteoarthritis usually begins gradually and is accompanied by joint swelling as well as joint pain and occasional muscle pain. The pain is usually aggravated by physical activity. The usual treatment for osteoarthritis is aspirin or a similar painkiller to ease the pain. Applications of heat and injections of anesthetic drugs may be recommended. In severe cases resulting in immobility, surgery or splints, braces, and other devices may be needed. Surgical replacement of hip and knee joints, utilizing plastics and metal alloys, has been very successful, particularly for older adults who are not likely to place great stress on an artificial joint. Plastic finger joints also have been developed for patients who have lost normal use of the hands due to osteoarthritis. For many patients, weight reduction often helps relieve the symptoms by decreasing the weight on the joint. *See also* **Orthosis.**

Osteolysis   The degeneration and loss of bone tissue due to infection or disorders that cause a disruption of blood flow to bone, as in **Raynaud's disease**. The bones of the hands and feet are usually affected, but the condition also can involve the teeth, resulting in dental caries.

Osteomalacia A bone disorder resulting from a deficiency of vitamin D, which is characterized by a loss of calcium from the bone matrix, resulting in a softening of the bone and spontaneous fractures. The pain may be vague and diffuse, usually involving the area of the hips, spine, and ribs, but aggravated in the pelvic area by body weight. Symptoms may also include weakness, loss of appetite, and weight loss. Causes can include a lack of calcium and phosphorus in the diet, a lack of vitamin D, inadequate exposure to sunlight, or a **malabsorption** disease. Other causes in older adults include kidney disorders, tumors, and medications that interfere with vitamin D metabolism. Treatment depends upon the underlying cause but often includes supplements of vitamin D, calcium, and phosphorus. Total recovery may occur in six months when other possible health factors, such as kidney impairment, or the use of harmful medications, are also corrected. *See also* **Osteoporosis.**

Osteomyelitis An inflammation of bone tissue, particularly bone marrow. The symptoms may include pain, fever, profuse sweating, and rigidity of the muscles overlying the affected bone. The skin over the area may appear inflamed, and the pain is usually aggravated by pressure on the diseased body part. Treatment consists of antibiotics, painkillers, and rest or immobilization of the inflammed body part. Surgery may be required if the inflammation leads to a bone **abscess**.

Osteoporosis A bone-loss disorder that affects mainly postmenopausal women and, to a lesser degree, sedentary men. Osteoporosis differs from **osteomalacia** mainly in that it involves a loss of total bone mass, whereas in osteomalacia the loss is primarily of the mineral portion of the bone. The total bone loss for postmenopausal women can be as much as 40 percent of the bone mass that was present between the ages of twenty-five and thirty, the period of skeletal maturity when a person's bone mass is normally at its maximum. For normal men, the rate of bone loss is much lower. Bone loss occurs in all parts of the skeleton, with the greatest loss tending to occur in spongy bone rather than compact bone. The exact cause of the loss of bone mass in older adults is unknown, but among the factors associated with osteoporosis in postmenopausal women are hereditary traits, the amount of bone mass at skeletal maturity, exercise, nutrition, and hormonal influences, particularly the loss of ovarian estrogen production. The woman with a greater amount of bone mass at skeletal maturity is less likely to be affected by osteoporosis than one with a smaller skeleton at the same age. Exercise seems to help in the development of the original bone mass and to retard its loss later in life. Some studies indicate that exercise can actually increase bone mass in older women. The role of nutrition is related mainly to the dietary intake of calcium, which tends to be lower in older adults and is usually aggravated by decreased intestinal absorption of what calcium is available in the foods eaten. Vitamin D availability also may affect calcium absorption. Research shows the risk of leg fractures in older women increases when calcium intake is reduced. The role of estrogen is shown by the fact that osteoporosis is rare among women before the menopause but increasingly common after menopause, with the risk of leg fractures doubling every five years after the age of sixty. The use of aluminum-based antacids, alcohol, tobacco, and caffeine have also been implicated as lifestyle factors that may contribute to a loss of bone mass.

Particularly serious are bone losses in the spinal column and the upper leg bone (femur). The vertebrae become compressed by body weight when weakened by osteoporosis; compression fractures of the vertebrae can reduce a person's height by several inches. Compression fractures can produce acute pain that lasts for several months. Therapy may include fluoride to harden the bones, steroid hormones, vitamin D and calcium, and estrogen. Because of the difficulty in consuming enough milk and dairy products to provide the recommended intake of calcium daily, many experts advise the use of calcium supplements (1 gram of calcium carbonate provides 400 milligrams of calcium). Administration of estrogen may require special precautions in postmenopausal women who may be vulnerable to cancer. Older men with osteoporosis may similarly be given a testosterone medication, with care taken to avoid the risk of cancer of the prostate from use of the sex hormone.

Otosclerosis A form of gradual hearing loss caused by the binding of one of the tiny middle ear bones (stapes) to the oval window of the inner ear, which contains the nerve tissues that help translate sound waves into hearing. The condition usually affects both ears, producing early symptoms of ringing in the ears (**tinnitus**) and progressive deafness, as the stapes become "frozen" to the inner ear and fail to transmit sound vibrations received from the other inner ear bones. Although it may develop in early adulthood, otosclerosis is the most common cause of hearing loss in middle-aged persons.

Ototoxic drugs Drugs that may affect the ear by interfering with hearing or the sense of balance. They include salicylates (aspirin), quinine, and certain antibiotics.

Outpatient A person who is examined or treated in a hospital or clinic but is not required to remain overnight.

Ovarian cancer   A carcinoma of the ovary, which occurs most frequently in women after the age of forty. Symptoms include abnormal vaginal bleeding, abdominal swelling and discomfort, weight loss, constipation, and change of urinary habits, such as an urge to urinate more frequently. Ovarian cancer accounts for nearly 25 percent of all cancers of the female reproductive tract and an even larger proportion of cancer deaths. Cancer of the ovary usually is not diagnosed until it has developed sufficiently to produce symptoms, by which time it is often far advanced. Treatment is by surgery, radiation, and chemotherapy.

Ovary changes with aging   Alterations in the size and function of the ovaries associated with the aging process. The ovary during and after **menopause** atrophies to less than half its previous size. The process begins with the approach of menopause, when the ovaries no longer react to the stimulus of hormones that trigger the maturation and release of an ovum. The myriad potential egg follicles that were present at the beginning of sexual maturity disappear as the menopause draws nearer. The ovaries may continue to produce and secrete a small amount of the female sex hormone estrogen for a few years after the menopause, but this activity increases the risk of cancer. A second female sex hormone, progesterone, is no longer secreted by the ovary, and only small amounts continue to be secreted by the adrenal gland. In the premenopausal woman, progesterone helps balance the activity of estrogen; after the menopause, there is not enough of the hormone to continue this activity. In the premenopausal woman, the ovary produces estrogens from the male sex hormone androgen secreted by the ovary and the adrenal gland. After the menopause, the ovary is no longer able to convert androgen, which continues to be produced, and this may result in the appearance of some male secondary sexual characteristics in some women, such as the appearance of small amounts of facial and body hair. Other effects include the cessation of menses and atrophic changes in vaginal and other tissues affected by sex hormones.

Overnutrition   An alternative term for **malnutrition**, usually associated with an excessive consumption of carbohydrates and reduced physical activity, and leading to obesity. *See also* **Nutrition.**

Overwear   Eye pain and sensitivity to light that sometimes occurs in persons from prolonged wearing of contact lenses. The contact lens may cause swelling and erosion of the surface of the cornea.

P

Pacemaker A battery-powered electronic device, implanted under the skin in the chest and connected to the heart by one or more electrodes, that maintains a normal rhythm of heart contractions by stimulating the heart muscle with electrical impulses at predetermined intervals. There are two basic types of pacemakers. One type emits a stimulus at a constant fixed rate; and the other, a newer and more commonly used synchronous design, functions only on demand of the heart muscle, as when the heart's natural pacemaker, a cluster of specialized cells in the sinoatrial node, fails to cause contractions at a particular rate per minute. The artificial pacemaker is used in the treatment of such disorders as **heart block** and severe **bradycardia**.

Paget's disease of the bone (osteitis deformans) A progressive bone disease that usually affects people after the age of fifty. The exact cause is unknown, although there is evidence that it may result from a viral infection. It also tends to occur in families, in men more frequently than in women, and in certain geographic areas, including North America. Paget's disease may or may not produce symptoms. When it is symptomless, its presence may be detected only through X-ray or radioisotope examination for the cause of fractures, bowing of legs, or other effects on the skeleton. The presence in the blood and urine of abnormal levels of substances associated with bone metabolism aids in the diagnosis. Most commonly affected bones are the pelvis, arms, legs, and skull, although the spinal column may become shortened due to softening of the vertebrae. This can result in loss of height, distorted posture, and arms that appear unusually long for the height of the individual. A sign that the skull may be affected is sometimes discovered when a person requires larger hat sizes. The disease occurs in two phases. The first phase is marked by **osteolysis** in which there is erosion of mineral from the bones, usually in specific areas of particular bones. In the second phase, new bone forms in more or less random patterns, with the result that some bones are misshapen or become larger or smaller than before onset of the disease. Paget's disease does not affect all people in the same way, and while more than half show no symptoms, others may have a wide range of symptoms that may not be identified with the disease. Frequently, symptoms that mimic osteoarthritis of the hip or knee, hearing loss, ringing in the ears, vertigo, double vision, neuromuscular disorders of the eye muscles, swallowing difficulties, loss of ability to speak distinctly, or loss of coordination are mistakenly attributed to the aging process or an inner ear disorder rather than to Paget's disease. Complications may include excessive levels of blood calcium, kidney stones, coronary artery disease leading to heart failure, and bone tumors. Treatment is with painkillers as needed, a high-protein, high-calcium diet, and drugs. Paget's disease of the bone should not be confused with Paget's disease of the breast, a form of breast cancer.

Pain A sensation of distress or discomfort resulting from stimulation of specialized cells within the nervous system. Pain may be described as burning, dull, sharp, piercing, mild or severe, diffuse or localized. Pain may evoke groans, cries, body movements, facial expressions, and changes in the tone of voice and pace of speaking. Severe pain can produce symptoms of pallor, sweat, "gooseflesh," dilated pupils, and increases in heart rate, blood pressure, respiration, and muscle tension. It can be *acute,* as pain caused by an injury, or *chronic,* as pain associated with one of the forms of arthritis. Pain is regarded as a protective mechanism of the body, a symptom of a disease or disorder prompting action by the person to withdraw from the cause of the pain, to seek relief from it, and to correct the condition causing the pain. In addition to the anguish it causes, pain can be debilitating, interfering with one's ability to work, play, or carry on the normal activities of daily living. Some pain may be psychogenic, continuing after treatment to relieve it. Treatment depends upon the severity of the pain and the underlying cause. Some mild pain may be relieved with aspirin, acetaminophen, or similar analgesics or by the use of narcotics in cases that fail to respond to ordinary painkillers. In some cases of severe pain, surgery may be used to sever associated nerve fibers. Narcotics are commonly used to reduce pain in surgical patients and in some cancer cases. Surgery may also be used to relieve the pain of certain cancers.

Palliation The use of drugs or other agents (palliatives) to relieve the symptoms of a disorder without actually curing it. Palliation may be used as a temporary measure, as when painkillers are used while a patient awaits surgery to treat an injury, or to diminish symptoms and discomfort of an incurable disease.

Papule A small, raised layer of skin or a pimple, formed of a solid mass of cells.

Paraplegia Paralysis of the lower part of the body, including both legs. When paralysis in the lower part of the body is partial, the condition is usually identified as *paraparesis. See also* **Hemiplegia.**

Parkinsonism Any disorder characterized by muscular rigidity and tremors that resemble those of **Parkinson's disease.** A parkinson-like syndrome can be caused by a brain injury, exposure to carbon monoxide gas, brain tumors, and the use of certain tranquilizers.

Parkinson's disease (shaking palsy, paralysis agitans) A chronic, progressive disorder of the central nervous system characterized by a slowness of movements, muscular rigidity, a tremor that occurs at rest, difficulties in speaking distinctly, drooling, and stooped posture. It usually begins in middle age. The most distinctive feature of the Parkinson's disease patient is a tremor of the thumb and fingers accompanied by wrist flexion, often described as a "pill-rolling" movement. The slow resting tremor is usually aggravated by fatigue or emotional stress, but it may stop with any voluntary movement and may disappear during sleep. Muscular rigidity in the Parkinson's disease patient involves the action and counteraction of opposing muscle groups, so that movements of a limb may appear to go through a series of starts and stops. The affected person walks with a propulsive "parkinson gait," beginning with hesitant steps that increase in speed, as if movement is needed to keep from falling forward. Speech may become impaired in ways analogous to gait changes, beginning slowly, softly, and monotonously but occasionally breaking into rapid, unintelligible sounds. Depression is a common complication. Patients often display a fixed expression with an unblinking stare due to **oculogyric crisis.** The exact cause of Parkinson's disease is unknown. Patients have a decreased level of a neurotransmitter (dopamine) in cells of the basal ganglia of the brain. The disease is not curable, but the symptoms are treated with drugs that increase levels of dopamine or other neurotransmitters.

Paronychia   An infection of the fold of the skin along the margin of a fingernail or toenail. A fungal infection along the edge of a nail, usually **monilial** paronychia, is characterized by a painful, red swelling. The nail may become thickened and hardened. This type of paronychia most often affects people whose work requires frequent immersion of the hands in water. Bacterial paronychia is similar to the fungal type, except that the condition is usually more acute and painful. Treatment usually requires the use of hot compresses, appropriate antibiotics or antifungal drugs, and, in some cases, removal of damaged portions of the nail. Persons can avoid aggravating the condition by wearing cotton gloves under rubber gloves when putting their hands in soapy water.

Patch   A discolored skin area, such as a flat mole or a freckle.

Pellagra   A deficiency of niacin affecting the skin, intestinal tract, and central nervous system. The cause may be a severe dietary deficiency of niacin, a B vitamin, or inability of the digestive tract to absorb niacin. It may also be caused by a deficiency of an amino acid (tryptophan) that can be converted by the body into niacin. Tryptophan is a component of proteins found in milk, eggs, and meat. Pellagra causes the skin to become thick, red, and cracked, particularly on the hands and arms. The tongue and mouth can develop a bright red coloration, ulcers, and cysts. Nausea, vomiting, diarrhea, and loss of appetite often accompany the skin symptoms. Central nervous system effects include confusion, disorientation, memory failure, depression, clouding of consciousness, insomnia, sucking and grasping movements, and, in severe cases, delirium. Older adults are susceptible to pellagra when their diets lack proteins and green leafy vegetables. Alcoholism and certain digestive diseases that interfere with absorption or utilization of niacin or tryptophan by the body may also cause pellagra. Treatment requires a balanced diet that includes ample protein and often supplementary doses of niacinamide.

Pelvic disorder   Any disease or abnormality involving the reproductive organs or other organs, including the urinary tract and the male prostate, in the lower abdomen. Pelvic disorders are a major cause of discomfort or disability in older women. Nearly one-fourth of women over the age of sixty experience some form of "pelvic relaxation," a weakening or failure of the muscles, ligaments, and other tissues that support the uterus, bladder, and rectum. The condition is most likely to affect women who have experienced multiple pregnancies. Symptoms may include pain, urinary **incontinence**, problems emptying the rectum, and uterine prolapse. A significant percentage of tumors of the ovaries, uterus, cervix, and external genitalia occur in older women. The most common disorder, cancer of the endometrial lining of the uterus, reaches a peak among women in their fifties. It is believed to be related to the continuing production of estrogen after the menopause. It may be present without any symptoms, or it can be a cause of abnormal vaginal bleeding. *See also* **Prostate disorders.**

Pemphigus   A serious disease of the skin and mucous membranes marked by eruptions of blisters on otherwise normal surfaces. The blisters occur most often on the scalp, hands, feet, and areas of skin folds. There may be redness at the base of the eruptions. The blisters, which contain a fluid with a foul odor, eventually rupture, leaving eroded areas on the skin. The eruptions sometimes disappear, but more frequently the condition worsens and can be fatal if not treated. Without treatment, the eruptions usually enlarge and spread. The person loses weight, becomes debilitated, and is susceptible to serious bacterial infections. Treatment is with corticosteroids and other medications. The cause is unknown. The disorder affects mainly men and women in their forties and fifties.

Peptic ulcer   A painful eroding sore in the mucous membrane lining the digestive tract caused by the action of the acid gastric juice of the stomach. The gastric juice, containing mainly hydrochloric acid and pepsin (an enzyme that breaks down proteins), is normally present in the stomachs of most individuals, although some people secrete much more acid than others. The stomach lining is normally protected against effects of the acid by a layer of mucus. Since only some potentially susceptible persons actually develop peptic ulcers, it is believed that certain factors such as stress or drugs may upset the balance between the acid gastric juice and the protective mucus layer. Aspirin, itself an acid, can increase the acidity of the gastric juice and interfere with blood clotting so that tiny bleeding wounds occur in the stomach lining. Peptic ulcers are identified by their location, such as in the stomach *(gastric ulcer)* or in the first segment of the small intestine (**duodenal ulcer**). A peptic ulcer usually causes pain, which may be mild or severe, and is usually described as a steady burning or gnawing sensation. The pain of a duodenal ulcer is usually relieved by food but may return two or three hours later. The pain of a gastric ulcer often is more severe after a meal. The pain produced by a peptic ulcer of the esophagus is generally more severe when swallowing or lying down. With age, the likelihood of developing a gastric ulcer decreases, while that of a duodenal ulcer increases. Careful diagnosis of a gastric ulcer is particularly important because, unlike a duodenal ulcer, a peptic ulcer of the stomach may become cancerous. Diagnosis is usually based on X-ray films made after a patient has swallowed a barium "meal" that coats the lining of the digestive tract so that any erosions or "craters" are highlighted. Doctors also may insert a lighted fiberoptic endoscope through the esophagus, permitting direct inspection of the stomach lining, and remove some of the gastric juice and mucous membrane cells for laboratory studies as part of the examination. Treatment includes medications, including antacids, a spice-free, caffeine-free diet, and sometimes surgery. The patient is often advised to avoid smoking and the use of alcohol, which may increase gastric acid secretion. *See also* **Duodenal ulcer, Ulcer.**

Perceptual defect Any loss of the normal ability to make conscious recognition of a sensory stimulus, such as sight, hearing, or touch, due to injury of disease affecting specific areas of the brain associated with the ability to identify sources of stimuli. Brain tumors, blood vessel disorders, exposure to carbon monoxide or industrial poisons, use of alcohol or other drugs, and brain infections are among possible causes of perceptual defects. Perceptual defects are often found in **Alzheimer's disease** and **Pick's disease** patients who, in the absence of deafness, fail to recognize sounds, or who can see but fail to recognize known objects.

Periarteritis *See* **Polyarteritis.**

Pericarditis An inflammation of the pericardium, the membranous sac that surrounds the heart. The cause is usually a viral, bacterial, or fungal infection; injury; **uremia**; **rheumatoid arthritis**; **myocardial infarction**; or a **tumor.** Symptoms include chest pain and tenderness, heart palpitations, dry cough, breathing difficulty, and fever. The pain may be deep and constant, resembling that of a heart attack in its location and degree of discomfort. A condition known as cardiac **tamponade** may develop if fluid accumulates within the membranous sac, resulting in alterations in normal heart and blood pressure functions. The person finds that the pain may be relieved by sitting up and leaning forward. If treatment is delayed, the person often experiences sweating, chills, pallor, and may go into shock. Treatment includes bed rest, diet changes, and drugs and other therapies to relieve the pain and underlying cause. Surgical drainage of the fluid accumulation may be needed in some cases.

Periodontal disease (pyorrhea) Inflammation and deterioration of the bone and soft tissues that support the teeth. The tooth structures affected, depending on the severity of the disease, include the gums (gingival tissues), the bone that forms the tooth socket, and the periodontal membrane that supports the tooth in its socket. Periodontal disease may begin as a gum inflammation (gingivitis) in adolescence and build toward a full-blown dental disorder in middle age. Causes include bacterial plaque that adheres to the sides of the tooth or to tartar in areas next to the soft tissues. The condition may be complicated by poor alignment of teeth (malocclusion), clenching or grinding of teeth, failure to clean the teeth and gums regularly, or a systemic disorder such as **diabetes mellitus**. Further complicating the disorder is periodontal **atrophy**, or recession, in which the gums and underlying bone gradually pull away from their normal attachment to the tooth. As the gums recede, the surfaces along the sides of the teeth become exposed to the air, heat, cold, and acidic foods, leading to the formation of abscesses along the sides of the teeth. Periodontal disease may be prevented or controlled by regular visits to a dentist and proper dental hygiene habits. Treatment includes cleaning out pockets of pus between gums and teeth, removal of plaque, surgery, and medications. The treatment must be followed by regular maintenance of the teeth and gums by a dentist.

Pes corvinius A medical term for "crows' feet," the wrinkles that often occur at the outer corners of the eyes with aging.

Petechiae Pinhead-size areas of bleeding in the skin or mucous membranes, such as may appear as a symptom of a vitamin C deficiency (scurvy).

Phantom pain Pain that is felt in a part of the body that has been amputated. It may begin as a sensation of numbness or "needles and pins" and gradually evolve into cramping, burning, or shooting pains that seem to come from the missing body part as if it were still there. The sensation is produced by irritation of endings of nerve fibers formerly connected to the amputated body part that still carry pain impulses to the brain. Some authorities contend the feeling is at least partly psychological in origin, an effort to resolve a body-image conflict. Person who are born with a body part missing do not experience the sensation. Phantom pain may be temporary or persist for years.

Phlebotomy The incision of a vein for the purpose of drawing blood. The procedure is used in blood donations and also to decrease the amount of circulating blood in certain disorders such as **porphyria cutanea tarda, polycythemia vera,** and some respiratory disorders.

Pick's disease   A degenerative brain disease characterized by a gradual, progressive loss of the ability to concentrate or think clearly, leading to **incontinence**, debility, and paralysis. The first signs of the disease often occur in the forties or fifties, and death follows in a few years after the onset of symptoms. Women are more likely to be affected than men. Some of the symptom are similar to those of **Alzheimer's disease**, although different areas of the brain may be affected. The disease evolves gradually, so that early symptoms of bewilderment, loss of ability to read and write, and rambling speech are followed by loss of control of the bladder and bowels. Unlike the Alzheimer's disease patient, who may appear restless in early stages of the disorder, the patient with Pick's disease may seem dull and apathetic. There is no known cure.

Pill-rolling tremor   An involuntary movement in patients with **Parkinson's disease** in which the thumb and fingers simulate the action of rolling a small ball or pill between them.

Pituitary gland changes with aging   Alterations in the function of the pituitary ("master") gland associated with the aging process. The pituitary is a small gland located at the base of the brain that secretes growth hormone; gonadotropic hormones that influence the production of sex hormones by other glands; the prolactin hormone that promotes milk secretion by the female breast; and hormones that stimulate activity by the thyroid and adrenal glands. One change that occurs in older adults is a decrease in growth hormone secretion. Pituitary disorders may be a cause of **hypothyroidism** and adrenal gland insufficiency in some older adults. Gonadotropic hormone levels may be at high levels in the older adult, but the gonads (sex glands) may fail to respond with the same degree of activity as in earlier years. One of the most serious effects of changes in the posterior pituitary gland is **inappropriate antidiuretic hormone (ADH) secretion**, resulting in **hyponatremia** or an abnormal loss of sodium in the tissues.

Pityriasis   Any of several skin diseases characterized by the formation of branlike scales. Some types of pityriasis are fungal infections, but others are of unknown causes. *Pityriasis rosea* tends to occur most frequently in the spring and autumn with eruptions mainly on the chest and trunk. Itching is generally mild but may range to severe. The eruptions usually disappear after several weeks without treatment, but medicated baths and lotions may help reduce symptoms earlier. Excessive use of medications may worsen the condition.

Plaque   Any flat area or patch of material on an otherwise relatively smooth surface of a tissue or organ. *Dental plaque* on tooth enamel is usually composed of mucus, food debris, microorganisms, and body tissue cells. An *atherosclerotic plaque* composed of cholesterol, fats, and cellular debris may be found on the inner surface of an artery. A *skin plaque* is an elevated area of skin cells, larger than a **papule** but smaller than a **tumor**. Examples of skin plaques include **moles** and **warts**.

Plummer-Vinson syndrome   An abnormal condition characterized by the growth of a thin membrane across the opening of the esophagus in certain patients with iron-deficiency anemia. The syndrome affects primarily middle aged women. The condition results in difficulty swallowing, especially of solid foods, but the web disappears when the anemia is treated. Other symptoms may be inflammation of the tongue, and dryness and atrophy of the mucous membranes of the throat.

Pneumoconioses   Respiratory diseases caused by inhalation of dust in the environment and reaction of the lung tissue to the dust. Persons most commonly affected are workers who have been exposed to asbestos, coal dust, cement, and dusts of aluminum, iron, silica (sand), or other materials. The term originally referred to lung disorders caused by inhalation of inorganic dusts but has been broadened in recent years to include dusts of organic materials. Pneumoconiosis is an insidious disease that often does not produce symptoms until twenty years after exposure to the dust that may have been inhaled in the workplace. Usually, only the smallest dust particles accumulate in the lungs; the larger particles become trapped in the respiratory passages and are expectorated or exhaled. The tiny particles irritate the lung tissue, which reacts by forming fibrous growths that diminish the lungs' elasticity and their ability to handle a normal exchange of oxygen and carbon dioxide. The affected person develops a cough and breathing difficulty, particularly with physical exertion. There may be tightness and pain in the chest, along with weakness and easy fatigability. There is no known cure for most pneumoconioses, though removal from exposure to dust may prevent the condition from worsening. Pneumoconioses from organic dusts are sometimes relieved by asthma medications.

Pneumonia   An acute inflammation of the lungs, usually due to inhalation of infectious bacteria, viruses, or other organisms. The microorganisms proliferate in the air sacs (alveoli) and small air passages, producing a thick mucus that blocks the movement of air into and out of the lungs. It has been identified as the most common fatal **nosocomial**

infection acquired in hospitals. The pneumonia patient usually has severe chills, a fever that may reach 105° Fahrenheit, a very rapid pulse, and difficulty in breathing. Other symptoms include chest pain and a cough that may produce a dark sputum, the result of red blood cells that have been destroyed by bacteria in the alveoli. Diagnosis is also based on specific sounds detected by an examining physician applying a stethoscope to the chest wall, and on X-rays.

Older adults are more susceptible to pneumonia than younger ones, and it is more often fatal, because of changes in lung structure and function that occur with aging. There is increased difficulty in expelling inhaled foreign organisms, either by exhaling or by coughing, as both functions become less effective as one grows older. Older persons are also more likely to develop pneumonia as a complication of a disabling disease or injury that causes them to be bedridden or immobile. Treatment includes bed rest, fluids, antibiotics for bacterial pneumonias, painkilling drugs, and oxygen, as needed. The length of recovery depends upon the condition of the patient and the severity of the infection. A vaccine is available to prevent infection by more than twenty strains of pneumonia bacteria. As pneumonia frequently follows an episode of influenza, older persons also are encouraged to obtain an influenza vaccination each year. The vaccine is changed annually to match new strains of influenza virus that develop with each new season. *See also* **Influenza, Legionnaire's disease.**

Pneumonitis   An inflammation of the lung tissue due to a hypersensitivity reaction to the inhaled material. Although the term is commonly applied to dusts of organic materials, the symptoms can also be produced by inhalation of various chemicals. Symptoms can include chills, fever, cough, and shortness of breath following exposure to the offending substance. The person may also experience nausea, vomiting, and loss of appetite. The symptoms are an allergic reaction to the inhaled substance. The substance is often a vegetable or animal protein, such as animal hair or dander, or a fungal spore from moldy hay, moldy cheese, or moldy sawdust. Relief from symptoms involves avoiding the sensitizing material and use of medications.

Podiatric disorders (foot problems)   Diseases and deformities of the feet, including bunions, corns, calluses, and nail problems. Podiatric disorders are a common cause of **immobility** and of instability leading to falls in older adults.

Polyarteritis   A serious disease characterized by the inflammation and destruction of small- to medium-sized arteries, resulting in oxygen starvation and death of tissues served by the affected arteries. The exact cause is unknown, but the disease has been associated with hypersensitivity reactions to drugs, vaccines, and bacterial and viral infections. The disease can affect persons of any age but tends to strike men in their forties. Diagnosis is often difficult because symptoms resemble those of numerous other diseases. The symptoms include fever, nausea, vomiting, diarrhea, weight loss, headache, muscle ache, breathing difficulty, and weakness. Pain may occur in the chest, abdomen, or at sites of interrupted blood flow. There may also be skin nodules, hypertension, blood in the urine or feces, confusion, and convulsions. The disease is often fatal, but the survival rate of patients is increased with early treatment that includes removal of any drug that may produce the reaction, steroid therapy, and other medications. Also called "periarteritis."

Polycythemia vera   A disease marked by an excess of red blood cells and hemoglobin, resulting in weakness, enlarged spleen, fatigue, disorders of hearing and sense of balance, headache, drowsiness, flushed face, and pain in the arms and legs. The underlying cause is an overproduction of bone marrow cells. Nearly all patients are over the age of forty, and the average age at the start of symptoms is sixty. Men are more often affected than women. Although the disease is life-shortening, the average patient survives about thirteen years with treatment, and many die of other age-related diseases. The usual treatment is **phlebotomy**, which is repeated from two to six times a year.

Polymyalgia rheumatica   A condition of muscle pain and stiffness, usually in the neck, back, shoulder, and pelvic areas. There may also be fever, loss of appetite, weight loss, general feelings of discomfort, and, in some cases, a severe headache. The stiffness is at a peak in the morning, occasionally making it difficult for the person to get out of bed. The symptoms may resemble those of **rheumatoid arthritis**. The condition is believed to be an inflammation of the arteries, which may be related to **temporal arteritis** since many persons develop both diseases. A complication is irreversible blindness that may develop suddenly. The disease affects mainly women over the age of fifty. Treatment includes painkilling drugs and corticosteroids.

Polymyositis   An inflammatory and degenerative disease of more than one muscle or muscle group. It is reported to be the most common disease of muscle tissue in older adults. The exact cause is unknown, but there is evidence of possible involvement of viruses, autoimmune reactions, and cancer. Symptoms include swelling and pain, which are sometimes accompanied by fever, weight loss, and muscle weakness. When the skin is also affected, with symptoms that include a rash and changes in skin pigmentation marked by either an increase in or patchy loss of skin pigment, the condition is usually identified as **dermatomyo-sitis**. Other systemic diseases such as **rheumatoid arthritis** and **systemic lupus erythematosus** are frequently associated with polymyositis or dermatomyositis. Polymyositis is often a sign of an underlying tumor; cancers are found in 15 to 20 percent of the polymyositis patients over the age of fifty. The tumors are commonly found in the lung, colon, ovary, or breast. Women are more likely than men to develop polymyositis. Treatment and prognosis depend upon the symptoms, the severity of the condition, and the probable underlying cause. Mild cases may receive little or no treatment, while more serious cases may be treated with corticosteroids, chemotherapy, and physical therapy.

Polyopsia   An abnormal condition in which two or more images of the same object may be seen because of defects in the cornea or lens of the eye. *See also* **Diplopia.**

Porphyria cutanea tarda   An inherited metabolic disorder that tends to produce symptoms in persons over the age of forty, with reddening of exposed skin surfaces, blisters, scabs, and scars. The skin eruptions often increase in late summer and early autumn after exposure to sunlight. There may also be liver disease in some patients. The underlying cause is the inactivity of an enzyme needed to break down and excrete certain nitrogen compounds in the body. The condition is activated by the use of alcoholic beverages, estrogen, oral contraceptives, and excessive iron intake. The incidence of the disease has increased as more women have begun taking iron medications and estrogens as well as alcohol. Treatment includes avoiding the factors that activate symptoms and reducing iron levels in the blood with medications or **phlebotomy.**

Postmenopausal   The period of a woman's life after the menopause. *See also* **Menopause, Osteoporosis.**

Postmyocardial infarction syndrome   A group of symptoms, including fever, inflammation in the area of the heart, pleurisy, and joint pain, that occurs occasionally in a patient several days or weeks after suffering a myocardial infarction (heart attack). Treatment usually consists of aspirin and other medications.

Presbycusis Loss of hearing that is associated with normal aging. The condition is marked by the loss of the hair cells that serve as sound receptors in the inner ear, degeneration of auditory nerve cells, and failure of the hearing centers of the brain that interpret nerve impulses transmitted from the inner ear. The first symptom is often a buzzing or ringing in the ears (**tinnitus**) or a need to turn up the volume on a radio or television set in order to hear words being broadcast. As presbycusis progresses, the person may have difficulty in hearing children or women with higher-pitched voices, as those are the sound frequencies that are first to be lost by the presbycusis patient. Because the hearing loss may increase gradually over a period of years, the affected person may not be aware of the problem and is likely to blame "background noise" or a failure on the part of another person to speak properly. Treatment usually requires a **hearing aid**, but many affected persons also learn lip-reading and rely increasingly on visual clues to communicate with others.

Presbyophrenia A form of psychosis marked by confusion, disorientation, memory impairment, **confabulation**, and mistakes in identification. The confabulations may be monotonous and lacking in imagination. Because the person tends to be amiable and euphoric, some social contacts are maintained.

Presbyopia A loss of the eye's ability to accommodate to near vision because of aging processes. The condition, caused by a loss of elasticity of the lens of the eye, occurs in almost all people in their fifties and sixties. Distant vision is not affected, hence the common term *farsightedness*. Reading glasses or bifocals are the usual remedy for presbyopia.

Presenile dementia An old term still sometimes used to identify conditions of progressive loss of intellectual ability, memory, judgment, and abstract thinking that begin in the forties and fifties, as distinguished from the "senile onset dementias" that usually do not appear until the person is over sixty years old. **Alzheimer's disease**, **Pick's disease**, and **Huntington's chorea** are among the disorders that may occur at an earlier or later age.

Pressure sores *See* **Decubitus ulcers.**

Primary biliary cirrhosis An inflammatory disease of the liver with symptoms of itching, weight loss, diarrhea, nosebleeds, bleeding under the skin, enlarged liver, jaundice, dark urine, and pale feces. It tends to affect women after the age of forty. **Osteoporosis** and **osteomalacia**

may also develop. The cause is unknown, but the condition is associated with **malabsorption** of calcium and vitamin D. There is no specific treatment for the condition, but the symptoms are relieved by a high-protein diet, medications, and vitamin supplements, particularly fat-soluble vitamins A, D, E, and K.

Progeria An abnormal condition of premature aging that begins in childhood with sparse, graying hair and dry, thin, wrinkled skin. The person acquires the posture and physique of an aged individual and usually dies before the age of twenty. The cause is unknown, but geriatricians study such cases in a search for clues that may lead to a better understanding of the processes involved in "normal" aging.

Prolapse The dropping down or falling of an organ, such as the downward displacement of the uterus, which in severe cases may protrude through the vagina. *See also* **Ptosis.**

Proprioceptive Pertaining to the sensation of an awareness of the position of the body and body parts in space. This awareness is compiled from inputs of vision and the sense of balance but also includes nerve impulses from the muscles, tendons, and joints, which allow the brain to judge body positions when they cannot be seen.

Prosopagnosia A loss of the ability to recognize familiar faces, such as may occur in some victims of **Alzheimer's disease** who fail to recognize old friends and co-workers.

Prostate disorders Abnormal structural and functional changes in the prostate gland that are generally associated with aging. The chestnut-sized gland in the lower male pelvis secretes various enzymes and other substances that form the liquefied semen ejaculated through the penis during orgasm. The most common prostate disorder is *benign prostatic hypertrophy,* which is enlargement of the prostate. *Cancer of the prostate* is the second most common cancer in men. Both conditions are uncommon before the age of fifty. Initial normal growth of the prostate gland, which encircles the male urethra immediately below the urinary bladder, occurs rapidly after puberty and then stops in early adulthood. Growth begins again in the late forties and continues for the rest of the man's life. The exact cause is not known, other than that it is related to male sex hormones. More than 80 percent of men over the age of seventy have some enlargement of the prostate, and the first signs of hypertrophy (overgrowth) are found in more than half of all men in their forties, even though first symptoms may not appear until ten years later. About 10 percent of the male population eventually undergoes surgery to correct the overgrowth, which results in obstruction of the flow of urine from the bladder. The enlarging gland gradually compresses the urethra, thereby blocking the flow of urine. Symptoms of an enlarged prostate include difficulty in initiating urine flow, decreased force and size of the urine flow, straining to void, dribbling after urination, and a feeling of incomplete emptying of the bladder. This feeling of urinary retention results in an urge to urinate more frequently, particularly at night. Treatment usually requires surgery (prostatectomy) to remove excess prostate tissue.

Cancer of the prostate, like enlargement of the prostate, is caused by unknown factors, but sex hormones and viruses may play a part. After its symptomless early stages, a cancer of the prostate produces the same symptoms as an enlarged prostate, when the growing tumor presses against the urethra, blocking the flow of urine. There may also be blood and pus in the urine. If the tumor growth results in obstruction of the ureters leading from the kidneys to the bladder, the person may experience symptoms of **uremia** or **congestive heart failure**. The cancer also may spread by **metastasis** to the skeleton, producing symptoms of bone pain, initially in the bones of the spine and pelvis. Treatment depends upon the degree of cancer growth and spread when it has been diagnosed, but in most cases it may consist of surgery to remove the gland, radiation, and, in advanced cases, hormonal therapy.

Prostatectomy   Surgical removal of all or a part of the prostate gland. In the treatment of benign prostatic hypertrophy (enlarged prostate gland), only the portion that causes obstruction to the flow of urine may be removed. Several surgical approaches are used. The most common surgical approach is *transurethral resection (TURP),* performed by inserting a tiny lighted scope with an attached knife blade through the urethra and snipping off bits of prostate tissue from the inside. When the gland has grown too large for this approach, a *suprapubic operation* is performed through an incision in the lower abdomen. A *perineal approach,* through the area between the anus and the genitalia, may be used when the objective is to obtain a small sample of prostate tissue to examine for possible cancer cells or when it is necessary to remove a stone trapped in the prostate. The entire gland is removed in cancer of the prostate, in a procedure called *radical prostatectomy.*

Pruritus   Severe itching. There are many causes, including dry or excessively sensitive skin, a fungal or other skin infection, a drug reaction, jaundice, or an allergy or reaction to substances in the home, work, or recreational environment. Scratching often aggravates the condition and increases the risk of bacterial infection if the skin is broken. Among recommended treatments are starch baths, antihistamines, alcohol baths, and various ointments to relieve itching, and lotions to restore skin moisture.

Pseudogout   A painful condition with symptoms very similar to **gout** but caused by deposits of crystals of calcium pyrophosphate in the joints, rather than crystals of uric acid. The patient experiences severe pain in red and swollen joints. Pseudogout tends to affect older adults, particularly if they already have **diabetes mellitus, hypothyroidism,** or excessive iron in the blood. The disorder is treated with anti-inflammatory medications while the underlying condition is also treated.

Psoriasis   A chronic, recurrent skin disease marked by thick, dry, silvery scales, usually covering reddish **plaques**. The lesions can occur anywhere on the body but usually appear on the scalp, back, elbows, knees, and buttocks. The lesions may be small and scattered or merge into large plaques. The exact cause is unknown, but the condition is associated with an overgrowth of skin cells, and there is often a family history of psoriasis. It often begins gradually, sometimes following sunburn, use of skin medications, or discontinuance of steroid hormone medications. There may be an itching sensation, and scratching or peeling the scales may result in pinpoint bleeding. Dry indoor climates in winter can worsen the symptoms. The health of the person, who may be of any age, is usually not affected, though some patients experience a complication of **rheumatoid arthritis**, primarily in the joints of the fingers and toes and occasionally the spine. Both skin and joint disorders are nearly always permanent once they become established, though there are unpredictable periods of remission. Stress sometimes seems to play a part in recurrences. There is no cure, and treatment is directed toward relief of the symptoms. Various medications are used, including those that reduce skin cell overgrowth, coal tar preparations, topical corticosteroids, and skin lubricants. When arthritis symptoms accompany psoriasis, they are treated in the same manner as rheumatoid arthritis.

Psychiatric disorder   Any neurotic or psychotic condition that impairs the normal functioning so that an individual is unable to meet the demands of activities of daily living, such as maintaining a home or job.

Psychic suicide   A term sometimes used to describe a loss of the will to live. In effect, the person terminates his own life passively and without the use of a lethal agent.

Ptosis The dropping or drooping of an organ or body part, such as the drooping of the eyelids in **myasthenia gravis**.

Pulmonary diseases *See* **Chronic obstructive pulmonary disease, Pneumoconioses, Pneumonia, Pneumonitis.**

Pulmonary hypertension An abnormal condition in which there is resistance to the flow of blood from the right ventricle of the heart to the arteries of the lungs. Causes of pulmonary hypertension may include emboli that block one or more of the artery branches, causing the right ventricle to work harder to push blood through the network of vessels, **chronic obstructive pulmonary disease**, and pulmonary fibrosis, such as develops from certain **pneumoconioses**. **Emphysema**, which can result in the loss of part of the network of blood vessels of the lung, also may be a cause. Symptoms can include pain or discomfort in the chest, particularly beneath the breastbone, breathlessness, cough, rapid breathing, and light-headedness. Analgesics (painkillers) and other types of medications are given while the underlying cause is treated.

Pustule A blisterlike elevation on the skin that contains pus. An acne eruption may be a pustule.

R

Radical mastectomy *See* **Mastectomy.**

Radiculopathy   Any disorder involving the nerve roots of the spinal cord. Examples may include **acroparesthesia, herniated disk,** and **spondylosis.**

Range of motion   A hypothetical arc or path through which a person is able to move a joint or body part, such as moving the head as far to the left and right and as far forward and backward as possible without moving the rest of the body. The range of motion for an arm, leg, or other body part is often limited by arthritis or other musculoskeletal disorders and is measured in degrees of arc as part of the diagnosis of a joint disease or disability. The range can also be extended in many cases by the use of therapeutic exercises.

Raynaud's disease (Raynaud's phenomenon)   A spastic disorder of the small arteries of the fingers and sometimes of the toes that impairs blood flow to the affected parts, resulting in pallor and numbness or a feeling of cold. The condition is often caused by exposure to cold temperatures or by emotional stress. It also may be associated with various circulatory or connective tissue diseases, or it may be a reaction to certain drugs or chemicals. The condition may be aggravated by the use of tobacco, which constricts blood vessels, and is relieved by medications and by avoiding exposure to cold temperatures.

RDA   Abbreviation for *recommended daily allowance,* the minimum amounts of vitamins, minerals, and other nutrients needed each day for normal healthy individuals, according to guidelines set by the National Academy of Sciences. RDAs do not provide guidance for variations in nutritional requirements due to aging, infections, metabolic disorders, or chronic illnesses.

Reactive depression   A form of depression that follows a severe disappointment or personal loss. It is ordinarily temporary, a reaction to the death of a loved one, loss of a job, financial loss, or a blow to the person's self-esteem. It may be marked by sadness, lack of initiative, feelings of worthlessness, discontent, loss of appetite or overeating, and insomnia or excessive sleeping. Treatment may involve psychotherapy. *See also* **Depression, Psychic suicide.**

Reality orientation   A type of therapy employed to counteract confusion and disorientation in adults who have suffered mental impairment as a result of brain injury or disease. It employs extensive use of clocks, calendars, and other devices to emphasize time, place, and other environmental facts, which are incorporated into the person's daily living activities.

Receptive aphasia (word deaf, word blind)   A mental disorder due to brain damage in which the affected person loses the ability to understand spoken or written language. The condition often results from a stroke that damages the dominant half of the brain. The person can recognize objects and their uses, but though he or she hears words, their meaning is incomprehensible. *See also* **Perceptual defect.**

Recurrent utterance   A symptom of some types of organic brain disease or damage in which the individual's conversation consists primarily of repeated words, phrases, or sentences. The condition also may occur in schizophrenia.

Referred pain   Pain experienced in a part of the body other than the localized area of disease, injury, or other cause of the pain. The transfer of the pain to another body area is due to a sharing by the two body areas of the same nerve pathways. A common example of referred pain is a headache caused by neck muscle strain. *See also* **Phantom pain.**

Reflex changes with aging   Variations in autonomic (involuntary) nerve reactions to stimuli that result from the normal aging process. The deep tendon reflexes, such as the knee-jerk reaction, generally remain unchanged as one grows older. However, some superficial reflexes diminish or disappear. These include an abdominal reflex, in which muscles of the abdominal wall contract in response to touch stimulation of the area; and the cremasteric reflex, which in men results in the drawing of the testes toward the abdomen when the skin of the inside of the thigh is stroked. The Babinski reflex, in which the toes of a healthy infant extend upward when the sole is stroked, is normally absent in an adult, but if present, it can be a sign of an abnormality in the brain or spinal cord. Some visual reflexes, including the reaction of the pupil to light stimulation and convergence of the eyes for binocular vision of close objects, may be impaired. Automatic nerve reflexes affecting blood pressure and bowel and bladder function may deteriorate in some individuals.

Reflux esophagitis *See* **Esophagitis, Hiatus hernia.**

Rejuvenation The process of restoring youthfulness. The concept is basically a myth that has been perpetuated since ancient times, when humans searched for a "fountain of youth" or a magic elixir that would roll back the years or restore youthful features and vitality. The myth has continued in modern times with claims for drugs, hormones, minerals, or health foods that presumably restore or prolong youth.

Relocation crisis A stressful condition associated with moving or being moved from one home or residence to another. Stress factors include loss of established personal relationships, disruption of services, difficulties in adjusting to a new environment, and the threat or loss of independence. Relocation crisis is reported to be a factor in the increased death rate of elderly persons who are forced to move from an established family home. A change of residence is one of the critical "life events" cited by psychologists as a cause of increased susceptibility to disease, anxiety, and disorganized behavior. Relocation often accompanies other life events such as death of a spouse, change in financial status, change in social activities, or trouble with in-laws and may trigger physical or emotional illness.

REM Abbreviation for *rapid eye movement,* which normally occurs during certain periods of sleep and is associated with dreaming.

Renal disorders *See* **Kidney changes with aging.**

Respiratory acidosis An abnormal condition caused by an excess of carbon dioxide in the lungs that combines with water in the body to form carbonic acid, thus altering the **acid-base balance** of the body. Symptoms include headache, breathing difficulty, tremors, and a rapid heartbeat. Untreated, the condition can lead to coma and death. Among its causes are obstruction of the air passages to the lungs, pneumonia, emphysema, chest injuries, fluid in the lungs, and neuro-muscular disease affecting respiration. Treatment may require oxygen therapy in some cases, intravenous medications, removal of any airway obstruction, and mechanical respirators.

Respiratory alkalosis An abnormal condition caused by a lack of carbon dioxide in the blood, leading to alteration of the **acid-base balance** with an excess of alkalinity (base) in the blood. Symptoms include deep, rapid breathing, dizziness or light-headedness, numbness or spasms in the hands and feet, abnormal heart rhythm, and muscle weakness. Causes can include a liver disorder, pneumonia, asthma, blood poisoning, fever, and a reaction to aspirin. Anxiety accompanied by hyperventilation is a common cause of respiratory alkalosis. Treat-ment may include sedatives to relieve anxiety and other therapies di-rected toward the underlying causes. Anxiety-induced hyperventilation is sometimes treated by having the person breathe into a paper bag so that exhaled carbon dioxide can be rebreathed, thereby raising the level of the gas in the bloodstream.

Respiratory disorders *See* **Lung changes with age, Pneumonia, Pneumoconioses, Pneumonitis.**

Respiratory system changes *See* **Lung changes with age.**

Restless legs syndrome A sleep disturbance that tends to affect some older adults with an intense uneasiness in the legs that prevents their falling asleep. The person may resort to stretching the legs, walking about, or even jumping in order to eliminate the feeling. In many cases, the sensation persists and the person must repeat several cycles of activity to relieve it. The feeling may be described as a tightness, jitteri-ness, itching, crawling, or pulling of the muscles anywhere from the calves to the thighs. If the legs are not exercised to reduce the tension, the person may experience involuntary contractions of the muscles.

Retinal detachment Separation of the retina from the blood-rich cho-roid layer at the back of the eye. It usually begins with a tear or hole in the retina that allows fluid to leak between the retinal and choroid layers. Causes include injury to the eyeball, cataract operations, inflam-mation, diabetes, or structural changes in the tissues due to aging that alter the shape of the eyeball and stretch the inner tissues. Most retinal holes develop on the outer edges of the retina, resulting in an early symptom seen as a flashing light at the edge of the normal visual field. A **floater**, caused by a piece of loose retinal tissue, may also appear. Actual detachment of the retina usually appears as a shadow that moves slowly across the visual field, obscuring vision. The condition is painless. A detached retina requires emergency treatment. If not corrected quickly, blindness results. The retinal detachment is corrected by laser treatment or by surgery under general anesthesia and is successful in 90 percent of cases.

Retrocollis Muscle spasms of the neck that cause the head to be drawn backward. *See also* **Wryneck.**

Retropulsion A symptom of **parkinsonism** characterized by a tendency to move rapidly backward with short steps, particularly when looking up. The action can be dangerous if it occurs while the person is on a stairway.

Rheumatic fever An acute inflammatory disease that commonly begins as an untreated streptococcal (bacterial) infection of the throat, which may spread to the joints, heart, brain, skin, and subcutaneous tissues. Although the disease usually attacks children under the age of eighteen, persons of any age, including older adults, may develop it, and attacks can recur. From one to four weeks after the initial infection, there is a fever, loss of appetite, fatigue, and general discomfort. There may also be nosebleeds and swelling of a large joint, which becomes very tender, red, and hot. Inflammation of the heart (carditis) also occurs in about half the persons who experience joint inflammation. Treatment usually includes aspirin or other painkillers and antibiotics. Patients with heart inflammation or arthritis may be restricted in activity, at least during the acute stages, and those with heart complications may be placed on a low-sodium diet. *See also* **Rheumatic heart disease.**

Rheumatic heart disease A complication of **rheumatic fever**. The heart is one of the five major sites in which infection lodges, and heart damage is a common aftermath of the disease. There may be symptoms of **pericarditis, murmurs**, and heart valve disorders, with chest and abdominal pain, abnormal pulse and heart rhythm, and breathing difficulties. **Mitral valve** stenosis, usually a result of the disease, is the most common form of rheumatic valvular heart disease in adults. *See also* **Heart changes with aging.**

Rheumatism A lay term for any of a variety of conditions of inflamed, sore, or stiff muscles or pain in the joints. There may be specific disorders that cause these conditions, ranging from **bursitis, myositis,** or **fibromyositis** to **rheumatic fever** and gonorrhea. Or rheumatism may be psychogenic, occurring during periods of mental stress. One form, *palindromic rheumatism,* affects a joint for a few hours to a few weeks from no known cause and then disappears without treatment. *See also* **Arthritis, Gout, Osteoarthritis, Rheumatoid arthritis.**

Rheumatoid arthritis (RA) A chronic inflammatory disease of the joints that results in progressive destruction of the tissues in and around the joints, including the synovial membranes. Though **osteoarthritis** is more prevalent, RA is the most common form of crippling arthritis. The exact cause is unknown, but **autoimmune** factors appear to play a significant part in the disease. The symptoms of swollen, tender, painful joints and fever may begin at any age, but the incidence of RA increases with age, peaking in the fifties among women and in the sixties in men. Women are two to three times as likely as men to develop rheumatoid arthritis. The disease may begin gradually, with symptoms of stiffness or pain on motion in a single joint, or suddenly, with a number of joints affected at the same time. In both types, the delicate synovial membranes thicken and develop folds. A substance called rheumatoid factor is produced as some joint tissues become fibrous and others die. Cartilage, ligaments, and other tissues of the joint erode. The overlying skin becomes smooth, thin, and shiny. Muscle fibers appear to become shorter and atrophied around the affected joints. Painless, firm rheumatic nodules form over joint prominences and tendon sheaths. As the disease progresses, there may be periods of remission, or reduction of symptoms, but the symptoms eventually return. In severe cases, the inflammation increases until the joint becomes permanently fixed, often in a distorted position.

The early symptoms of rheumatoid arthritis so closely resemble those of other diseases, such as gout or rheumatic fever, that a diagnosis may take several months of observations and laboratory tests. Numerous clinical signs and symptoms must be continuous for at least six weeks for a definite or even probable diagnosis of rheumatoid arthritis. Treatment may include complete bed rest during the most painful period of the disease. Therapy also consists of an adequate diet, anti-inflammatory and antipain medications (usually aspirin unless it causes adverse side effects), plus exercises, physical therapy, and surgery, as needed. In some cases, hip or knee joints severely damaged by RA may be replaced with artificial joints so that normal activities of daily living can be resumed. When older adults develop rheumatoid arthritis, it usually begins gradually and involves the small joints of the hands, wrists, and feet at first, later spreading to other larger joints. The disease also is generally milder and less disabling when it begins in an older adult.

Right bundle branch block   A heart disorder in which the electrical impulse from the heart's pacemaker is unable to transmit its signal on the right side of the heart. In persons over the age of forty, the defect is usually associated with **coronary artery disease**. It may cause a fraction of a second delay of the contraction of the right ventricle. Right bundle branch block usually does not require treatment, but it is often an early sign of an underlying heart disease. In certain complicated cases, the condition may be controlled by surgical implantation of an artificial **pacemaker**.

Rigidity   A personality trait of "rigid ego," sometimes observed in older adults and expressed in four possible ways. The person may exhibit a diminished capacity for learning new things; may appear to be in a rut that has developed through the safe practice of old, established habits; may protect against the fear of changes in life by blocking out thoughts about such changes; or may display the rigidity of a perfectionist. Some psychiatrists believe that persons who exhibit a rigid ego actually have a personality weakness and display rigidity in an effort to conceal an inability to cope effectively with changes encountered in later years.

Root entrapment   A condition in which a nerve root is caught between displaced pieces of bone resulting from degeneration of the spinal column or a herniation of a vertebral disk. The nerve roots are small nodes next to the spinal cord through which nerve branches carrying impulses to and from the extremities of the body are attached to the spinal cord. Blood vessels accompany the nerve root attachments to the spinal cord. Root entrapment results in pain and numbness in the part of the body, usually one side only, served by the attached nerves. Muscles served by the affected nerve may atrophy, and associated reflexes may be lost. The person may be unable to feel a pinprick in the affected body segment. Specific treatment varies with the part of the spine that has been damaged, but root entrapment usually requires painkillers and sedatives as well as **laminectomy** to restore the spinal column and the functions of the affected body areas.

S

Salicylism (aspirin poisoning)   Adverse effects that result from taking excessive doses of aspirin (acetylsalicylic acid) or related medications containing salicylate. Because aspirin is used so widely, it is not surprising that salicylates may be the most common cause of adverse effects from medications in the United States. Among older adults, the condition often develops from excessive doses of aspirin taken for rheumatic disorders. The amount of aspirin that can result in an overdose depends in part on several individual factors, such as body weight, and the general health of the person, including possible kidney disorders and dehydration. A person who weighs 120 pounds could be poisoned by the same number of aspirin tablets that would be safe for a heavier person. The symptoms of a salicylate overdose are a ringing or buzzing in the ears, hearing impairment, rapid breathing, and agitation that may progress to **stupor** or **delirium**. Since it is an acid, aspirin can increase the acidity of gastric juices in the stomach, leading to the erosion of the stomach lining and the formation of **peptic ulcers**. Aspirin even in small doses can prevent normal blood clotting, and thus can interfere with healing of bleeding ulcers or other wounds in the digestive tract. Aspirin also can disrupt normal **metabolism** of carbohydrates, so that symptoms of **hypoglycemia** or **hyperglycemia** result. Severe salicylate intoxication can result in coma, depressed breathing, and other emergency medical conditions. In addition to aspirin, a common cause of salicylate poisoning is the use of oil of wintergreen (methyl salicylate), which can be absorbed through the skin. On the positive side, aspirin is an inexpensive and effective analgesic (pain-killer), antipyretic (fever-reducer), and anti-inflammatory drug when used as directed. Persons taking aspirin regularly should consult a physician about the size and frequency of doses. In some instances, the physician may advise an alternative medication. The physician also may recommend taking adequate amounts of water or milk with aspirin tablets or using "buffered" or specially coated aspirin products that reduce acid side effects in the stomach or delay tablet dissolving until it reaches the small intestine.

Scaling   A skin disorder characterized by the sloughing off of surface skin cells. The condition is seen in dandruff and **psoriasis**.

Scar   An abnormal area of skin in which connective tissue has formed to replace tissue destroyed by a wound, burn, or other injury. A **keloid** is a scar that is raised above the surrounding skin surface.

Sciatica   A severe pain along the path of the sciatic nerve, from the lower back as far as the lower leg or foot. The pain may be felt in the pelvis, buttock, thigh, calf, or foot. It is caused by any of several degenerative disorders of the lower spinal column area, such as a herniated disk that compresses the sciatic nerve. Sciatica also may result from infection, diabetic neuritis, alcoholism, or other disorders that cause irritation of the nerve. Sciatica sometimes mimics the symptoms of **intermittent claudication**, producing pain on walking, running, or ascending stairs. Treatment usually requires bed rest, painkillers, muscle relaxants, and, if necessary, traction and **spinal fusion** surgery.

Scleroderma   A chronic disease in which the skin becomes tough and leathery and firmly bound to underlying tissues. The disease may spread to internal organs such as the heart, lungs, and digestive tract, which also undergo sclerosis. The early symptoms of scleroderma are similar to and sometimes confused with those of **Raynaud's disease, rheumatoid arthritis**, or other disorders marked by fibrous degeneration of tissues. The skin changes occur first, often causing the patient to seek medical care before the internal organs become involved. After the initial swelling and hardening of the skin, the joints of the fingers become deformed and painful. As the skin acquires a leathery texture, the face becomes a taut, shiny mask that impairs the flexibility needed for chewing and swallowing. The disease can be fatal if internal organs become involved, but patients have survived thirty or more years with mild forms. Persons most likely to acquire scleroderma are middle-aged women. The cause is unknown, and there is no specific treatment.

Sclerosis   Any hardening of tissue, as from infiltration of fibrous material, deposits of calcium or other minerals, or inflammation. The term is often accompanied by a modifying word that identifies the affected tissue, as **arteriosclerosis** refers to sclerosis of the arteries.

Scotoma   A defect within the field of vision that leaves a blind area, often the result of damage to the retina or to some fibers of the optic nerves. There is a natural blind spot in the part of the retina that is the site of the optic nerve. Some people have a comma-shaped extension of this physiological blind spot. Scotomas also may be caused by **glaucoma**, exposure to solar eclipses, or wearing glasses with high-powered lenses that create blind spots.

SDAT   Abbreviation for *senile dementia of the Alzheimer type.*

Seborrheic keratosis   A small yellow skin **plaque** that gradually enlarges, thickens, and darkens to a brownish black color. It may resemble a **wart** or **mole** but acquires a greasy, velvety texture. **Keratoses**, which usually appear on the trunk and head, are generally harmless. Sometimes, but not always, they produce itching and irritation. The cause is unknown. They are common in nearly all older adults. They do not need to be removed unless they are disfiguring.

Secondary cancer (metastatic carcinoma)   A cancer that develops from malignant cells that have traveled through the blood or lymph vessels from a primary cancer in another part of the body. The process of spreading is called **metastasis**.

Sedative   Any drug that reduces excitement or nervousness by depressing the nervous system. Examples of sedatives include *alcohol, barbiturates,* and *minor tranquilizers.* Larger doses of barbiturates and certain other sedatives may be used to induce sleep. Drowsiness and confusion may be adverse side effects of sedatives when they are not given to induce sleep.

Self-medication   The practice of determining for oneself which remedies are appropriate for treating certain symptoms and administering the remedies by oneself. Taking aspirin for a headache is an example of self-medication. The remedies chosen are generally nonprescription (over-the-counter) drugs.

Senescence   The process or the time period of aging.

Senile angioma (cherry angioma, ruby spot)   A small, bright red skin tumor that may appear anywhere on the body. It consists of a small compressible mass of capillaries and tends to occur most frequently in persons after the age of forty-five. The tiny red spots are not considered dangerous, and there is no recommended treatment, although surgical removal of a senile angioma may be desired if it is disfiguring.

Senile cataract   *See* **Cataract.**

Senile delirium   A psychological disorder in older adults, marked by restlessness, insomnia, disorientation, wandering, and occasional hallucinations. The symptoms usually follow a head injury, infection, or other disturbing event, such as surgery, and often can be relieved with tranquilizers while the underlying disease or injury is treated. Older adults are more prone to delirium as a reaction to physical or psychological stress than younger persons.

Senile dementia   Mental deterioration associated with atrophy or degeneration of brain tissues. The condition is usually irreversible and may produce symptoms of memory loss, impaired judgment, loss of abstract thinking ability, confusion, **confabulation**, and irritability. The term is sometimes applied to organic brain disorders that develop in persons over the age of sixty, to distinguish the condition from the **presenile dementias**, which may begin in middle age.

Senile freckle   *See* **Lentigo.**

Senile involution   A term applied to any progressive shrinking, degeneration, or other loss of structure or function of tissues due to the aging process. Initial signs of senile involution, such as skin wrinkles, joint degeneration, and atherosclerotic plaques, begin to appear between the ages of twenty and twenty-five.

Senile keratosis (actinic keratosis)   A thickened lesion of the skin that appears as a flat or slightly elevated brownish or tan scaly spot, measuring up to one-half inch in diameter. The growths usually appear in groups and may merge. Skin areas generally affected are the face, ears, neck, and the back of the hands. The lesions are caused by excessive exposure to sunlight. They are most commonly seen on persons with outdoor jobs, such as farmers and sailors. Fair-haired, thin-skinned individuals with blue eyes are most vulnerable to the damaging effects of sun exposure. A senile or actinic keratosis is considered precancerous and should be removed early.

Senile lentigines (liver spots)   Pigmented patches of skin that appear on surfaces often exposed to the sunlight, such as the forearms, face, and backs of the hands. They are produced by skin pigment cells that increase in number as one grows older. Despite the popular term, they have nothing to do with the liver. They can be prevented by protecting exposed skin from excessive sunlight exposure and may be removed with bleaching creams or minor surgery.

Senile muscular atrophy   A series of natural aging changes in skeletal muscle tissue that begins after the age of fifty and results in a gradual loss of strength and physical endurance. Skeletal muscle tissue of older individuals is darker than that of young adults, in part as a result of deposits of a brownish pigment (lipofuscin) and in part an accumulation of fat and connective tissue fibers between the muscle cells. Individual muscle fibers become smaller and lose their connections with nerve fibers that normally stimulate muscle contractions. Senile muscular atrophy begins in the extremities, affecting the hands and feet first, and gradually spreads through all of the voluntary muscles of the body. Senile muscular atrophy appears to occur independently of other factors such as nutritional status or the presence of inflammatory muscle diseases, including **polymyositis** or dermatomyositis, associated with aging.

Senile pruritus   A common form of **pruritus** associated with changes in the structure of the aging skin, particularly diminished secretion of oil by the sebaceous glands. It is not associated with the time of year or dryness. Treatment is often difficult.

Senile psychosis   *See* **Senile dementia.**

Senile vaginitis   An inflammation or irritation of the vagina due to effects of the aging process. The mucous membranes of the vagina become thinner and drier and secrete less mucus after menopause and are therefore more susceptible to infection. Symptoms may include itching and an odorous discharge. The cause of infection is most often a fungus or bacteria, and it can be controlled by appropriate oral or topical medications. Senile vaginitis increases in frequency after the age of seventy.

Senile venous lake   A type of "blood blister" that sometimes appears as a dark bluish spot on the skin of older adults, most frequently on the face, neck, or lip. Men are affected more often than women. The lake can be removed for cosmetic reasons by draining the blood.

Senile wart *See* **Senile keratosis.**

Senility A popular term used for any degenerative mental condition that is associated with the aging process. Similar physical or mental changes that occur before the age of forty are sometimes identified as *premature senility.* Many of the typical signs of senility, such as memory impairment, a decreasing interest in physical appearance, inattention, and irritability, are the results of organic brain disease or damage. When the same symptoms occur at an earlier age, they usually stem from other causes.

Septic arthritis (infectious arthritis) A form of **arthritis** in which a joint is infected by bacteria or other agents. A wide range of infectious agents may enter a joint through the bloodstream or as a result of injury or a medical or surgical procedure involving the joint. Persons with **rheumatoid arthritis** or other forms of joint inflammation are particularly susceptible to infection. Symptoms can include pain, stiffness, fever, chills, swelling, and tenderness. Treatment is with antibiotics. If untreated, the infection can destroy the joint.

Sexual function changes with aging Alterations in sexual activity associated with the aging process. The male may continue to achieve an erection in his seventies or eighties, although the amount and force of ejaculate during orgasm may be diminished. The refractory period, or temporary state of physiological resistance to sexual stimulation, may last from eight to twenty-four hours in an older man, as compared to a refractory period of thirty minutes for a thirty-year-old man. Reasons given for reduced female sexual activity in later life include a lack of sexual partners, physiological changes that include diminished vaginal lubrication and atrophy of the mucosal lining of the vagina, and less vigorous contractions of the pelvic platform during orgasms.

Shingles *See* **Herpes zoster.**

Shoulder girdle A **skeletomuscular** unit formed by the two collarbones, the two shoulder blades, the top of the breastbone, and the various muscles and other tissues linking these bones. The shoulder girdle forms a fender-shaped guard, attachment, and support for the arms. *See also* **Limb girdle-trunk paresis.**

Shoulder pain Any pain that occurs in the shoulder joint or that may be referred to the shoulder from another part of the body. Pain involving the shoulder structures may be caused by **arthritis, bursitis, aneu-**

rysm, rupture of a tendon, muscle strain, fracture of a bone, or compression of a nerve. Pain may be referred to the shoulder by **angina pectoris, pleurisy, tuberculosis, cancer, peptic ulcer** or **herpes zoster**. An enlarged spleen may result in pain in the left shoulder. The range of motion of the arm at the shoulder is sometimes a clue to the cause of shoulder pain. An arm that can be raised through a half-circle without pain gives evidence that no joint is involved; if the arm can be raised through a half-circle although the movement is quite painful, the cause may be arthritis. A fracture or a tendon rupture may also limit the range of motion.

Shy-Drager syndrome   A neurological disorder marked by orthostatic **hypotension**, bladder and bowel **incontinence**, tremors, muscle wasting, and loss of muscle coordination. Loss of nervous system control over the arteries and veins occurs gradually, moving upward through the legs toward the trunk. There may also be a loss of hair, beginning on the legs, and eventually decreased sweating, salivation, and tearing. In advanced cases, there may be loss of visual accommodation and the ability to constrict the pupils of the eyes. Treatment involves drugs to relieve symptoms. Special antigravity stockings are recommended to prevent the accumulation of blood in the legs, a result of hypotension and loss of muscle tone in the blood vessels in the legs.

Silicosis   A lung disorder caused by the inhalation of dust containing silica, a mineral component of sand and other substances. The symptoms include breathing difficulty on exertion, a mild, unproductive cough, and breath sounds. In acute cases there may also be fever and weight loss. Chest X-rays show an accumulation of nodules throughout the chest. The nodules are formed by fibrous tissue that forms over the silica particles, as if to wall them off from the normal lung tissue. The nodules collapse and destroy the tiny air sacs of the lung, resulting in a condition similar to **emphysema**. Chest expansion for breathing becomes increasingly difficult, and affected persons eventually become incapacitated. They may also develop an enlarged heart or heart failure. Persons most often affected are those exposed to silica in industry, such as those working with abrasives, abrasive soaps, foundry castings, or cement products; or those involved in sandblasting, lens grinding, quarrying and tunneling, or coal mining. For most workers the symptoms do not appear until after many years of industrial exposure, at a time of life when lung function is declining naturally because of the aging process. There is no cure for silicosis, and patients are treated as cases of **chronic obstructive pulmonary disease**. Because silicosis disrupts the lungs' normal processes that protect against disease, persons with silicosis are more susceptible to tuberculosis and other respiratory infections.

Sinoatrial (S-A) block   A heartbeat abnormality in which the electrical impulse from the heart's natural pacemaker (sino-atrial node) fails to trigger contraction of the upper chambers (atria) of the heart. The condition occurs mostly in persons with **coronary artery disease** or chronic **rheumatic heart disease** and produces a symptom of "skipped" heartbeats. If uncorrected at an early stage, the S-A block may result in light-headedness and loss of consciousness. The effect, which tends to occur most frequently in older adults, can be caused by certain medications and is treated by surgical implantation of an electronic **pacemaker**.

Sitophobia   A morbid fear of food or eating. It occurs most often in older adults, usually as a result of pain or discomfort that may follow a meal.

Sjögren's syndrome   An inflammatory disease characterized by dryness of the mouth, eyes, and other mucous membrane surfaces. It usually affects women over the age of forty, has **autoimmune** causes, and is often associated with **rheumatoid arthritis, scleroderma**, and other disorders. Joint inflammation is a common complaint, and more than two-thirds of the patients show positive results in a test for the rheumatoid factor, which sometimes indicates the presence of rheumatoid arthritis. Almost any system of the body can be involved. There may be damage to the corneas of the eyes, increased dental caries, dryness of the vagina, loss of scalp hair, atrophy of digestive system tissues, inflammation of the pancreas, or complications of the heart, lungs, kidneys, and nervous system. The dominant feature of these effects is tissue dehydration, and treatment is directed toward relieving this by sipping fluids frequently. A frequent complication is a proliferation of lymphatic cells into the affected tissues, leading to **lymphoma**.

Skeletomuscular system   The bones, muscles, ligaments, tendons, and other related tissues that provide the human body with the means of movement and locomotion, while also affording protection for many vital organs. **Arthritis, osteoporosis, spondylosis, limb girdle-trunk paresis**, and fractures are among the disorders that interfere with normal functioning of the skeletomuscular system.

Skin cancer   Any cancer that appears on the surface of the body, often beginning as a **plaque, mole**, pimple, or ulceration. The most common type of skin cancer is *basal cell carcinoma,* which arises from the basal cells at the base of the epidermis. These cancers tend to develop on the face, neck, and head and are associated with exposure to sunlight, radiation, heat, and certain chemicals such as tar. Light-skinned persons and those who work outdoors are most likely to be affected, and the risk of developing a basal cell carcinoma increases after middle age. Basal cell cancer usually appears first as pearly nodules that ulcerate and form a crust. It may also begin as a shiny brown or black sore. The cancer is treated by surgical removal. Less common is *squamous cell carcinoma,* which tends to develop in skin areas previously damaged by sunburn, contact with chemicals such as tar, or an **actinic keratosis**. A squamous cell carcinoma also tends to favor persons who are middle-aged or older. It may begin as a wartlike lesion on the skin, with or without a small red area caused by dilated capillaries. A squamous cell carcinoma can metastasize (spread), whereas a basal cell carcinoma rarely does. If it is found early and removed surgically, it can be cured. The third type type of primary skin cancer is a *malignant melanoma,* which is much more dangerous than the other two forms. A malignant melanoma appears as a light tan to black flat or slightly raised skin lesion or a pigmented mole. It can develop anywhere on the body. A dark mole that suddenly changes size, shape, or other characteristics should be suspected of being a malignant melanoma. The exact cause is unknown. Early detection and surgery are important because a malignant melanoma can metastasize through the lymphatic system. Although a malignant melanoma may affect a younger person, most cases develop between the ages of fifty and seventy.

Skin changes with aging   Alterations in skin structure and function associated with the aging process. Among noticeable changes in the skin of older adults are loss of fat layers beneath the skin, increased pigmentation, decrease in sweat glands and hair follicles, and thickening of the blood vessels. The number and distribution of oil glands remains about the same, but they no longer secrete oil. The skin becomes thinner, drier, and more wrinkled as subcutaneous fat disappears. Graying of hair often accompanies skin changes in most people. Skin blemishes that occur more frequently in older adults include **senile keratosis, senile purpura**, liver spots, and cherry angiomas. The changes in skin structure make older adults more susceptible to lesions that can evolve into **skin cancers**. The loss of fat layers makes the person more vulnerable to temperature extremes, and deterioration of oil and sweat glands can make the skin dry and itchy. For bedridden persons, **bedsores** (decubitus ulcers, or pressure sores) can develop in the skin and penetrate deeper soft tissues and bone. There is also a decline in the number of nerve receptors for the senses of touch and pressure in the skin of the fingers, and an estimated 30-percent decline in the smaller blood vessels of the skin. One of the more obvious effects of age-related changes in skin tissues is the appearance of "bags," "double chins," and "love handles," due to a redistribution of fat cells and fibrous tissue.

Sleep changes with aging Alterations in sleeping patterns that are associated with the aging process. In general, older adults spend less time in deep sleep and more in nighttime wakefulness than younger adults. Some studies show that an older person needs less sleep than in earlier years. Sleep-disturbance complaints can be due to the pain of **arthritis**, the discomfort of **hiatus hernia**, or heart-rhythm disorders, such as those related to temporary breathing interruptions (**apnea**) during sleep. **Nocturia**, or the need to urinate at least once during the night, is a common cause of interrupted sleep. Insomnia can also have emotional sources such as **depression**, the most frequent cause of insomnia among older adults. In severe cases of insomnia or disturbed sleep, an older adult may find the day-night cycles reversed and will spend much of the night wandering about. Chronic sleep disturbances may require consultation with a physician, who may prescribe a medication. However, many physicians object to the use of drug therapy as a permanent solution for sleep disturbances. *See also* **Insomnia.**

Snoring Noisy breathing during sleep, caused by the vibration of the soft palate and other structures in the mouth and throat.

Sodium balance *See* **Hypernatremia.**

Solar keratosis *See* **Actinic keratosis.**

Spinal fusion A surgical procedure in which two or more vertebrae are fused or joined, sometimes with a bone graft, to provide greater stability to a weakened or damaged spinal column. The operation is most often performed on the lower back region but also may be done on the vertebrae in the neck. *See also* **Herniated disk, Sciatica.**

Spondylosis A form of **osteoarthritis** involving the vertebrae. The condition tends to occur in the neck vertebrae after the age of fifty, and the frequency increases with age. As in other parts of the spinal column, the vertebral bones and the intervertebral disks may degenerate. These changes cause deformities of the spine with compression of the spinal cord or attached nerve roots, producing pain, numbness, or tingling.

The pain or numbness may radiate from the neck down the arm to the hands. The person may hear or feel a crackling or grinding sound when turning the head. In some cases, the condition may be relatively pain-free except under certain circumstances, such as coughing. Treatment depends upon the extent of the injury. In relatively mild cases, symptoms may be relieved by bed rest, painkilling drugs, and wearing a cervical collar that restricts sudden movements of the neck. For other cases, it may be necessary to place the patient in head traction until a **laminectomy** can be performed to remove offending pieces of bone from the spine and fuse remaining vertebrae to ensure stability of the spinal column. *See also* **Root entrapment.**

Squamous cell carcinoma *See* **Skin cancer.**

Stapedectomy A surgical procedure for correcting a hearing loss due to a defect in the stapes, one of the three tiny bones in the middle ear. The stapes helps transmit sound vibrations from the eardrum to the inner ear. If it becomes rigidly fixed due to **sclerosis**, the stapes is unable to transmit the vibrations, resulting in a form of conductive deafness. In the operation, the stapes and the inner ear window attached to it are removed under a local anesthetic. A new oval window is grafted from a piece of skin, and an artificial stapes of plastic or stainless steel is attached to the graft.

Stasis dermatitis A skin condition that develops around the feet and ankles of older adults as a result of impaired blood circulation. The disorder, which frequently occurs in people with varicose veins, begins with red, scaly, itching patches that become blisters. Scratching usually leads to infection, ulcerations, and increased brownish pigmentation of the affected skin area. The condition is generally complicated by fluid accumulation about the ankles, obesity, infections, and a form of eczema that spreads over other areas of the body. Treatment may include elevation of an affected leg above heart level and the application of wet compresses, medicated ointments or creams, and, when appropriate, antibiotics.

Stiffness An abnormal condition in which movement of a joint is limited or contraction of a muscle is difficult or mildly painful. The condition usually is noticed after a period of sleep or rest ("morning stiffness") which, in mild cases, is relieved after about fifteen minutes of activity. In cases of degenerative joint disease, such as **arthritis**, the pain and discomfort of stiff joints or muscles may persist for two hours or more after a period of inactivity.

Stress Any environmental factor that can cause a strain or disruption in the body's mental or physical resources. The term is also used to describe the effect of a disruptive organic or psychological force. *Physical stress* can be produced by extremes of heat or cold, a serious infection, or adverse drug reaction. *Psychological stress* may occur in pressures of competition, frustrations, or loss of income or loved one. Stress is not necessarily harmful if the individual is able to adjust to or cope with the particular stressor. Vigorous physical exercise, for example, may exert a beneficial type of stress on the heart, lungs, and muscles. Certain types of mental stress, similarly, can be psychologically beneficial, as in negotiating the purchase or sale of property. Tension, panic, anxiety, or use of alcohol are common adverse reactions to stress when a person fails to adjust to or cope with a stressor effectively.

Stridor An abnormal noise made during inhalation by a person whose voicebox (larynx) is obstructed. It is usually a high-pitched sound caused by the force of incoming air on the vocal cords.

Stroke Any of several types of circulatory disorders of the brain, caused by an insufficiency or interruption of blood flow to the brain area. It results in abnormal functioning of the body area influenced by the affected brain tissues. Brain injury can result from a reduced flow of blood or interruption of blood flow to a brain area due to an obstruction in an artery or the rupture of an artery (brain hemorrhage). A stroke can occur suddenly, with results that range from a relatively mild interruption of normal brain function to death. Factors that contribute to stroke include **hypertension, arteriosclerosis**, cigarette smoking, **diabetes mellitus, obesity**, lack of physical activity, heart disease associated with an **embolus**, a family history of strokes, or a personal history of **transient ischemic attacks** (temporary mild strokes). Symptoms of a stroke usually develop within a few minutes of the event and may increase over a period of several hours or several days. There may or may not be headache, pain, or fever. There may be loss of vision in one eye or both eyes, numbness or weakness in one arm or leg, paralysis, confusion, vertigo, or slurred speech, or the affected person may collapse without losing consciousness. The precise symptoms are often clues as to the type and location of brain damage as brain area "maps" can trace a function in one part of the body to a particular segment of brain tissue, which may be on the opposite side of the body. Any stroke, like a heart attack or serious injury, is an emergency that requires immediate medical care in order to save the life of the victim or prevent irreversible brain damage.

Stupor   A mental state in which a person is generally unresponsive, though not unconscious. The person may respond to painful stimuli by partial arousal, may or may not respond to questions or commands, and may give inconsistent or vague responses, as with grunts, moans, or "body language" actions. The stuporous person does not converse or make other meaningful speech sounds.

Subluxation   A partial or incomplete dislocation. A subluxation of the spine as a result of **arthritis** or **spondylosis** can result in compression of the spinal cord and paralysis of much of the body.

Sundowning   A term used to describe the confusion that overtakes some older adults as evening approaches. If their vision is impaired, the gradual darkness blots out important visual cues that help them maintain their orientation. The condition may be aggravated by other sensory deficits such as hearing loss.

Sympathetic nervous system   A part of the **autonomic nervous system** that controls a number of the body's involuntary functions, such as dilation of the eyes, constriction of the blood vessels, and control of glandular secretions. It is this system that causes sweat glands to secrete perspiration and hormones to be released. Sympathetic nervous system functions help mobilize the body's physical and mental resources to meet increased demands of physical or mental effort.

Symptom substitution   The development of a new symptom when an earlier symptom has been treated successfully. The situation frequently occurs in the psychotherapy of a neurotic person, who may, for example, be weaned from chain-smoking cigarettes but become a binge eater.

Syncope   A temporary loss of consciousness (fainting) caused by an interruption of blood flow to the brain. An attack of syncope usually follows a feeling of dizziness or light-headedness and may be insignificant or be caused by a number of heart and circulatory disorders. In some instances, a coughing spell can lower the blood pressure in the arteries so that the brain is temporarily deprived of oxygen. Other factors causing syncope can be a sudden change of body position from sitting or reclining to standing (orthostatic hypotension), emotional stress, profuse sweating, or **hypotension**. Men are more commonly affected than women, and the risk of attacks increases with age as the body's receptors for detecting and compensating for sudden changes in blood pressure gradually diminish.

Systemic   Pertaining to the entire body or to one or more body systems, as distinguished from a body part or localized condition.

Systemic lupus erythematosus (SLE)   A serious chronic inflammatory connective tissue disease that involves the skin, mucous membranes, joints, kidneys, and nervous system. SLE is an **autoimmune** disease, and a specific antibody (LE factor) is present in the blood of most patients. The disease may be marked by a wide variety of signs and symptoms that may suggest involvement of almost any body system. They include **Raynaud's disease**, hair loss, skin lesions, **arthritis**, photosensitivity, and ulcers of the mouth and throat. A rash or area of redness in the shape of a butterfly extending across the bridge of the nose is a clinical sign that usually identifies the disease. Although SLE is usually regarded as a disease that affects mostly young women, studies show that in about 15 percent of all cases, the first symptoms appear in persons of both sexes after the age of fifty. Symptoms also appear with a different frequency in older adults; they are likely to experience photosensitivity and skin lesions more often but have a decreased incidence of other symptoms. Kidney involvement, a common effect of the disease in young patients, is rare in older individuals. Treatment depends upon the severity of the disease and the specific symptoms. Mild cases are usually treated with large doses of aspirin or similar drugs and other medications, including corticosteroids, if needed. Corticosteroids are the main form of therapy for severe cases. SLE is a less severe disease in older adults, but it is easily complicated by respiratory and other infections, and it is recommended that patients receive vaccinations against influenza and pneumonia.

Systole   Contraction of the heart. Systole is that part of the heart rhythm in which the heart muscle exerts maximum pressure to force blood out of the ventricles and into the aorta and pulmonary arteries. The blood pressure measured at systole is the first number in a blood pressure reading. The second number is the blood pressure at **diastole**, or relaxation of the heart muscle.

T

Tachycardia A cardiac **arrhythmia** marked by an abnormally rapid heartbeat, usually in excess of 100 contractions per minute. The heartbeat in some cases of tachycardia may exceed 200 per minute. Tachycardia is experienced as a rapid fluttering sensation in the chest, often accompanied by a feeling of faintness, weakness, and breathing difficulty. There may be a tightness or pain in the chest. The condition is most commonly associated with arteriosclerotic heart disease, but it may also be caused by anemia, hemorrhage, shock, or congestive heart failure. Abnormally rapid heartbeats also can result from fever, exercise, or nervous excitement. The rapid contractions can involve either the upper heart chambers *(atrial tachycardia)* or the lower chambers *(ventricular tachycardia)*. Atrial tachycardia is less likely to be a life-threatening event, but ventricular tachycardia is very dangerous as it may progress to ventricular **fibrillation**, which is frequently fatal. The heart cannot function effectively for prolonged periods at such a rapid rate, and emergency treatment, with hospitalization, is usually required to stabilize the heart rhythm. *See also* **Fibrillation, Flutter.**

Tachypnea Abnormally rapid breathing, sometimes measured at more than forty respirations per minute. Tachypnea is sometimes a symptom of an **embolism** or **infarction** of the lung. It can cause hyperventilation, with carbon dioxide depletion and **alkalosis**.

Tamponade The use of pressure to stop the flow of blood. The term also may identify the application of a tampon, or roll of absorbent material, to control blood flow by absorbing the blood or compressing a leaking blood vessel. The term is commonly used to refer to *cardiac* *tamponade,* an abnormal condition in which blood or fluid leaks into the membrane (pericardium) surrounding the heart. The cause is usually the rupture of a blood vessel of the heart, but cardiac tamponade can also result from an injury to the heart, such as a knife wound. If enough blood or fluid accumulates, it can produce pressure against the heart that interferes with normal heart functions. Symptoms are engorged neck veins, breathing difficulties, and "pulsus paradoxus" (a pulse that decreases each time the person takes a deep breath). Treatment involves keeping the patient in bed with the head of the bed raised at a 45-degree angle, insertion of a hollow needle into the pericardium to drain accumulated blood or other fluid, and surgery to repair the ruptured blood vessel or other damaged heart tissue.

Tardive (late) dyskinesia A medication-induced neurological disorder characterized by repeated involuntary contractions of muscles of the face, arms, legs, and trunk. The symptoms may resemble those of **Huntington's chorea.** Persons most commonly affected are older adults who have been treated with major tranquilizers such as phenothiazines, haloperidol, or similar medications for symptoms of **parkinsonism** or psychiatric disorders. Treatment is difficult because the symptoms may fluctuate between remission and recurrence for months or years. More than half of all cases require more than fifteen months of treatment. Mild cases may be relieved with sedatives such as barbiturates that reduce the involuntary movements to the point where they can be tolerated. Severe cases may be treated with reserpine or other drugs, but some patients with well-established tardive dyskinesia fail to respond to treatment. Drug-induced tardive dyskinesia is an example of an **iatrogenic** disease.

Tardy peroneal nerve palsy A type of **neuropathy** marked by numbness in the legs that is produced when they are crossed. The pressure of the upper leg compresses the peroneal nerve in the leg beneath it. *See also* **Acroparesthesia.**

Tardy ulnar nerve palsy Numbness or a loss of sensation in the hands caused by compression of the ulnar nerve of the arm, a common result of resting one's weight on the elbows. Repeated or prolonged compression of the ulnar nerve can result in nerve damage, leading to atrophy of the muscles controlling the fingers and loss of the ability to perform activities that require fine finger movements.

Taste changes with aging Alterations in taste sensations that may occur as part of the natural aging process. There may be less diminishment of taste acuity in older adults in good health than has been thought. Most information suggesting a loss of taste buds and a decreased sense of taste has been based on studies of institutionalized elderly individuals, who may be ill or disabled or on medications that can affect the sense of taste. When taste acuity changes in older adults, it is likely to affect only some of the four basic taste sensations: sweet, sour, salty, and bitter. A contributing factor to diminished taste acuity in some cases may be a lower level of saliva secretion, as the presence of saliva is generally necessary for the detection of flavors.

Tectal midbrain syndrome   A loss of the ability to move the eyes up or down, usually due to a disease or damage affecting the brain stem.

Telangiectasia   Small red marks that appear in the skin in increasing numbers after middle age. They are caused by permanent dilations of capillaries beneath the skin.

Temperature regulation   The ability of the body to adapt to variations in the temperature of the environment. Normal automatic body responses to changes in room or outdoor temperatures include sweating, shivering, dilation and constriction of blood vessels, and some physiological reactions such as alterations in metabolism. This responsiveness diminishes with age, so many older adults are less able to adapt to wide ranges of heat and cold, making them more vulnerable to **hypothermia**, heat exhaustion, and **heat stroke**. They are less capable of sensing temperature changes, have an impaired ability to shiver when it is cold, and usually require higher temperatures than younger persons before the body's sweat glands begin to react. Many older adults are unable to detect temperature differences smaller than nine degrees Fahrenheit. If the older adult uses any of a wide variety of drugs, ranging from alcohol and aspirin to sedatives and tranquilizers, he or she is more susceptible to **hypothermia**, may experience a greater body heat loss in cold weather because of less fat beneath the skin, or may be less able to produce needed body heat because of **hypothyroidism, hypoglycemia**, or disorders that disrupt the temperature-regulating mechanism in the brain. Loss of ability to respond properly and rapidly to temperature extremes makes older adults more susceptible to effects of stroke or heart attacks during heat waves, or pneumonia and other respiratory infections in cold weather.

Temporal arteritis   An inflammatory disease of an artery, usually a cranial or temporal artery of the head. The inflammation causes the artery walls to thicken, narrowing the opening through the blood vessel and restricting blood flow. The disease affects mainly people over the age of fifty, especially women. Symptoms are severe headaches, usually around the temple or the back of the head, depending upon which artery is inflamed, difficulty in chewing, weight loss, loss of appetite, low-grade fever, weakness, and rheumatic pains. Among possible complications are loss of vision, stroke, heart attack, and impaired circulation of the arms and legs. Sudden blindness is the most serious threat, caused when arteries supplying blood to the eye become involved. Early treatment with steroids and other drugs is essential to avert visual damage. Also called "giant cell arteritis."

Tennis elbow   *See* **Epicondylitis.**

Tension headache   *See* **Headache.**

Terminal drop   A marked decline in certain mental functions that frequently precedes the death of an older person. The drop is independent of any serious physical illness. Several medical researchers have reported that intelligence and coping ability often begin to decline, along with personality changes, within a five-year period prior to the death of an aged person. The initial studies were conducted among elderly people in institutions, but similar changes in mental performance were found later in elderly persons living independently in the community.

Testes changes with aging   Alterations in the structure and function of the male gonads (sex glands) as a result of the aging process. Changes in the reproductive capacity of the male occur much more slowly than in the female, and some men remain fertile into their nineties. There is degeneration of the seminiferous tubules of the testes, resulting in sperm that have failed to mature or that are produced in reduced quantities, compared to the activity in the testes of younger men. But about 50 percent of the seminiferous tubules of the average male at age sixty are still producing sperm, and the rate is around 40 percent at eighty years of age. Studies show that half of the semen samples taken from men in their seventies contain mature spermatozoa. There does, however, appear to be an increase in the percentage of spermatozoa with chromosomal abnormalities.

Thiamine deficiency (beriberi)   An abnormal condition caused by a lack of vitamin B$_1$ (thiamine), due to of a lack of the vitamin in the diet or as a result of other factors, such as impaired absorption from the digestive tract, liver disease, or **hyperthyroidism**. Symptoms include loss of appetite and stamina, depression, memory defects, inability to concentrate, and lack of motivation. Untreated, the condition progresses to **neuritis**, muscle wasting, breathing difficulty, and heart disorders. Use of diuretics may cause increased excretion of thiamine. The condition is also aggravated by alcohol abuse. If a diet is high in carbohydrates, as is often the case with older adults, thiamine need is greater for proper carbohydrate **metabolism**. Thiamine is present in nearly all foods, but the best sources are whole grains, pork, beans, and peas. The need for thiamine is increased with a fever, cancer, and use of intravenous (IV) fluids. *See also* **Vitamin deficiency, Wernicke-Korsakoff syndrome.**

Third-degree (complete) heart block A heart rhythm disorder in which the impulses for heart contractions are no longer conducted from the upper heart chambers (atria) to the lower chambers (ventricles). As a result, the atria and ventricles of the heart tend to beat independently. The affected person may experience **syncope** with a risk of sudden, fatal heart failure. Treatment is by surgical implantation of an electronic **pacemaker**. *See also* **Heart block.**

Thrombocytopenia A decrease in the number of platelets in the bloodstream. One function of blood platelets is to form blood clots and prevent or stop hemorrhages. Thus, an early sign of thrombocytopenia is bleeding that results from insignificant injuries or for no apparent reason. There may be bleeding under the skin, nosebleeds, bleeding from the vagina, or into the digestive or urinary tracts. The blood loss may result in **anemia**, fatigue, weakness, and **congestive heart failure**. The usual cause is a disorder of the blood-forming tissues of the bone marrow, frequently due to an adverse drug reaction. In a number of cases, however, the cause is unknown. Treatment usually requires replacement of the missing platelets with blood transfusions or injections of platelet concentrates. As any medication may be a contributing factor, use of drugs is curtailed until it has been determined which medication, if any, has interfered with the person's normal platelet production.

Thrombophlebitis An inflammation of a blood vein, accompanied by a blood clot, or **thrombus**. It occurs most frequently in a leg and can have a number of possible causes, including injury to the vein, infection, chemical irritation, a disorder that encourages blood clot formation, pooling of the blood following surgery, or immobility that includes prolonged sitting or standing in the same position. If the affected vein is near the surface, it may appear hard and cordlike and be very sensitive to pressure. The surrounding skin may be red and warm, but the rest of the leg may be cold, pale, and swollen. There is usually a cramping pain, which may be aggravated if weight is placed on the leg. *Deep venous thrombosis (DVT)* may develop without symptoms, or it may be marked by pain, tenderness, heat, fluid accumulation (edema), and a bluish coloration of the skin. Acute DVT is usually a more serious condition because of the ever-present threat that a clot may break loose and be carried into the lungs, resulting in a fatal pulmonary **embolism**. Treatment is directed toward prevention of pulmonary embolism and usually requires hospitalization, bed rest with the legs elevated, nonaspirin painkillers, and anticoagulant drugs to dissolve the clot. Surgery to remove the clot may be recommended in some cases. Elastic stockings may be worn to prevent fluid accumulation in the leg.

Thrombosis   A condition in which there is a **thrombus**, or blood clot, in a blood vessel. The clot poses a serious risk if it breaks loose and is carried by the bloodstream into the smaller arteries of the heart, lung, brain, or other organs, obstructing the normal flow of blood and causing the death of the tissue deprived of its blood supply. A thrombus in a coronary artery usually causes a **heart attack**; a thrombus in a cerebral artery usually produces a **stroke**. Other diseases that are associated with thrombosis include **atherosclerosis**, which narrows the lumen, or opening, through a blood vessel; **diabetes mellitus; intermittent claudication**; and **coronary artery disease**. Although such factors increase the risk of thrombosis, there is no way to predict when such an event may occur in a susceptible person.

Thrombus   A blood clot that forms within a blood vessel. It consists of various blood elements, including platelets, fibrin, and clotting substances. *See also* **Embolus.**

Thymus changes with aging   Alterations in the lymphatic gland, located behind the breastbone above the heart, associated with the natural processes of aging. After reaching its maximum size at puberty, the thymus becomes smaller and less active, eventually appearing only as small islands of tissue in older adults. As thymic tissue diminishes, it is replaced by fat. The gland plays an important part in the immune system's defenses against infection, and atrophy of the thymus is believed to be linked to the deterioration of the immune system that occurs with aging.

Thyroid cancer   Carcinoma of the thyroid gland. There are five different forms of thyroid cancer, each with somewhat different symptoms and rates of growth. The first symptom is usually enlargement of the gland in the front of the neck. Most thyroid cancers do not cause discomfort initially but can be tender and painful when pressed. An exception is *anaplastic carcinoma of the thyroid gland,* a relatively rare form of the disease that is marked by rapid, painful enlargement of the gland. The anaplastic form of thyroid cancer accounts for more than half of all fatal cases of the disease. Other symptoms of thyroid cancer may include hoarseness, difficulty in swallowing, and breathlessness. The prevalence of thyroid cancer increases with age, until nearly half of the patients are in their seventies. Older adults with thyroid cancers include some persons who received radiation treatment for enlarged tonsils or adenoids or other disorders several decades before, when the adverse effects of radiation were not known. Thyroid cancers, particularly anaplastic carcinomas, tend to develop in persons who have a history of **goiter**. Women are more susceptible to thyroid disorders than men, and they are twice as likely to develop a cancer of the thyroid gland. Thyroid cancer is treated by surgical removal of all or a part of the thyroid gland, radioactive iodine, thyroid hormone, and other appropriate drugs.

TIA *See* **Transient ischemic attack.**

Tic A muscle spasm involving repeated contractions of a group of muscles, usually in the upper part of the body, from the shoulders to the face. Tics are generally involuntary, may be psychological in origin, and increase when the person is frustrated, anxious, frightened, or annoyed. A tic may occur as blinking, shrugging of the shoulders, or jerking of the facial muscles. In some cases it may be accompanied by a vocalization in the form of a gasp or a grunt. A tic can sometimes be cured by psychotherapy, but it is often replaced by a different tic, as in **symptom substitution**. Also called "habit spasm."

Tic douloureux *See* **Trigeminal neuralgia.**

Tinnitus A ringing or buzzing in the ears. Different individuals describe the sound in various ways, from a hissing sound to a bell-like tinkling. The effect is associated with a number of disorders of the external, middle, or inner ear, including earwax, middle ear infection (otitis media), **otosclerosis, Ménière's disease**, a tumor of the nerve leading from the ear to the brain, and a reaction to certain drugs. Tinnitus is a frequent symptom of excessive aspirin use. *See also* **Salicylism.**

Tongue coating   A condition in which the tongue has the appearance of being coated with a whitish foreign matter. It can be caused by an infection of a yeastlike fungus, **leukoplakia** lesions that may become cancerous, or it may simply be a result of breathing through the mouth or of a decreased flow of saliva. Coated tongue can also be caused by antibiotics, tobacco, fever, and certain mouthwashes.

Tonometry   Measurement of the pressure within the eyeball (intraocular pressure) is a test for **glaucoma**. Two basic methods are used: *applanation,* in which pressure is determined by the amount of force required to flatten a specific area of the cornea, and *indentation,* a method in which a fixed weight is applied to the cornea. With the second method, the pressure is calculated from the amount of indentation produced by the weight. The eye is anesthetized so that no pain or discomfort is experienced during the test. An instrument called a pneumotonometer measures intraocular pressure by blowing a puff of air against the cornea and flattening it slightly. It does not require any instrument contact with the eye but may not be as accurate as other methods.

Tonus (muscle tone)   The degree of tension of a muscle or muscle fiber, usually measured by its resistance to being stretched. Tonus may be abnormally low as a result of diseases of the brain or peripheral nerves that cause muscles to be flaccid. In other conditions, such as muscle spasticity or rigidity, tonus may be abnormally high. In some types of organic brain disease, such as **dementia**, the individual may be unable to relax during attempts to stretch a muscle.

Torticollis   *See* **Wryneck.**

Toxic amblyopia   An abnormal condition in which there is some loss of vision without any measurable changes in the structures of the eyeball. However, the optic nerve may be affected. Tobacco, alcohol, or other potentially toxic substances may be causes of the condition. When it is associated with a B vitamin deficiency or other form of malnutrition, toxic amblyopia may be correctable by diet if the optic nerve has not been permanently damaged. More often, it is irreversible. The impaired vision cannot be corrected by eyeglasses.

Toxic multinodular goiter   An enlarged thyroid gland, or **goiter**, that is marked by many nodules. The condition is often associated with **hyperthyroidism**. Symptoms include nervousness, irritability, tremor, weight loss, weakness, and easy fatigability. The patient also may experience heart rhythm disorders or **congestive heart failure**. Thyroid nodular diseases affect women much more frequently than men. Treatment includes radioactive iodine and sometimes surgery.

Transient ischemic attack (TIA)   A temporary, usually brief, episode of impaired brain function caused by partial obstruction of an artery serving the brain tissues. Causes include an **embolus** or deposits (**atherosclerosis**) on the lining of the artery that restrict the blood flow. The symptoms, similar to those of a **stroke**, include visual disturbances in one or both eyes, fainting spells, weakness, loss of sensation in an arm or other body part, or slurred speech. The symptoms depend on the degree of blockage and the area of brain tissue deprived of oxygenated blood. Narrowing of the carotid artery in the neck is a frequent cause of interrupted blood flow to the brain. The symptoms may be present so briefly that the person may not even realize what has happened, or they may last an hour or more. TIAs that last for several hours are generally caused by an embolus. A TIA is often a forewarning of a major stroke, and the chances of a future stroke are increased if the person experiences several TIAs within a short period of time, particularly if obstruction of a carotid artery is involved. Treatment includes anticoagulant and other medications or surgery.

Tranquilizer   *See* **Major tranquilizer, Minor tranquilizer.**

Trauma   Any physical injury caused by an external force, such as a wound, blow, accident, injection of a poison, amputation, burn, or electric shock. The term also is used to identify a severe emotional experience that may result in a neurosis or other change in behavior. Experiencing a natural catastrophe or terrorist attack can be a psychic trauma.

Tremor   Spontaneous, involuntary rhythmic movements of body parts, usually involving alternate contractions of opposing groups of muscles. Tremors may be classified as to whether they occur at rest or during motion, according to the type of **neurological disorder** involved, and as either "coarse" or "fine," depending upon the number of muscle contractions per second. A "rest," or passive, tremor occurs when the involved part of the body is at rest and diminishes when the body part moves, while an "intention" tremor tends to occur or increase when the affected body part is in motion. An intention tremor generally is caused by a neurological disorder in the cerebellum, a part of the brain stem. The tremor of **Parkinson's disease** is a rest tremor that often diminishes when body movement occurs. A rest tremor is usually due to a disorder involving a part of the brain that normally controls contractions of muscles throughout the body. Rest tremors can affect the hands, legs, head, or trunk. They may also occur in the muscles of the mouth and lips without interfering with speech or swallowing. Action tremors are caused by the simultaneous contractions of opposing muscles and can occur during activity or rest. Senile tremors and **essential tremors** are action tremors. Static tremors are rhythmic involuntary muscle contractions that may develop when a person tries to hold a part of the body in a steady position without support. Most tremors are treated with drugs that affect the nervous system.

Tricyclic antidepressant   A family of drugs used to treat depression. They act in the same general manner as a **monoamine oxidase inhibitor (MAOI)**, another class of antidepressant drug, by increasing the amount or activity of neurotransmitters in the brain. The choice of a specific antidepressant drug depends upon the nature of the condition and individual patient factors. A particular drug may act adversely on conditions such as heart ailments, glaucoma, urinary retention, and other problems. Prescriptions for such drugs should be for the lowest dosages that are effective because diminished liver and kidney function in older adults, affecting drug metabolism and excretion, makes them particularly susceptible to adverse side effects.

Trigeminal neuralgia (tic douloureux)   A severe facial pain caused by irritation or inflammation of the fifth (trigeminal) cranial nerve, which supplies the face, forehead, temple, and eye. The disorder generally affects only one side of the face and may be experienced as a brief but severe lancinating pain that is triggered by some stimulus. A dull, continuous, painful sensation may precede the severely "hot" pain episode, and there may be repeated episodes of the more intense pain, which is often accompanied by flushing and a flow of tears. The triggering stimulus may be something as simple as a breeze, a tickling sensation, chewing, or a light touch. The problem initially involves only one branch of the trigeminal nerve, most commonly one innervating the upper lip and teeth and eye on one side of the face. The disorder affects mainly older adults, and women are affected more frequently than men. In most cases, no cause can be found, but some cases have been attributed to multiple sclerosis, a tumor, viral infection, or a drug reaction. The condition is initially treated with drugs for the pain. If drug treatment is unsuccessful, surgery by electrocoagulation may be performed on the nerve.

Triglyceride   A chemical molecule formed naturally in the body from three molecules of fatty acids and a molecule of glycerine. It is a major form of fat in the human body. Levels of triglycerides and cholesterol usually increase with age but do not seem to be associated with an increased risk of heart disease after the age of sixty.

Trochanteric fracture   A common type of hip fracture in older adults. It may involve either of two bony projections (trochanters) at the top of the upper leg bone (femur) that serve as attachments for various muscles of the hip joint. *See also* **Hip fracture.**

Truncal ataxia   A loss of coordination of the muscles of the trunk, making it impossible to stand or walk normally. In extreme cases, the person may even have difficulty in sitting in a chair without support. It is caused by damage to a nerve center in the brain.

Tuberculosis   An infectious disease, caused by the tubercle bacillus (a bacterium), that most commonly affects the lungs, causing inflammation and the formation of tubercles, or nodules; the destruction of normal tissue; and formation of abscesses, fibrosis, and calcium deposits. Although the lungs are the usual target area for tuberculosis, nearly any organ or system of the body may be affected. The disease is acquired by inhalation of contaminated salivary droplets or dry tuberculosis bacteria in the air. The incidence of tuberculosis in most industrialized countries has been decreasing in recent years but at a slower rate among older adults. The chance of acquiring tuberculosis in the United States is about six times greater for a person over the age of sixty than for one under the age of thirty and is more likely to be found among underprivileged populations. Tuberculosis may cause no symptoms at first. It usually begins in lower lung tissue and spreads through the lymphatic system to other body areas. Several months or years may elapse before the first signs of lung inflammation develop, with fever, cough, chest pain, and breathing difficulty. There may be weight loss that is so gradual as to be unnoticed. Coughing at first occurs in the morning, as a result of secretions that drain into the bronchi during the night. The early coughing produces little sputum, but as the disease progresses, coughing is more frequent and more productive, eventually yielding sputum that is tinged with blood. The appearance of blood is a sign that tissue erosion has opened a blood vessel in the lung, and sometimes large amounts of blood are coughed up. The diagnosis of pulmonary tuberculosis is based on chest X-rays and laboratory tests. Treatment for most tuberculosis patients involves the use of the drug isoniazid, which is taken daily for eighteen to twenty-four months. Other drugs, including rifampin, are also used. Follow-up medical checkups are required to ensure that the disease is under control and also to make sure that the patient has not suffered any adverse effects from the medications.

Tumor   Any new growth of tissue, usually marked by a swelling or enlargement. A tumor may be a solid mass that began as a pimple or **nodule** and gradually expanded in size and depth. It may be identified by the type of cells it contains, such as an *epithelioma,* which is composed of epithelial cells, or its location, such as a *splenoma,* which is a tumor of the spleen. A tumor may be noncancerous (benign) or cancerous (malignant).

Tunnel vision   The loss of peripheral vision, the outer portion of the visual field, while some degree of central vision remains. The condition occurs in advanced cases of **glaucoma.**

Twenty-twenty (20/20)   The standard notation for normal visual acuity, meaning a person is able to read letters or other symbols on a chart twenty feet away. It is sometimes noted as 6/6, which is the 20/20 equivalent in the metric system.

U

Ulcer Any craterlike lesion or sore on the skin or a mucous membrane, such as the lining of the stomach. It usually results from an inflammation, infection, irritation, or cancerous process. An ulcer may be shallow, involving only the surface layer of the skin, or deep, as when a **peptic ulcer** penetrates the wall of the stomach.

Ulcerative colitis A serious, recurrent inflammatory disease of the colon, or large intestine, marked by degeneration of the lining and bloody diarrhea. The diarrhea may begin with a sudden and violent attack. Accompanying symptoms include a cramping pain in the lower abdomen, chills, and fever. The condition leads to anemia and weight loss, and there may be perforation of the bowel wall resulting in peritonitis. Because of blood loss, blood poisoning, and other complications, an attack of ulcerative colitis can be fatal. Although the disease may begin at any age, the outlook is particularly serious for persons who develop the first symptoms after middle age. Ulcerative colitis patients are very susceptible to colon cancer, and the risk of cancer increases with the length of time the person has been afflicted with the disease. Treatment is with corticosteroid drugs, fiber-free (and in some cases milk-free) diet, and surgery, depending upon the severity of the colitis.

Ulnar tunnel syndrome A condition of pain or loss of feeling in the forearm and hand, with a wasting or weakness of the involved muscles. The cause is a compression, at either the elbow or the wrist, of the ulnar nerve, which originates from the spinal cord near the level of the shoulder. The condition tends to affect persons who continually lean on their elbows, have a displacement of the nerve from repeated arm movements in work such as carpentry, have a slight deviation of the forearm, or have an injury to the elbow from fractures or dislocations. *See also* **Acroparesthesia, Carpal tunnel syndrome.**

Unconsciousness   A condition characterized by the inability of a person to respond to usual sensory stimuli, such as sound, light, or touch. An unconscious person does not, for example, react to voice commands or tapping or pinching. There may be many causes, including damage to the brain, such as **stroke**, a blow to the head, concussion, brain tumor, epileptic seizure, or severe infection of the central nervous system. Loss of consciousness also can result from a spinal cord injury, cardiac arrest, hemorrhage with serious loss of blood, or a decrease in the amount of oxygen reaching the brain due to an obstruction in the respiratory airway. Poisons and drugs, including carbon monoxide gas, methane, alcohol, tranquilizers, sedatives, narcotics, and some antihistamines also can produce unconsciousness. Still other causes are an **electrolyte** imbalance, kidney or liver failure, hormonal disorder, blood sugar imbalance, or diabetic acidosis. A state of unconsciousness is a medical emergency requiring professional health care.

Unilateral   Pertaining to a condition that occurs on only one side of the body, such as unilateral conjunctivitis caused by an infection in one eye.

Unimodal progeroid syndromes   A medical term for a group of hereditary diseases that cause a person to age faster than the average individual. Examples include certain forms of **amyloidosis** and hypercholesterolemia. Familial hypercholesterolemia is marked by premature **atherosclerosis,** and Type III amyloidosis results in an accumulation of starchlike fibers in the heart and aorta that may impair normal function by the age of forty. An inherited factor causes **progeria,** a disease associated with premature aging in early childhood. Other progeroid syndromes may also involve inherited factors that "accelerate" the aging process.

Uninhibited bladder   A urinary **incontinence** problem that is due to a failure of a site in the brain that is normally able to delay urination when there is an urge to empty the bladder. The failure may be due to a stroke or other central nervous system disorder. The effects of this failure vary. A person who is able to recognize the urge and is agile enough to reach a bathroom quickly can usually avoid incontinence, whereas one who suffers from confusion or disorientation or is immobilized is likely to urinate involuntarily.

Uremia An abnormal condition marked by the kidney's inability to excrete waste products and the resulting presence in the bloodstream of nitrogen compounds, such as urea, that are normally excreted in the urine. The condition is associated with kidney failure. The nitrogen compounds are produced by the metabolism of proteins, which, unlike fats and carbohydrates, cannot be broken down into water and carbon dioxide and excreted through the lungs or skin if kidney function is impaired. Symptoms include nausea, vomiting, diarrhea, headache, visual difficulties, loss of appetite, restlessness, and depression. The person may also have fetid breath, nosebleeds, breathing difficulties, muscle twitching, convulsions, and dehydration, leading to delirium and coma. The condition usually requires treatment by **dialysis**. *See also* **Kidney changes with aging.**

Uremic encephalopathy A type of brain disorder associated with **uremia**. Symptoms include an inability to concentrate, personality changes, confusion, drowsiness, stupor, tremors, and coma. Treatment requires correction of the underlying uremia, usually by **dialysis**, and medications.

Uremic neuropathy A form of peripheral nerve disorder that results from **uremia**, usually affecting the legs and arms with severe, sometimes incapacitating, pain. Treatment requires the use of medications to relieve pain and correction of the underlying condition, which may involve **dialysis** or a kidney transplant. *See also* **Burning feet syndrome.**

Urethritis An inflammation of the urethra. The disorder, frequently associated with **dysuria**, may be caused by the irritating effects of urine passing through the urethra. The condition may also be due to an infectious disease or **diabetes mellitus**. There is often a puslike discharge when the cause is a bacterial infection. Treatment is with antibiotics and correction of any contributing condition.

Urinary system changes with aging Alterations in the structure and function of the organs of the urinary system that occur with aging. The major changes are a shrinking of the capacity of the bladder by as much as 50 percent, an increase in involuntary bladder contractions, and a decrease in the urethra pressure that normally helps keep urine within the bladder. Automatic contractions of the muscles of the bladder are controlled by nerve centers in the lower spinal cord. Contractions of the urethra and the muscles of the pelvis that restrain emptying of the bladder are also controlled by nerve centers in the spinal cord. There are brain-controlled mechanisms that can override these spinal nerves, which is what occurs in childhood toilet training. Any malfunction in the coordination of the different nerves and their attached muscle groups can contribute to urinary incontinence. It is not uncommon for the brain function that controlled toilet training in childhood to be lost with increasing age. More than half the cases of urinary incontinence in older adults are associated with **uninhibited bladder**, which, in turn, may be due to stroke. The decline in urethral pressure also contributes to urinary incontinence. The reduced size of the bladder diminishes its maximum capacity. The condition may be complicated further by drugs such as diuretics that result in increased urine volume and frequency. *See also* **Incontinence.**

Urinary tract disorders   Various abnormal conditions of the kidney, ureters, bladder, and urethra. Urinary tract disorders are among the most common health problems of older adults and a common cause of death in elderly people. One study found that 97 percent of all elderly men and women have some degree of kidney degeneration. In addition, urinary disorders are frequent complications of diseases such as diabetes and enlarged prostate in the male. Urinary disorders include increased urine excretion or urge to urinate; a frequent urge to urinate at night (**nocturia**); pain or burning sensation (**dysuria**); urinary retention or **incontinence**; blood in the urine (**hematuria**); bladder inflammation (**cystitis**); and the presence of urea and related urinary waste products in the blood (**uremia**). Prostate enlargement or other obstructions in the urinary tract below the kidney level can result in a back-pressure effect of urine accumulation above the bladder, causing irreversible damage to the kidneys. An infection, inflammation, tumor, or stone in the urinary tract can be both an obstruction and a cause of blood in the urine. Increased fluid intake results in increased urine production and frequency of urination, but a failure to drink enough fluids results in reduced kidney filtration activity and the retention of waste products in the blood. Increased fluid pressure can lead to bulges (diverticula) in the wall of the bladder. Bladder diverticula become increasingly common in older men and are also found in older women. *See also* **Dribbling, Inappropriate antidiuretic hormone secretion, Kidney changes with aging, Natriuresis, Nephrotic syndrome.**

Urticaria (hives)   An allergic skin condition characterized by the eruption of pale, irregularly shaped **wheals**, or fluid-filled blisters. They are caused by the release of histamine from damaged cells surrounding blood vessels in the skin. Itching usually accompanies the eruptions. Acute cases often disappear without treatment in a few hours or days, but chronic urticaria may persist for months or years with cycles of recurrence. Treatment includes medicated baths, sedatives, and other drugs, and a diet that eliminates certain foods to test whether they are the cause of the allergic reaction.

Uterine cancer   Any malignancy of the uterus, which is the third most common site of cancer in women, after breast cancer and cancer of the bowel. Uterine cancer begins in the lining of the uterus (endometrium) and usually affects women after the **menopause**. Its development is linked to estrogen-producing tumors of the ovary, postmenopausal intake of unopposed estrogen products, delayed menopause, a history of menstrual disorders, infertility, obesity, diabetes, hypertension, or a family history of cancers of the breast or ovary. The most frequent symptom is vaginal bleeding after the menopause. The Papanicolaou ("Pap") test, which is extremely helpful in detecting **cervical cancer** at a very early stage, usually does not detect uterine cancer. Diagnosis usually requires a tissue sample obtained by biopsy or a D & C (dilatation and curettage) procedure that permits removal of some cells from the endometrium. Untreated uterine cancer spreads to the other reproductive organs and may also metastasize through the bloodstream and lymph system to distant body tissues. Treatment usually requires **hysterectomy** and often removal of the ovaries and fallopian tubes in the woman. The five-year survival rate for women undergoing hysterectomy for uterine cancer before it spreads to other areas approaches 90 percent.

V

Vaccination Inoculation of a vaccine, a substance containing living or killed microorganisms that cause specific diseases, in order to generate immunity to the disease. The vaccine triggers the formation of antibodies that will resist any future infection by the same organism. Some vaccines confer a permanent immunity; others must be repeated periodically. Vaccines recommended for older adults include: pneumococcal pneumonia, the sixth leading cause of death in the United States with the highest death rate among persons over the age of forty; and influenza, a particularly high-risk disease for older adults. Diphtheria and tetanus require booster shots every ten years. More than 65 percent of all tetanus cases involve persons over the age of fifty.

Vaginal cancer A cancer that generally affects women from their middle years into their sixties, with symptoms of vaginal bleeding or discharge, **dyspareunia**, and increased urinary frequency as the initial symptoms. Daughters of women who were treated with the hormone diethylstilbestrol during pregnancy, between the 1940s and 1960s, are especially vulnerable to vaginal cancer. Treatment involves surgery or radiation, or both, depending upon the severity of the case. Vaginal cancer is relatively uncommon, but it is a dangerous form of cancer and the long-term survival rate is low.

Vaginitis *See* **Senile vaginitis.**

Vagotomy A surgical procedure sometimes performed in the treatment of a **peptic ulcer**. It consists of severing those fibers of the vagus nerve that normally stimulate the secretion of gastric juices in the stomach.

Valsalva maneuver   An attempt to force an exhalation against a closed airway, as when one takes a deep breath, then holds the breath while tightening the abdominal and other muscles. The procedure is commonly used in trying to force a bowel movement or when straining to move a heavy object. While a healthy young person can perform the Valsalva maneuver without harm, it should be done with caution by older adults with heart or circulatory problems because of its effect on the cardiovascular system. The increased pressure in the chest causes the pulse to slow, while blood pressure in the major veins is increased. When the pressure is relaxed, blood rushes to the heart, potentially overloading it and perhaps causing **cardiac arrest**.

Valvular heart disease   Any heart disorder caused by a defect in one of the heart's four valves. The mitral, or bicuspid, valve between the left upper chamber (atrium) and left lower chamber (ventricle), is most commonly affected. A mitral valve defect can allow a regurgitation of blood from the left ventricle back into the left atrium during heart contractions. The aortic valve, between the left ventricle and the aorta, and the tricuspid valve, between the right atrium and right ventricle, also may become impaired, allowing regurgitation of blood. Causes of valve failure include accumulations of calcium deposits on the small flaps, or leaves, of the valves, interfering with their closure, and damage to the tiny muscles inside the heart that control the opening and closing of the valves. The heart valve damage often is secondary to an episode of **rheumatic fever**. Pulmonary heart valve disease is relatively uncommon and usually is due to a congential defect. Many patients with heart valve disease show no symptoms; others may experience chest pains, breathing difficulty, palpitations, fainting spells, or become easily fatigued. The condition is treated by surgery.

Varicella-zoster virus   The virus that causes shingles (**herpes zoster**) in adults and chickenpox in children.

Varicose veins   Veins that become excessively dilated, a condition usually accompanied by defective valves that allow blood to accumulate in the legs or lower trunk. Varicose veins can develop spontaneously in the middle years and later, or they may be the result of any of several abnormal conditions, such as injury, congestive heart failure, a tumor or **thrombophlebitis. Obesity** may contribute to their development. They occur in women more often than in men. Varicose veins that develop near the skin surface are highly visible and are usually seen before they cause discomfort. Symptoms may vary from pain and pulsations to orthostatic **hypotension** and fainting, particularly in severe cases involving pooled blood in large veins of the leg. Methods of treatment include elevating the affected leg occasionally to allow the blood to drain toward the trunk of the body, wearing elastic stockings, exercise, and surgery.

Vascular disease   Any disease of the blood vessels, such as **aneurysm, atherosclerosis, thrombosis,** or **Raynaud's disease**.

Vasculitis   An inflammation of the blood vessels.

Vasoconstriction   A narrowing (constriction) of a blood vessel.

Vasodilation   An expansion (dilatation) of a blood vessel.

Vasospasm   A spasm of the muscles in a blood vessel. Vasospasm can result in a constriction of arteries and lead to a heart attack if it involves the coronary arteries. A **stroke** may occur if the spasm is in an artery supplying the brain. Vasospasms may also occur in the brain several days after a brain hemorrhage; this is a compensatory action by body chemicals that normally constrict arteries to prevent further bleeding. Spasms may cause symptoms of drowsiness or other neurologic disorders, and in severe cases can interrupt the blood supply to a vital area of brain tissue, causing permanent disability or death.

Ventricular fibrillation   *See* **Fibrillation**.

Ventricular gallop   An abnormal extra heartbeat that is usually not important when heard in a child or young adult but which may be a sign of a heart disorder when detected in an older adult.

Vertebrae   Any of thirty-three bones that form the spinal column, from the base of the skull to the tailbone. The vertebrae protect the spinal cord and help support the body. These bony segments are separated by intervertebral disks of fibrous cartilage and are held together by various ligaments that permit a limited range of motion. Individual vertebrae vary somewhat in size and structure, depending upon their location and function. *See also* **Herniated disk, Spondylosis.**

Vertigo   A sensation of spinning or whirling and falling. It may be accompanied by nausea, vomiting, profuse sweating, **tinnitus,** and difficulty in walking in some but not all cases. Some persons may also experience sensations of movement while lying on their back, and in another variation the person has the sensation of standing still while objects in the environment move. Vertigo is sometimes distinguished from dizziness by the sensation of movement, whereas dizziness is described as faintness or light-headedness without the sensation of movement. Although both disorders may be caused by a disturbance in the inner ear's sense of balance, this problem usually results in vertigo. *See also* **Ménière's disease.**

Verrucae *See* **Warts.**

Vesicle A small, blisterlike collection of fluid in the outer skin layers, as may occur in a reaction to a mild burn or contact with poison ivy. If the blister becomes filled with pus, it is called a **pustule**.

Vestibular neuronitis A severe form of **vertigo** that is accompanied by nausea and vomiting. It is believed to be caused by a viral infection of the inner ear. Some but not all persons experience **tinnitus** and a feeling of fullness in the affected ear. The attacks of **vertigo** are frequent at the onset of the disorder, then become less frequent with time and eventually disappear. The disorder affects mainly adults after the age of forty. Treatment may include drugs that are often used to combat motion sickness, such as antihistamines.

Visual accommodation The ability of the eye to maintain a clear image of objects at various changing distances from the eye. Accommodation is possible because of contractions and relaxations of the ciliary muscle that changes the shape of the lens and varies its optical power, as needed, to keep an object in focus. Accommodation declines with increasing age as the lens loses its elasticity and becomes hard and inflexible.

Visual field loss A complication of eye injury, brain injury, or **glaucoma**. In glaucoma, there is usually a loss of the peripheral, or outer, portions of the field of vision first. If uncorrected, the condition advances progressively toward a gradually smaller visual field, and total blindness then ensues. *See also* **Tunnel Vision.**

Vital capacity The amount of air that an individual can expel from his lungs after taking a deep breath. Vital capacity varies with sex, age, posture, physical fitness, and other factors. The average maximum breathing capacity usually peaks at around 4,000 to 5,000 milliliters of air at about the age of twenty-one, and then declines at a rate of nearly 30 milliliters a year.

Vitamin Any of several chemical compounds, generally present in foods, necessary as coenzymes, or catalysts, for one or more bodily functions. Because they cannot be produced by the body's own tissues, vitamins must be obtained through food in the diet or by taking vitamin supplements.

Vitamin deficiency An insufficiency or lack of any of the vitamins, essential chemical compounds present in foods, that results in signs or symptoms of a disease. Many of the substances identified as vitamins are needed for one or more vital body functions. It is generally necessary to meet the body's daily needs for vitamins by eating foods that contain them or by taking vitamin supplements, or both. While vitamin needs apparently do not increase with age, vitamin intake may sometimes become a problem. Decreased vitamin intake, and thus deficiencies, can arise when foods are eliminated from the diet because of tooth or gum problems, digestive disorders, or low-calorie weight-loss plans. Certain medications, such as **diuretics** or anticonvulsant drugs, can also deplete vitamin levels. Vitamin deficiencies can result in visual disorders and diseases of the skin and mucous membranes (vitamin A); digestive disorders (niacin); pernicious anemia (vitamin B_{12}); scurvy (vitamin C); bone defects (vitamin D); hemorrhage (vitamin K); or beriberi (thiamine). *See also* **Nutrition, RDA, Thiamine deficiency.**

Vitiligo An irregular area of abnormally pale skin caused by a loss of normal pigmentation. It can occur anywhere on the body but appears most often on the face and the backs of the hands. The condition is generally progressive, with expanded areas of depigmented skin, though there also may be periods in which pigmentation returns. The loss of pigment is most obvious during the summer when lesions become sunburned or the skin becomes tanned in patches. Causes include exposure to certain industrial chemicals, various skin infections, and autoimmune processes. In many cases, the exact cause is unknown; in others, there is a hereditary factor.

W

Waddle gait (duck gait)   A walking pattern characterized by excessive side-to-side tilting. It may be a sign of weakness of the gluteus muscles of the hip or of the **pelvic girdle**. If there is a tendency for the pelvis to tip forward because of this weakness, the trunk may be thrown backward to compensate, producing a swayback appearance. *See also* **Gait disorders.**

Walking problems   *See* **Gait disorders.**

Wallenberg syndrome   A condition caused by the most common form of **stroke** involving the brain stem. The neurologic damage is usually on the same side of the body as the brain tissue damage. Symptoms include decreased facial sweating, drooping eyelid, a pupil that is smaller than the pupil in the normal eye, involuntary eyeball movement, and abnormal pain and temperature sensations.

Warts   Noncancerous, contagious skin tumors caused by viruses. They may occur in many areas of the body but tend to appear most often on exposed body surfaces, such as the face, hands, feet, and neck. They may vary in size, shape, and pigmentation. However, they require no treatment unless they are annoying or need to be removed for cosmetic reasons. *See also* **Senile keratosis.**

Water balance   *See* **Fluid balance.**

Water intoxication   A condition in which a fluid imbalance with **electrolyte** disorders results from compulsive water drinking, **inappropriate**

antidiuretic hormone (ADH) secretion, certain kidney disorders, **dialysis,** or the use of **diuretics** that may cause a sodium deficiency. Symptoms may include lethargy and confusion, progressing to **neuromuscular disorders, stupor,** convulsions, and coma. Water intoxication, with symptoms resembling those of alcohol intoxication, sometimes develops in alcoholics who drink excessive amounts of water to soothe inflammation of the stomach lining. Some persons also may drink excessive amounts of water in attempting to compensate for fluid losses due to diarrhea or vomiting. Treatment is directed toward restoration of a normal fluid and electrolyte balance.

Water retention A condition that tends to occur in older adults, particularly in association with oversecretion of the antidiuretic hormone (ADH). It may also occur in diseases such as **pneumonia, tuberculosis, stroke,** impaired kidney function, **congestive heart failure,** and various disorders of the hormonal, respiratory, and central nervous systems. Water retention may result in **edema, water intoxication,** and a decreased concentration of sodium in the blood.

Watershed infarction An interruption of blood flow to an area of the brain that may be located in between branches of major artery systems serving that organ. Watershed areas are often first to be deprived of blood and oxygen when there is a brief interruption of circulation to the brain. While brain tissues on either side receive oxygen, tissue between arterial branches may die. As a result, a **transient ischemic attack (TIA)** may result in a temporary loss of neurologic function to certain parts of the body, while neighboring parts are not affected. *See also* **Multi-infarct dementia.**

Weakness A lack of strength or vigor. It may be manifested in symptoms of fatigue, poor muscle tone, weariness, or exhaustion. Although the condition is often associated with the aging process, weakness may also be due to a metabolic or other disorder that could affect younger persons, such as parathyroid disease, anemia, hypothyroidism, and poor eating habits leading to malnutrition. *See also* **Muscle changes.**

Wear-and-tear theory A theory to account for the aging process that is based on observations that aging may be a matter of gradual accumulated damage to tissue cells from internal and external influences, such as simple repeated use of muscle or connective tissue fibers.

Weaver's bottom A popular term for ischial bursitis, or chronic inflammation of the hip joint.

Weber-Christian disease A skin disorder marked by tender areas of **nodules** and **scales**, mainly on the thighs and buttocks. The disorder tends to affect overweight middle-aged women and follows a period of fever and a feeling of discomfort. The eruptions eventually subside but leave areas of darkly pigmented skin. Treatment of symptoms usually consists of rest, heat, and aspirin.

Weber test A hearing test in which a vibrating tuning fork is placed on the midline of a person's head. If the loudness of the sound is equal in both ears, it is assumed there is no conductive hearing loss. If there is a conductive hearing loss in one ear, the tone will be louder in that ear, although the reason for the effect is unknown. The same test may be used to detect a sensorineural hearing loss, in which case the tone will be heard in the normal ear but not in the impaired ear. *See also* **Hearing loss.**

Wernicke-Korsakoff syndrome (cerebral beriberi) A thiamine (vitamin B_1) deficiency disease affecting specific areas of the brain that may be caused by alcoholism, malnutrition, or both. Symptoms include failure of recent and new memory, confusion, disorientation, **confabulation**, and drowsiness. There also may be loss of muscle coordination, **stupor**, double vision (**diplopia**), and other visual difficulties. Early treatment with thiamine can usually correct visual symptoms, including paralysis of the eye muscles, but loss of memory and confusion may be irreversible when brain areas controlling those functions are damaged. *See also* **Thiamine deficiency.**

Wheal A slightly raised, localized patch of **edema** in the skin that is the typical lesion of hives (**urticaria**) caused by an allergic reaction to food or drugs. The lesions are usually transient, may change shape and size, disappear without marking the skin, then reappear in another location. The pressure from the swelling usually makes the patch white with a red outline. The lesions usually cause intense itching.

White blood cell changes with aging Alterations in the structure and function of white cells (leukocytes) associated with the aging process. The number of white blood cells in the circulatory system does not change significantly as one grows older, but certain white cells are no longer as active in resisting or suppressing infections as in earlier years of life. The most important change involves the lymphocytes, one of the five types of white blood cells, which include the "T cells" that normally destroy substances identified by the body's immune system as "nonself," or foreign matter. It is believed that atrophy of the **thymus** gland, which begins soon after sexual maturity is reached, leads to a depletion of thymic hormone needed to make these white cells active in the defense of the body. The white cell changes may not only account for the increased susceptibility of older adults to new infections, such as **pneumonia**, but may explain why some previous infections, such as **tuberculosis** and **varicella-herpes zoster,** can resurface in later years when the person's immune defenses have become weakened. *See also* **Immune deficiency.**

Winter itch   An intense itching sensation that may develop in the skin of older adults during winter months when humidity of the home is low. The itching tends to affect the legs more than other body areas. The skin is naturally dry because of a loss of oil and water from the skin cells. Frequent bathing in wintertime aggravates the condition. The recommended treatment is less frequent bathing and use of ointments to reduce skin dryness.

Withdrawal reaction   A form of psychological defense in which a person pulls back from social contact and involvement in situations that he finds threatening. The reaction may be observed in an older adult who has lost a spouse or contact with old friends or family members and is reluctant to join in community activities to meet potential new friends.

Wound healing changes with aging   Alterations in the rate of healing of open wounds as a result of the aging process. Skin-cell reproduction and replacement are slower in an older adult so that open wounds contract more slowly and require more time for closure. The rate of healing can be complicated by factors such as malnutrition, particularly protein deficiency, as certain amino acids in proteins are needed for wound healing. Vitamins A and C and copper, iron, and zinc found in an adequate diet are also involved in the chemistry of new tissue formation and rapid wound healing.

Wrinkles   The accumulation of folds and furrows of skin due to the loss of tone and elasticity. In addition to the effects of aging, wrinkling is accelerated by exposure to excessive sunlight. The effects generally appear first in the late twenties and are noticeable on the forehead, eyelids, and the area of the lips and nose. So-called crow's feet next develop at the angles of the eyes; then wrinkles spread to the ears, neck, and chin. Loss of fat beneath the skin and atrophy of muscle tissue, absorption of underlying bone, and loss of water and oil from the skin contribute further to the formation of wrinkles.

Wryneck (torticollis) An abnormal condition in which the head is twisted and tilted to one side, usually as a result of injury or congenital defect in the spinal column. The condition also can be caused by a reflex spasm or a contracture of the neck muscles, a "stiff neck" associated with a rheumatic disorder, a defect in the inner ear causing a distorted sense of balance, or an eye abnormality that encourages the person to tilt the head in order to obtain binocular vision. Abnormal postures of the head and neck are sometimes identified as *static torticollis,* to distinguish them from *spasmodic torticollis,* in which involuntary muscle contractions cause movements of the neck backward, forward, or to one side. Wryneck may be a symptom of a defect of the muscles of the **shoulder girdle**, central nervous system infection, psychological disorder, tumor in the bones or soft tissues of the neck, or a muscle tone disorder marked by slow, writhing contractions of muscles of the neck and shoulders.

X

Xanthelasma Soft yellow to brownish plaques that appear on the upper eyelids of middle-aged persons. They are associated with disorders of the liver or gallbladder, diabetes, and certain disorders of fat metabolism. The plaques can be removed surgically or with medications.

Xanthoma A noncancerous fatty tumor or plaque that develops below the surface layer of the skin, usually near a tendon. Xanthomas are yellowish in color and may be flat or slightly raised. They may begin to form in middle age and are commonly associated with lipid disorders. Xanthomas usually do not require treatment but may be removed surgically or with drugs if they are disfiguring.

Xanthopsia A visual abnormality in which objects in the environment appear to have a yellowish coloration. It is a side effect of the drug digitalis, experienced by some persons who take it for heart trouble.

Xeroderma A mild form of skin disease that affects middle-aged or older persons who have dry skin, bathe frequently, and have a sensitivity to detergents and other potential irritants. It tends to occur on the lower legs, with moderate itching. The condition is usually more severe in winter weather when the humidity is low.

Xerophthalmia A drying of the eye surfaces, marked by a loss of the luster normally seen on the surfaces of the cornea and conjunctiva. It is usually the result of a vitamin A deficiency or a condition in which the eyelids fail to close completely. *See also* **Vitamin deficiency.**

Xerosis A medical term for abnormal dryness of the skin.

Xerostomia Dryness of the mouth, a symptom of **Sjögren's syndrome**, mouth breathing, or the use of certain medications. Because patients with xerostomia often suck on hard candies to relieve the discomfort of mouth dryness, the condition is sometimes identified by a more popular term, "sourball sign."

Xiphisternal arthritis A form of arthritis of the bones forming the breastbone (sternum). The main symptom is a pain in the area of the breastbone or upper abdomen that radiates to the back. Because of the location of the pain, the condition is often mistaken for **angina pectoris, hiatus hernia**, or **peptic ulcer**. The disorder may be diagnosed by gently pressing on the joint between the bone segments of the sternum, which may produce the symptoms.

Y

Yeast infections (thrush)   Diseases such as Candidiasis (moniliasis) that can produce sores or lesions about the mouth, vagina, skin, nails, and other body areas. *Oral moniliasis* commonly occurs in some older adults with poorly fitted dentures. Such yeast infections of the mouth may appear as creamy white flakes on a reddish inflamed background. The condition also may be accompanied by cracks or fissures at the corners of the mouth (perlèche), and the disorder may be complicated by poor eating habits that result in nutritional deficiencies. Yeast infections also may be aggravated by the presence of diseases such as **diabetes mellitus**. Other yeast infections include *athlete's foot* and *intertrigo.* They may develop in the groin, under the breasts, and on the glans penis. Yeast infections are usually treated with medications and nutritional supplements, as needed.

Yellow-nail syndrome   An abnormal condition of the nails, which acquire a yellowish coloration and thicken as nail growth slows. There also may be increased curvature and ridging of the nails. The condition is associated with a defect in lymph circulation and may be a sign of edema of the lymphatic system.

Yellow spot   A common term for macula lutea, the yellowish central area of the retina and point of acute central vision. It is the area of **macular degeneration,** which is the most common cause of blindness in persons over the age of fifty.

Young-old   A term sometimes used to identify persons in the age group of early retirement, or between sixty-five and seventy-five. Those between seventy-five and eighty-five are designated as middle-old, and those over eighty-five as old-old.

Z

Zenker's diverticulum   A herniation of the mucous membrane lining the esophagus through the wall of the esophagus. The disorder tends to occur most frequently in persons over the age of sixty. Symptoms may include regurgitation of food, swallowing difficulty, and the appearance of a mass in the neck as the pouch gradually enlarges. Temporary relief may be obtained by careful chewing of bland low-residue foods and drinking adequate amounts of water after a meal to flush out any food that may have become trapped in the pouch. Permanent treatment requires surgery. Because the herniation usually occurs near the throat, the condition may be complicated by the accidental aspiration (inhalation) of food particles from the pouch, leading to aspiration pneumonia. *See also* **Diverticulosis, Esophagitis.**

Zollinger-Ellison syndrome   A peptic ulcer condition caused by a tumor of the pancreas that stimulates an excessive secretion of hydrochloric acid in the stomach. Ulcers may develop anywhere from the esophagus to the small intestine. Symptoms may include pain in the upper abdomen, nausea, vomiting, and diarrhea. Most affected persons have more than one tumor. Although the tumors are small, usually benign, and grow slowly, they can be malignant. Treatment involves drugs to reduce gastric acid production and to relieve symptoms plus nutritional supplements. Surgery may be advised in some cases. *See also* **Acute abdomen.**

Zoster   *See* **Herpes zoster.**